New polymers for encapsulation of nutraceutical compounds

New polymers for encapsulation of nutraceutical compounds

EDITED BY

Jorge Carlos Ruiz Ruiz
Maira Rubi Segura Campos

WILEY

This edition first published 2017 © 2017 by John Wiley & Sons, Ltd.

Registered Office
John Wiley & Sons, Ltd, The Atrium, Southern Gate, Chichester, West Sussex, PO19 8SQ, UK

Editorial Offices
9600 Garsington Road, Oxford, OX4 2DQ, UK
The Atrium, Southern Gate, Chichester, West Sussex, PO19 8SQ, UK
111 River Street, Hoboken, NJ 07030-5774, USA

For details of our global editorial offices, for customer services and for information about how to apply for permission to reuse the copyright material in this book please see our website at www.wiley.com/wiley-blackwell.

Library of Congress Cataloging-in-Publication data applied for

9781119228790

A catalogue record for this book is available from the British Library.

Wiley also publishes its books in a variety of electronic formats. Some content that appears in print may not be available in electronic books.

Cover image: Peter Chadwick LRPS/Gettyimages

Set in 9.5/13pt Meridien by SPi Global, Pondicherry, India

10 9 8 7 6 5 4 3 2 1

Contents

List of contributors

Nicolas Anton
Faculté de Pharmacie
Laboratoire de Conception et d'Application de Biomolécules
Université de Strasbourg
Strasbourg, France

Maria Filomena Barreiro
Polytechnic Institute of Bragança
Campus Santa Apolónia
Bragança, Portugal

Artur Bartkowiak
Center of Bioimmobilisation and Innovative Packaging Materials
Faculty of Food Sciences and Fisheries
West Pomeranian University of Technology
Szczecin, Poland

Miles C. Braithwaite
University of the Witwatersrand
Johannesburg, South Africa

Cristina Caleja
Polytechnic Institute of Bragança
Campus Santa Apolónia
Bragança, Portugal

María Chávarri
Bioprocesses and Preservation Area
Health Division
Tecnalia Spain
Parque Tecnológico de Álava, Spain

Yahya E. Choonara
University of the Witwatersrand
Johannesburg, South Africa

Lorena Deladino
Centro de Investigación y Desarrollo en Criotecnología de los Alimentos
Consejo Nacional de Investigaciones Científicas y Técnicas
Facultad de Ciencias Exactas
Universidad Nacional de la Plata
La Plata, Argentina

Maria Inês Dias
Polytechnic Institute of Bragança
Campus Santa Apolónia
Bragança, Portugal

Alicja Federowicz
Center of Bioimmobilisation and Innovative Packaging Materials
Faculty of Food Sciences and Fisheries
West Pomeranian University of Technology
Szczecin, Poland

Isabel C. F. R. Ferreira
Polytechnic Institute of Bragança
Campus Santa Apolónia
Bragança, Portugal

S. K. Giri
APPD, Central Institute of Agricultural Engineering
Bhopal, Madhya Pradesh, India

Mershen Govender
University of the Witwatersrand
Johannesburg, South Africa

Wioletta Krawczyńska
Center of Bioimmobilisation and Innovative Packaging Materials
Faculty of Food Sciences and Fisheries
West Pomeranian University of Technology
Szczecin, Poland

Agnieszka Krudos
Center of Bioimmobilisation and Innovative Packaging Materials
Faculty of Food Sciences and Fisheries
West Pomeranian University of Technology
Szczecin, Poland

Pradeep Kumar
University of the Witwatersrand
Johannesburg, South Africa

Zheng Li
Food Science and Human Nutrition Department
Institute of Agricultural and Food Sciences
University of Florida
Gainesville, FL, USA

Antonio Diego Molina García
Instituto de Ciencia y Tecnología de Alimentos y Nutrición
José Antonio Novais
Madrid, Spain

Alba Sofía Navarro
Centro de Investigación y Desarrollo en Criotecnología de los Alimentos
Consejo Nacional de Investigaciones
Científicas y Técnicas
Facultad de Ciencias Exactas
Facultad de Ingeniería
Universidad Nacional de la Plata
La Plata, Argentina

Thi Thrinh Lan Nguyen
Faculté de Pharmacie
Laboratoire de Conception et d'Application
de Biomolécules
Université de Strasbourg
Strasbourg, France

Cheng Peng
University of Auckland
Auckland, New Zealand

Adrián A. Perez
Área de Biocoloides y Nanotecnología
Instituto de Tecnología de Alimentos
Facultad de Ingeniería Química
Universidad Nacional del Litoral
Santa Fe, Argentina

Viness Pillay
University of the Witwatersrand
Johannesburg, South Africa

Siew Young Quek
University of Auckland
Auckland, New Zealand

Jorge Carlos Ruiz Ruiz
División de Estudios de Posgrado e Investigación
Instituto Tecnologico de Mérida
Mérida, México
Facultad de Ingeniería Química
Universidad Autónoma de Yucatán
Yucatán, México

Liliana G. Santiago
Área de Biocoloides y Nanotecnología
Instituto de Tecnología de Alimentos
Facultad de Ingeniería Química
Universidad Nacional del Litoral
Santa Fe, Argentina

Maira Rubi Segura Campos
División de Estudios de Posgrado e Investigación
Instituto Tecnologico de Mérida
Mérida, México
Facultad de Ingeniería Química
Universidad Autónoma de Yucatán
Yucatán, México

Katarzyna Sobecka
Center of Bioimmobilisation and Innovative Packaging Materials
Faculty of Food Sciences and Fisheries
West Pomeranian University of Technology
Szczecin, Poland

Osvaldo E. Sponton
Área de Biocoloides y Nanotecnología
Instituto de Tecnología de Alimentos
Facultad de Ingeniería Química
Universidad Nacional del Litoral
Santa Fe, Argentina

Aline Schneider Teixeira
Centro de Investigación y Desarrollo en Criotecnología de los Alimentos
Consejo Nacional de Investigaciones Científicas y Técnicas
Facultad de Ciencias Exactas
Universidad Nacional de la Plata
La Plata, Argentina

M. K. Tripathi
APPD, Central Institute of Agricultural Engineering
Bhopal, Madhya Pradesh, India

Thierry F. Vandamme
Faculté de Pharmacie
Laboratoire de Conception et d'Application de Biomolécules
Université de Strasbourg
Strasbourg, France

María Carmen Villarán
Bioprocesses and Preservation Area
Health Division
Tecnalia Spain
Parque Tecnológico de Álava, Spain

Wissam Zam
Department of Analytical and Food Chemistry
Faculty of Pharmacy
Al-Andalus University for Medical Sciences
Qadmus, Syrian Arab Republic

Preface

Microencapsulation has been widely used as a system of controlled release in the pharmaceuticals industry. However, it also has a great potential to be used in the area of functional foods for protecting nutraceutical ingredients. It is an interdisciplinary field that requires knowledge of the field of pure polymer science, familiarity with emulsion technology, and an in-depth understanding of stabilizing bioactive compounds.

In the 21st century, many polymers have been proposed for producing capsules. Examples include the natural polymers alginate, agarose, chitosan, cellulose, collagen, and xanthan and synthetic polymers polyethylene glycol, polyvinyl alcohol, polyurethane, polyether-sulfone, polypropylene, sodium polystyrene sulfate, and polyacrylonitrile-sodium methallylsulfonate. However, the use of novel or nonconvectional polymers as coating materials is a field that still needs study.

The present book provides an approach to the characterization of novel polymers and their use in encapsulation processes, the stability of nutraceutical compounds encapsulated with novel polymers, and the application of encapsulated compounds with novel polymers in functional food systems. These polymers could present many advantages in terms of cost and ability to protect and stabilize the nutraceutical compounds compared to those already used by the food industry to develop functional food systems.

Jorge Carlos Ruiz Ruiz

TOPIC 1

Characterization of modified polymers and their use in encapsulation processes

CHAPTER 1

Tailor-made novel polymers for hydrogel encapsulation processes

Artur Bartkowiak, Katarzyna Sobecka, and Agnieszka Krudos
Center of Bioimmobilisation and Innovative Packaging Materials, Faculty of Food Sciences and Fisheries, West Pomeranian University of Technology, Szczecin, Poland, Ul. Klemensa Janickiego 35 71-270

1.1 Introduction

Natural polymers are materials of large molecular weight and natural origin such as plants, animals, or microorganisms. They have been known for centuries and have found widespread use in various industries, such as food, cosmetics, pharmaceuticals, textiles, plastics, and paper. They are of considerable importance because they are generally biodegradable and are generally recognized as safe (GRAS), which is a significant advantage, especially in recent times, when "pro-nature" policies and goals to reduce "chemicals" and synthetic materials in our lives, including food, have become popular. This makes the interest in natural polymers unabated and still increasing. One successful way of using these materials is in encapsulation processes, including spray-drying, emulsion techniques, coacervation, and ionotropic gelation. The utility of polymers as encapsulants is determined by their specific properties. These can include film-forming properties, emulsifying properties, high resistance to the environment of the gastrointestinal tract, biodegradability, low viscosity at high solids contents, low hygroscopicity, and availability and low cost (Özkan and Bilek, 2014).

Generally, among the natural polymers two main groups can be distinguished: polysaccharides and proteins. The next section presents the most popular polymers, commonly used as materials to form capsule matrix (Table 1.1 and Table 1.2). Despite the many well-known encapsulants, there is still a need to look for novel polymers and new means to use the old ones in other ways to create ideal capsules with excellent resistance and mechanical properties and wide applicability; this topic is also presented in this chapter.

New Polymers for Encapsulation of Nutraceutical Compounds, First Edition.
Edited by Jorge Carlos Ruiz Ruiz and Maira Rubi Segura Campos.

Table 1.1 Selected carbohydrate polymers commonly used for hydrogel encapsulation processes.

		Properties							
Origin/ Isolation	**Structures**	**Solubility in Water**	**Viscosity**	**Gel Formation/ Gelation**	**Synergistic Effects with**	**Other**	**Micro-encapsulated Active Substances**	**Micro-encapsulation Techniques**	**References**
Alginate Mainly from marine brown alga Also from exocellular material of some bacteria	Linear anionic polysaccharide Copolymer with homopolymeric blocks of (1-4)-linked β-D-mannuronate and α-L-glucuronate residues	Depends on the rate of dissociation and the type of the counter-ion Alginic acid: insoluble Salts of alginic acid (sodium alginate): soluble	High viscosity at relatively low concentration Exponential increase with the molar mass Highly dependent on ionic strength	Ionotropic gels in the presence of polyvalent cations (Ca^{2+} most commonly used) The α-L-glucuronate blocks are responsible for gelation	—	—	Folic Acid (Alginate-Starch) *Lactobacillus Acidophilus, Bifidobacterium lactis* (Alginate/ Hi-Maize Starch) *Lactobacillus, Acidophilus* (Alginate, $CaCl_2$, chitosan)	Coacervation Emulsion	Madziva *et al.* (2006) Kailasapathy (2006) Krasaekoopt *et al.* (2006)
Carrageenan Red seaweed (Rhodophycae) *Chondrus crispus, Gigrtina, Furcellaria* (κ, ι) *Eucheuma cottoni* (K) *Euchema spinosum* (ι)	Anionic polyelectrolytes Structure can vary with the source and extraction and purification conditions Three types of carrageenan are commercially available: ι- (iota), κ- (kappa), λ- (lambda) chains contain alternating (1-3)- linked β-D-galactopyranosyl and (1-4)-linked α-D-galactopyranosyl units	Depends on the carrageenan type Solubility in cold/hot water: ι-Carrageenan: Na-salt soluble; K-, Ca-, ammonium salts from limited to high swelling/ soluble >70 °C κ-Carrageenan: Na-salt soluble; Ca-salts give thixotropic dispersions, soluble >70 °C		ι-Carrageenan: thermo-reversible gels during cooling in the presence of specific counter-ions; strongest gels are obtained with Ca^{2+} Gels are elastic, have high freeze–thaw stability, do not undergo syneresis	Other gums, e.g., κ-carrageenan brittle gels became softened with locust bean gum	—	*Bifidobacterium longum*	Two-phase (water/oil) system	Adhikari *et al.* (2003)

	Some (1-3)-linked units are like the 2- and 4-sulfates Some (1-4)-linked units are like the 2- and 6-sulfates, the 2,6 disulfates, the 3,6-anhydride, the 3,6-ahydride-2-sulfate	λ-Carrageenan: All salts soluble, create viscous, pseudoplastic solutions/ soluble		κ-Carrageenan: thermo-reversible gels during cooling in the presence of specific counter-ions; strongest gels are obtained with K^+ Gels are brittle, have low freeze–thaw stability, undergo syneresis λ-Carrageenan: non-gelling					
Xanthan									
Produced by bacteria (*Xanthomonas campestris*) in aerobic fermentation	Anionic polyelectrolyte mixed salt of sodium, potassium and calcium Main chain consists of β-(1-4)-D-glucuronosyl units Every second unit at 3C position has the trisaccharide side chain (one D-glucuronosyl unit between two D-mannosyl units	Soluble in cold water	Progressive reduction with increasing shear stress; reversible after eliminating shear stress Stable in a broad range of pHs (2–12) and temperatures Increases after salt addition to a salt-free xanthan solution in concentration >0.15% Increases during heating salt-free xanthan solution	—	Guar gum: enhancement of viscosity Locust bean gum and konjac mannan: obtain soft, elastic thermo-reversible gels at higher concentration	Undergoes cryogelation Not degraded enzymatically	*Bifidobacterium lactis*	Extrusion	McMaster *et al.* (2005)

(*Continued*)

Table 1.1 (Continued)

Origin/ Isolation	Structures	Properties					Micro-encapsulated Active Substances	Micro-encapsulation Techniques	References
		Solubility in Water	Viscosity	Gel Formation/ Gelation	Synergistic Effects with	Other			
Gellan									
Produced by some bacteria strains (e.g., *Sphingomonas elodea*)	Linear, anionic polyelectrolyte Tetrasaccharides repeating unit consisting of one rhamnose and glucoronic acid unit, and two glucoses The 3-linked glucose unit is substituted with glyceryl and acetyl at O(2) and O(6), respectively Designated → 4)-L-rhamnopyranosyl-A-(1 → 3)-D-glucopyranosyl-B-(1 → 4)-D-glucuronopyranosyl-B-(1 → 4)-D-glucopyranosyl-B-(1 →	Depends on the degree of acetylation and the type and amount of ions Low acyl gellan depends more on the ion concentration (needed sequestrant addition) High acyl gellan depends less on the ion concentration Generally in hot water (85–95 °C)	Increases with the degree of acetylation	Thermo-reversible gels during cooling Low acyl gellan: needed gelling cations High acyl gellan without cations Low acyl gellan gels: hard, non-elastic, brittle High acyl gellan gels: soft, elastic, flexible, transparent	—	Resistant to heating to 120 °C	*Bifidobacterium lactis* (hydrated gellan) *Lactobacillus* sp.	Extrusion Interfacial polymerization	Mcmaster *et al.* (2005) Yáñez-Fernández *et al.* (2008)
Chitosan									
Main source of chitosan is chitin Mainly obtained by alkaline deacetylation of shrimp and other crustacean shells Isolation from fungi has been carried out	Linear, polyelectrolyte composed of randomly distributed β-(1-4)-linked D-glucosamine and n-acetyl-D-glucosamine (deacetylated and acetylated unit, respectively)	Depends on degree of acetylation Chitosans with acetylation <40% are soluble in acidic pH		With tripolyphosphate and alginate	—	Film-forming properties Antimicrobial activity	Astaxanthin/ multiple emulsion Tuna o/w emulsion (lecithin-chitosan)	Solvent evaporation layer-by-layer deposition + spray-drying	Higuera-Ciapara *et al.* (2004) Klinkesorn *et al.* (2006)

Gum Arabic									
Obtained from stems and branches of *Acacia senegal* or *Acacia seyal*	Branched neutral or slightly acidic compound of arabinogalactan oligosaccharides, polysaccharides, glicoproteins Composition is highly variable due to climate, source, season, rainfall, etc. Generally the main chain contains β-(1-3)-linked D-galactopyranosyl units Side chains contains two to five β-(1-3)-linked D-galactopyranosyl units combined with the backbone by 1,6-linkages Main and side chains consist of α-l-arabinofuranosyl, α-l-rhamnopyranosyl, 4-*O*-methyl-β-glucuronopyranosyl	Highly soluble in cold and hot water to 50 wt%	Depends on gum arabic type, pH, ionic strength Maximum viscosity is noted between 6 and 7 pH 40 wt% solutions behave like Newtonian liquids <40% solutions are pseudoplastic	—	Majority of plant hydrocolloids, proteins, modified starches Gum tragacanth: lowering the viscosity	Creation of a strong protective film around oil droplets because of presence in the branched structure both protein (hydrophobic) and polysaccharide (hydrophilic) moieties Obtained film/layer protect against, e.g., aggregation, oxidation, evaporation, and moisture absorption	Betacyanin	Spray-drying	Pitalua *et al.* (2010)
							Betalain	Spray-drying	Janiszewska & Włodarczyk (2013)
							Lycopene	Spray-drying	Shu *et al.* (2006)
							Turmeric	Spray-drying	Martins *et al.* (2010)
							Limonene (gum arabic-sucrose-gelatin)	Freeze-drying	Kaushik & Roos (2007)
							Lactobacillus sp./	Interfacial polymerization	Yáñez-Fernández *et al.* (2008)
							Linoleic acid	Spray-drying	Fang et al., (2005)

(*Continued*)

Table 1.1 (Continued)

Origin/ Isolation	Structures	Properties							
		Solubility in Water	Viscosity	Gel Formation/ Gelation	Synergistic Effects with	Other	Micro-encapsulated Active Substances	Micro-encapsulation Techniques	References
Gum Karaya (Sterculia Gum)									
Dried exudate from the stems and braches of *Sterculia* or *Cochlospermum* spaces (e.g., *Sterculia urens*)	Compound partly acetylated polysaccharide received as Ca- and Mg-salts Branched structure Main chain contains α-D-galacturonic acid and α-L-rhamnose units Side chains are linked to the galacturonic acid of the backbone by (1-2)-linkage of β-D-galactose or (1-3)-linkage of β-D-guluronic acid Half of the backbone rhamnose units are (1-4)-linked to β-D-galactose units	Native gum soluble up to 10%/up to 30% Deacetylated gum soluble up to 90%	—	—	Other plant hydrocolloids, carbohydrates, proteins	—	—	—	—
Mesquite Gum									
Obtained from mesquite tree (*Prosopis* spp.) or shrub	Neutral salt of a composite acidic polysaccharide Branched structure Main chain contains (1-3)-linked β-D-galactose units	Comparable to gum arabic Possible concentration of solution up to 50%	Increases with concentration	—	—	Good film-forming properties	Cardamom oil *Lactobacillus* sp.	Spray-drying Interfacial polymerization	Beristain *et al.* (2001) Yáñez-Fernández *et al.* (2008)

	Side chains are linked with backbone by (1-6) bond Side chains consist of single sugar or oligosaccharide such as ʟ-arabinose (pyranose and furanose ring forms), l-rhamnose, β-ᴅ-glucuronate, and 4-*O*-methyl β-ᴅ-glucuronate Small amount of proteins								
Pectin									
Main sources: citrus fruits and apples	Hetero-polysaccharide Presents a highly complex, nonrandom structure with linear homo-poly(galacturonic acid) blocks) (smooth regions) and strongly branched blocs (hairy regions) Contains at least 65 wt% α-(1-4)-linked ᴅ-galacturonic acid–based units units can occur as free acid or salts (Na-, K-, Ca-, ammonium), naturally methanol esterified or as acid amide in amidated pectins	Soluble Possible concentration at range of 6%–12% Most stable at pH 3–4	Low viscosity in comparison with plant gum Close to Newtonian flow at low concentration Pseudoplastic behavior at higher concentration	Depends on the degree of esterification *HM pectins:* Gel in the presence of sugars and low pH range Gel strength is inversely related to pH level *LM pectins:* Gel in the presence of calcium ions	—	—	Fish oil and fish oil–extra virgin olive oil	Spray-drying	Polavarapu *et al.* (2011)
							Lycopene (complex with gelatin)	Coacervation	Silva *et al.* (2012)

(*Continued*)

Table 1.1 (Continued)

		Properties							
Origin/ Isolation	**Structures**	**Solubility in Water**	**Viscosity**	**Gel Formation/ Gelation**	**Synergistic Effects with**	**Other**	**Micro-encapsulated Active Substances**	**Micro-encapsulation Techniques**	**References**
	Polymer chain contains some neutral sugars (e.g., L-rhamnose, D-galactose, L-arabinose, D-xylose) L-Rhamnose unit exists only as (1-2)-linked in the backbone Other sugar units preferably at the rhamnose and galactose residues to the backbone Two types of pectin depending on the esterification degree: high methocylated (HM) >50% esterification and low methoxylated (LM) <50%			Gelation depends also on the proportion and arrangement of the carboxyl groups in the pectin chain Ca^{2+} with pectin interaction increases with decreasing esterification degree Amide groups increase the range of the calcium ion concentration where the LM pectins form gel					
Starch Produced by most green plants as an energy store	Polymer of α-D-glucose Two architecturally different molecules in the structure: linear (amylose) and branched (amylopectin)	Insoluble in cold water Swelling Swelling power decreases with decrease in granule size and increased amylose content	Amylose is responsible for the solution's high viscosity	*MC:* Occurs on heating above 50 °C Reversible on cooling substitution	—	—	*Bifidobacterium* PI1 Fish oil Chlorophyll	Spray-coating, spray-drying Spray-drying Spray-drying	O'Riordan *et al.* (2001) Tan *et al.* (2005) Porrarud and Pranee (2010)

Commercial sources: cereal grain seeds (corn, wheat, rice, sorghum), roots and tubers (potato, tapioca, arrowroot), stems and pith (sago)	Generally the content of amylose is about 20%–30% and amylopectin 70%–80% *Amylose* contains from 500 to 6000 D-glucose units, which are linked by α-(1-4)-glycosidic bond *Amylose* occurs in the form of a double helix *Amylopectin* contains up to 2 million D-glucoses Side chains include about 30 D-glucoses and occur approximately every 20 to 30 glucose units along the chain The point of chain branching has α-(1-6) glycosidic bond Present in small grains of different shapes (spherical or lentil-shaped) and size (e.g., 1–100 μm, 5–900 μm)	Crystalline becomes amorphous in water at 60–70°C *Amylose:* Specific dissolution behavior because of helical structure Soluble in hot water In dilute solution it can bind with itself in a double helix Undergoes retrogradation and, as a consequence, after drying it becomes insoluble Retrogradation is faster with lower concentration, temperature, molar mass; the fastest is between pH 5 and 7 *Amylopectin:* Insoluble in cold and hot water No tendency to retrogradation and crystallization		Gelation temperature decreases with high degree of substitution *HPMC:* Creating thermo-reversible gels Gel transition temperature is in range of 50 to 90 °C and depends on the ratio of methyl to hydroxypropyl derivatization Gel texture is changeable with increasing hydroxypropyl substitution

(Continued)

Table 1.1 (Continued)

Origin/ Isolation	Structures	Properties: Solubility in Water	Viscosity	Gel Formation/ Gelation	Synergistic Effects with	Other	Micro-encapsulated Active Substances	Micro-encapsulation Techniques	References
		Derivatives of native starch: Modification of structure (in chemical, biological, biochemical way) and controlled effect on hydrogen bonding to improve starch properties, e.g., improvement of heat and shear stability, inhibition of swelling, reduction of retrogradation							
Cellulose and Derivatives (Methylcellulose (MC), Hydroxypropyl Methyl Cellulose (HPMC)									
Major structural plants material Sources: wood, cotton, straw, flax, jute, hemp Other: acetic bacteria and many algae synthesize cellulose	Linear polymer of β-D-glucose Chain units are bonded by β-(1-4)-glycosidic linkage	Native cellulose: Insoluble Crystalline become amorphous in water at 320°C And 25 MPa Derivatives: Swelling and soluble Decreases with increase in polymerization and substitution degrees Solutions are surface active	MC solutions are stable from 3 to 11 PH Mixture of MC and HPMC exhibit pseudoplastic non-thixotropic flow properties Deviation from Newtonian behavior increases with molar mass			MC and HPMC have good film-forming properties	Fish oil/spray-drying		Kolanowski *et al.* (2007)

From Wandrey et al., 2010; Milani & Maleki, 2012.

Table 1.2 Selected proteins commonly used for hydrogel encapsulation processes.

		Properties						
Origin/Isolation	**Structures**	**Solubility in Water**	**Viscosity**	**Gel Formation/ Gelation**	**Other**	**Microencapsulation of Active Substances**	**Microencapsulation Techniques**	**References**
Gelatin								
Produced from collagens by destruction of their secondary and higher structures Main sources of collagen to gelatin production: skin, hides, bones of cattle, pigs, horses; skin of fish Depending on the using processes are obtained two types of gelatins: type A by acid treatment (pH 1.5–3.0) and type B by alkaline treatment (pH 12) of collagens	Heterogeneous mixture of single- or multistranded polypeptides consisting of 300 to 4000 amino acids Each polypeptide has extended left-handed proline helix conformations Generally, every third unit in all chains is glycine then proline and 4-hydroxyproline as next often occurring residues *Type A gelatin (obtained from pigskin):* Typical composition of amino acids (residues per 100 units): glycine 33, proline 13, alanine 11, hydroxyproline 9, arginine 5, serine 3.5, aspartic acid 3, lysine 3, glutamic acid 2.5, and further leucine, valine, phenylalanine, threonine, isoleucin, hydroxylysine, methionine, histidine, and tyrosine *Type B gelatin:* Aspargine and glutamine are conversed into aspartic acid and glutamic acid	Soluble in hot water In cold water, swelling to an elastic mass after 5–10 min	Solutions characterized by high viscosity, viscoelastic flow, streaming birefringence	Thermo-reversible, elastic, transparent gels Mammalian gelatins gel below 35–40 °C Fish skin gelatins gel at 5 °C Or 12 °C, depending on the fish type from which skin originated: cold-, warm-water fish respectively	Amphiphilic nature Good emulsifying properties	Lycopene	Spray-drying	Rocha *et al.* (2012)
						Fish Oil (Fish Gelatin/Corn Starch)	Spray-drying	Kolanowski *et al.* (2007)

(Continued)

Table 1.2 (Continued)

		Properties						
Origin/Isolation	**Structures**	**Solubility in Water**	**Viscosity**	**Gel Formation/ Gelation**	**Other**	**Microencapsulation of Active Substances**	**Microencapsulation Techniques**	**References**
Whey Proteins								
Obtained from whey As powders of different quality (demineralized, delactosed, and demineralized-delactosed), whey protein concentrate (WPC: low level of fat and typically 35%–80% protein), whey protein isolate (WPI: fat and lactose removed, >90% protein), lactalbumin, individual whey protein fractions -β-lactoglobulin isthe most important whey protein	Globular proteins Main components: α-lactoalbumin (0.07%–0,15%), β-lactoglobulin (0.2%–0.4%), immunoglobulins (0.06%–0.1%), serum albumin (0.01%–0.04%) α-Lactalbumin: calcium metalloprotein with four intramolecular disulfide cross-links β-lactoglobulin has two intramolecular disulfide cross-links and one free SH group	Depends On pH Insoluble at isoelectric point at about pH 5 and also after denaturing at >70°C	Less viscous than caseinate solutions Newtonian flow at concentration from 4%–12% exhibit pseudoplastic behavior in the range of 18%–29%	Thermally irreversible gels after denaturing (>70°C) Cold-induced gelation of preheated mixture in presence of calcium	Form films after thermally induced disulfide cross-linking Films 'tensile strength is like synthetic films Good surface-active properties Amphiphilic Ability to be adsorbed at the emulsion interface and coat oil droplets, preventing coalescence and floculation	Astaxantin *Bifidobacterium. breve* (milk fat, denaturated whey proteins) Conjugated linoleic acid (CLA)/	Multiple emulsion/solvent evaporation Emulsion, spray-drying Spray-drying	Higuera-Ciapara *et al.* (2004) Picot and Lacroix (2004) Jimenez *et al.* (2006)

Caseins								
Obtained from skim milk by destabilizing of micelles Main products: mineral or lactic acid casein, rennet casein Possible fractionation Most commonly used is Na-caseinate	Heterogeneous group of phosphoproteins Distinguishes the following four main groups: A_{s1}-casein (0.9%–1.5%) A_{s2}-casein (0.3%–0.4%) Β-casein (0.9%–1.1%) Κ-casein (0.3%–0.4%) In milk they occur in the form of micelles	Depends on pH Varies according to the fractions Generally insoluble in isoelectric point, at about pH4.6	Solutions of 10%–15% prepared at pH6–7: high viscosity At pH <3.5: solution highly viscous, even gel-like	Only Ca-salt of caseins exhibit reversible thermal gelation	Film-forming properties Na-caseinate And β-caseinate surface of films have the lowest viscoelasticity and best flexibility: highly heat-stable, no coagulation by heat Good fat emulsifiers	Curcumin	Spray-drying	Pan *et al.* (2013)

From Wandrey *et al.* (2010).

1.2 Well-known and commonly used polymers

1.2.1 Carbohydrate polymers

Carbohydrate polymers are described as natural homo- and copolymers that consist of sugar residues and/or their derivatives. Characteristic linkages that bond specific monosaccharides together in this polymeric structure are the O-glycosidic linkages. The interaction can occur between any of the hydroxyl groups of sugar monomers, resulting in polysaccharides presenting linear or branched-chain construction. The character of a polymer's structure determines its functional properties, such as solubility, gel-forming, and surface properties. Table 1.1 gives an overview of the origin and physicochemical properties of selected carbohydrate polymers. Figure 1.1 shows the principal chemical structure of selected carbohydrate polymers.

1.2.2 Proteins

Proteins are large molecules composed of linear long chains of amino acids that are bonded by amide (or peptide) linkage. The compositions of protein polymers are various combinations of 20 amino acids that give an enormous variety of sequences. These polymers have a natural origin, but some of their properties, such as fibers and hydrogels, can be compared to those of synthetic materials. Table 1.2 gives an overview of the origin and physicochemical properties of selected protein-based polymers used especially in the food industry.

1.3 Novel polymers

1.3.1 Zein

1.3.1.1 Origin and structure

Zein is a major storage protein obtained from natural, sustainable and renewable source of corn or maize seeds (*Zea mays* L.), accounting for 35% to 60% of total proteins present in corn (Luo and Wang, 2014; Patel *et al.*, 2014). Commercial zein is currently separated from corn gluten meal, a coproduct of corn wet milling, and is a mixture of at least four types of proteins: α-, β-, γ-, and δ-zein, each with a different amino acid sequence, molecular weight, and solubility (Shukla *et al.*, 2001; Zhu *et al.*, 2007; Zhong *et al.*, 2009).

1.3.1.2 Properties

Zein is one of the few hydrophobic water-insoluble biopolymers that have been approved for oral use by the U.S. Food and Drug Administration (FDA). Zein is considered a prolamine due to its characteristic solubility. It is insoluble in water unless specifically defined conditions are applied, such as a certain concentration of alcohol, high concentrations of urea, extreme alkaline condition (pH >11), and/or anionic detergents. This unique solubility behavior of zein is attributed to

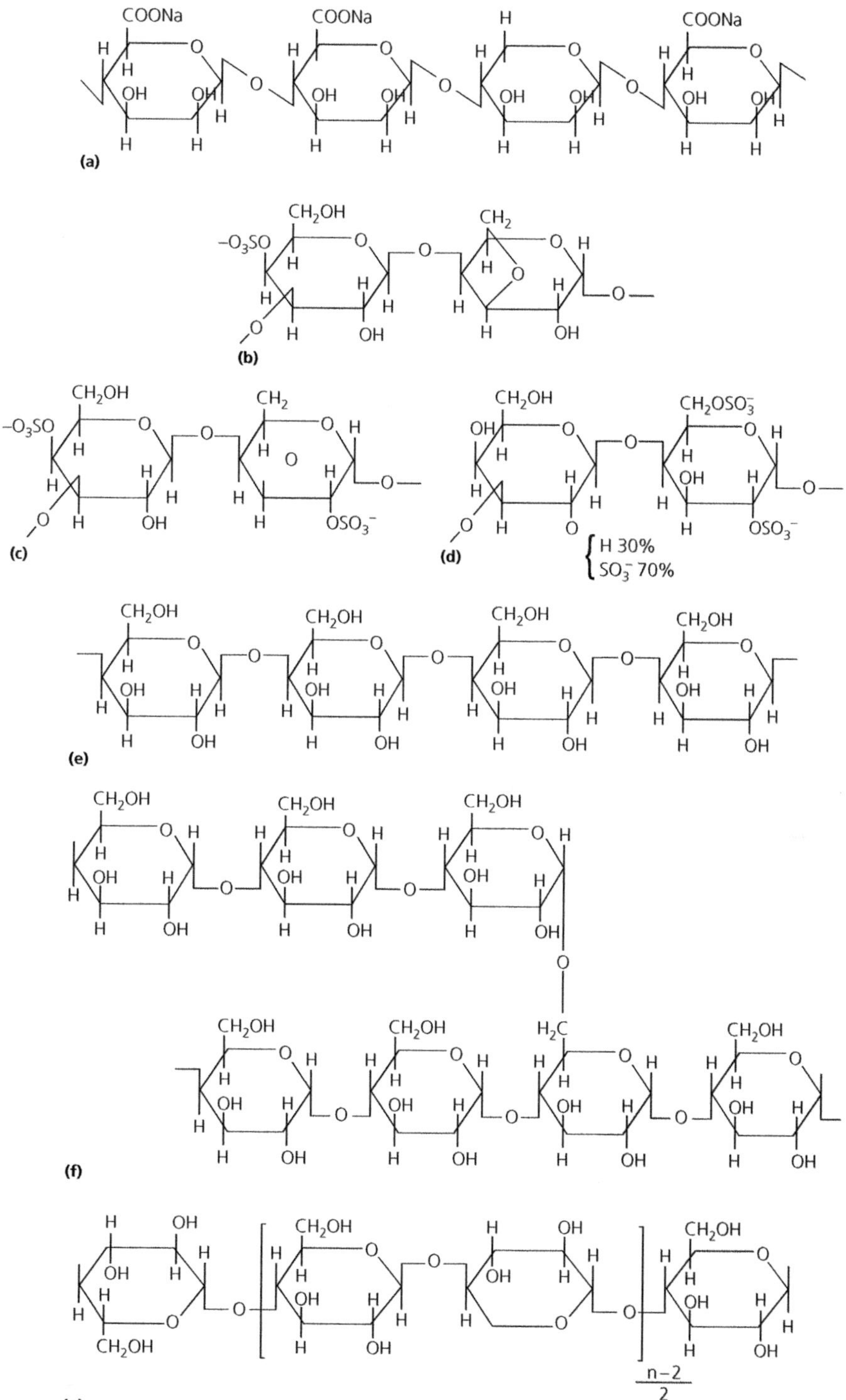

Figure 1.1 Principal chemical structure of selected carbohydrate polymers. **a,** sodium alginate; **b,** κ-carrageenan; **c,** ι-carrageenan; **d,** λ-carrageenan; **e,** amylose starch; **f,** amylopectin starch; **g,** cellulose.

the high percentage of nonpolar amino acids, with more than 50% being nonpolar, including leucine, proline, alanine, phenylalanine, isoleucine, and valine (Luo and Wang, 2014; Lawton, 2002; Shukla and Cheriyan, 2001; Patel *et al.*, 2014). The protein structure allows zein to function as a polymeric amphiphile (as it contains nearly an equal amount of hydrophilic and lipophilic amino acid residues), which has been observed to facilitate the encapsulation and dispersion of oil-based microspheres (Torres-Giner *et al.*, 2010; Wang *et al.*, 2008).

Because zein is hydrophobic, this protein can be easily transformed into colloidal particles by simply changing the solubilizing capacity of the primary solvent through dilution with a nonsolvent, the process commonly known as the antisolvent precipitation method. This is achieved due to excellent miscibility of ethanol and water, where the water is not a good solvent for the dissolved material such as zein (Torres-Giner *et al.*, 2010). Zein micro- and nanoparticles have been studied as promising delivery systems, especially for hydrophobic nutrients or drugs. Generally, the hydrophobic bioactives are dissolved together with zein in aqueous ethanol binary solvent and then mixed with an antisolvent, such as water, to coprecipitate bioactives with zein (Luo and Wang, 2014).

Zein has long been a subject of research for scientific interest, as well as industrial applications (as material used in production of coatings, fibers, and printing ink) (Hamakar, 1995; Lawton, 2002; Patel *et al.*, 2014), and it has been employed as an edible coating for foods and pharmaceuticals because it shows low water-uptake values, high thermal resistance, and good mechanical, oxygen, and aroma barrier properties (Shukla and Cheriyan, 2001; Patel *et al.*, 2014). Zein can create a protective layer because of its extremely high surface area and trapping efficiency (Torres-Giner *et al.*, 2010). Zein is also known for its resistance to digestive enzymes, resulting in a slower digestibility in the gastrointestinal tract, which can be exploited for a controlled release of functional components loaded in zein colloidal particles (Patel *et al.*, 2014).

Taken together, these properties make zein an attractive novel material that is used in a wide range of protecting applications of bioactive components such as polyphenols, vitamins, and omega-3 fatty acids. Because zein used in the preparation of colloidal particles is edible (GRAS), encapsulation in zein colloidal particles exhibits potential in the design of novel functional foods or bioactive packaging strategies to enhance the long-term stability of bioactive functional ingredients.

1.3.1.3 Application of zein in the encapsulation process

1.3.1.3.1 Zein–chitosan complex nanoparticles

A water-soluble chitosan derivative, carboxymethyl chitosan (CM-chitosan), is used to form coatings on the zein surface. CM-chitosan forms a gel at an acidic pH and thus provides greater protection of zein protein against enzymatic degradation. A CM-chitosan coating also confers thermal stability to zein nanoparticles, so that the complex nanoparticles can provide excellent protection of labile nutraceuticals against thermal degradation and oligomerization (Luo and Wang, 2014).

The zein–chitosan complex nanoparticle is a specific design for encapsulation and delivery of nutrients or drugs and can be tailored in two ways for different applications. The first example of the zein–chitosan complex delivery system is in the design of chitosan nanoparticles as hydrophilic core and zein coating as hydrophobic shell. In this method, chitosan–tripolyphosphate (TPP) nanoparticles are first fabricated through ionic gelation, and then zein (predissolved in 70% ethanol aqueous solution) is added into nanoparticles, dispersing with gentle stirring. Because of the acidic condition (pH <5.5) of chitosan–TPP nanoparticles, zein forms films spontaneously upon removal of ethanol by nitrogen stream or rotary evaporation under reduced pressure. When compared with chitosan nanoparticles without a zein coating, the zein–chitosan complex nanoparticles provide significant improvement in functionalities, namely, higher encapsulation efficiency and slower sustained release of hydrophilic nutrients or drugs in the gastrointestinal tract, owing to the hydrophobic zein shell, which prevents dissolution of chitosan in the acidic condition of the stomach and helps the complex maintain its structure. The second example of a zein–chitosan complex delivery system is encapsulating and delivering hydrophobic drugs and nutrients, where zein nanoparticles, along with hydrophobic bioactives such as fat-soluble vitamins, are poured into chitosan solution to induce phase separation and form zein–chitosan complex nanoparticles (Luo and Wang, 2014).

Vitamin E (α-tocopherol) is the main dietary fat-soluble antioxidant and is widely considered to help reduce the risk of many chronic diseases, such as cardiovascular diseases (Herrera and Barbas, 2001; Tucker and Townsend, 2005; Luo *et al.*, 2011). This vitamin, like other lipophilic nutraceuticals, is poorly soluble in water and is biologically unstable when exposed to environmental factors, such as light, high temperature, and oxygen (Miquel *et al.*, 2004; Sabliov *et al.*, 2009; Luo *et al.*, 2011).

Physicochemical analyses suggest that electrostatic interactions, hydrogen bonds, and hydrophobic interactions are the main forces in an α-tocopherol–zein–chitosan complex. Chitosan coating does not affect the encapsulation efficiency but greatly improves the controlled-release properties of α-tocopherol in release profile in the presence of enzymes. This result indicates that α-tocopherol–zein–chitosan complex can be developed as a novel nano-scale delivery system of α-tocopherol supplementation or treatment (Luo *et al.*, 2011).

In the case of encapsulation of vitamin D_3 into zein–chitosan complex nanoparticles prepared by phase separation, it was possible to achieve a controlled-release property and improve the stability of labile nutrients (Luo *et al.*, 2012). Vitamin D is one of the fat-soluble vitamins and has two major physiologically active forms, vitamin D_2 (ergocalciferol) and vitamin D_3 (cholecalciferol). Dietary sources of vitamin D_3 are very limited, and only fish are an abundant source. Vitamin D is an essential nutrient for human health, not only for calcium absorption and homeostasis regulation but also for the prevention of many chronic diseases, such as type 2 diabetes, hypertension, and cardiovascular disease (Picciano, 2010; Pittas *et al.*, 2010; Luo *et al.*, 2012). Vitamin D_3 was first encapsulated into zein nanoparticles, and then chitosan was applied to coat zein nanoparticles and hardened by calcium ions. Photostability of vitamin D_3 against ultraviolet (UV) light was significantly improved after encapsulation of hydrophobic nutrients in zein nanoparticles with chitosan coatings (Luo *et al.*, 2012).

1.3.1.3.2 Zein–polyphenol composite colloidal particles

Polyphenols are known to strongly interact with proline-rich proteins via non-covalent interactions such as H-bonding and hydrophobic interactions. Moreover, polyphenols have excellent solubility in lower alcohols, and thus they can be encapsulated in zein colloidal particles using the process of antisolvent precipitation (Zhang *et al.*, 2008; Zheng *et al.*, 2005; Patel *et al.*, 2012; Patel *et al.*, 2014).

Quercetin is a natural flavonol known to possess a wide range of physiological benefits in humans, including antioxidant, anticancer, and antiviral activities (Zheng *et al.*, 2005). Use of this polyphenol for food and clinical applications is limited due to its low oral bioavailability, owing to its limited aqueous solubility and degradation in the physiological alkaline pH of the intestinal tract (Zhang *et al.*, 2008).

Novel zein–quercetin composite colloidal particles were prepared by simultaneous precipitation of zein and quercetin by adding their hydroalcoholic solution to aqueous solution in the presence of sodium caseinate as an electrosteric stabilizer. Electrosteric stabilization of zein colloidal particles using an oppositely charged protein (sodium caseinate) results in the surface interaction between positively charged zein particles and negatively charged caseinate and provides protection against aggregation in physiologically relevant conditions and due to the hydrophilic nature of sodium caseinate (Patel *et al.*, 2014).

The precipitation of quercetin from an organic solvent generally results in the formation of needle-like crystals. Incorporation of quercetin in zein matrix results in the formation of spherical particles, with complete disappearance of needle-like particles at a zein-to-quercetin ratio of 25:1 wt/wt, suggesting effective encapsulation of quercetin. The entrapment of quercetin in zein colloidal particles led to its enhanced molecular stability to alkaline pH and UV irradiation. The positive effect of encapsulation was successfully demonstrated by comparing the antioxidant activity of quercetin in alkaline medium (Patel *et al.*, 2012; Patel *et al.*, 2014).

Curcumin is a natural polyphenol that exhibits a range of pharmacological activities including antioxidant, antiinflammatory, antiproliferative, and antiangiogenic activity (Patel *et al.*, 2010; Aggarwal and Sung, 2009). It is a very powerful antioxidant, but the formulation and delivery of curcumin in oral products is a very challenging task due to a combination of factors including low solubility in aqueous medium, photodegradation, susceptibility to enzymatic degradation, and instability in alkaline intestinal conditions (Patel *et al.*, 2014; Patel *et al.*, 2010). Zein–curcumin composite colloidal particles were successfully prepared using an antisolvent precipitation method. Encapsulation of curcumin in zein colloidal particles was carried out by coprecipitating different ratios of zein to curcumin (50:1 to 5:1 wt/wt) in the presence of sodium caseinate as a stabilizer. Curcumin in colloidal particles showed enhanced water dispersibility. Zein colloidal particles led to enhanced stability of curcumin at all physiologically relevant pH levels and to UV irradiation (Patel *et al.*, 2010; Patel *et al.*, 2014).

Procyanidins are known to have antioxidant capacities and might reduce the risk of chronic diseases, such as cardiovascular diseases and cancers (Lou *et al.*, 2012), and cranberry procyanidins exhibit preventive effects against urinary tract infections. Cranberry procyanidins have been encapsulated in zein colloidal particles using a modified liquid–liquid dispersion method to enhance their stability as well as improve their bioavailability through controlled *in vivo* delivery (Lou *et al.*, 2012; Patel *et al.*, 2014).

1.3.1.3.3 Zein–protein nanoparticles and microparticles

Zein–β-lactoglobulin nanoparticles

To design a colloidal delivery system to encapsulate the poorly water-soluble bioactive flavonoid tangeritin, a hydrophobic protein (zein) was used as a core for forming protein nanoparticles based on antisolvent precipitation (Chen *et al.*, 2014).

Tangeritin is a flavonoid found in citrus fruits and has beneficial effects that include anticarcinogenic activity and antiinflammatory effects (Li *et al.*, 2009). However, the extensive application of this flavonoid is currently limited because of its low water solubility, which means it may be present in foods as crystals, making it difficult to incorporate into many aqueous-based foods and beverages (Li *et al.*, 2009; Patel *et al.*, 2012; Chen *et al.*, 2014).

Tangeritin-loaded protein nanoparticles were produced by mixing an organic phase containing zein and tangeritin with an aqueous phase containing β-lactoglobulin, then converting it into powder by freeze-drying. When dispersed in water, this powder formed a colloidal suspension that was relatively stable to particle aggregation and sedimentation. To the authors' knowledge (Chen *et al.*, 2014), this was the first time that zein nanoparticles had been used as a delivery system for tangeritin, which is an important nutraceutical. Thus, bioactive flavonoid tangeritin incorporated into small protein nanoparticles that consisted of a hydrophobic zein core and an amphiphilic β-lactoglobulin shell could be used in various food products as a functional ingredient. These zein–protein nanoparticles behaved similarly to β-lactoglobulin–coated fat droplets under different environmental conditions: They were stable at low salt concentrations at pH values far from the isoelectric point, but they aggregated at higher salt levels and pH values near the isoelectric point. In addition, they were stable to aggregation at temperatures below the thermal denaturation temperature of β-lactoglobulin, but they aggregated at higher temperatures, particularly in the presence of salt (Chen *et al.*, 2014).

Zein–soy protein microparticles

A novel technique, the cold gelation method, has been reported to produce zein–soy protein isolate (SPI) complex microparticles for delivery of hydrophilic nutraceuticals, such as riboflavin (vitamin B_2) (Chen and Subirade, 2009). In this method, zein was dissolved at pH 11.0 in the absence of alcohol and then mixed with preheated SPI and calcium carbonate. The mixture was then emulsified in soybean oil to form a water-in-oil emulsion, followed by addition of acetic acid to lower the pH and induce the gelation of the zein–SPI matrix. Blending of SPI and zein provides a convenient method of adjusting the hydrophobicity and crystallinity of the protein matrix. Interestingly, in this process without any alcohol involvement, phase separation did not occur between zein and SPI, which suggested excellent compatibility and miscibility.

When compared with pure SPI microparticles that showed first-order release kinetics of riboflavin, zein–SPI microparticles demonstrated a zero-order release kinetics in simulated gastric and intestinal conditions. Microspheres with zein–SPI blended at ratios of 5:5 and 7:3 displayed near-zero-order release kinetics, and less than 20% of the riboflavin was released from the microspheres after 30 minutes in gastric fluid, which is the expected time for a food product to pass from the stomach into the intestine and suggests that most of the capacity could reach the intestine without being exposed to gastric conditions. The remaining riboflavin was analyzed after complete enzymatic degradation of the protein matrices and found to be 91% to 96% active, indicating that the nutrient was well preserved in the zein–SPI microspheres (Chen and Subirade, 2009).

Research results showed that zein–SPI microparticles were surprisingly better than pure zein or SPI microparticles in terms of slowing the release rate and increasing the absorption availability of riboflavin in the jejunum, the main site of absorption. Zein–SPI complex microparticles encapsulating riboflavin were further tested in a food product (yogurt). Suspending microparticles in yogurt significantly delayed nutrient release, which would increase the likelihood of gastric-sensitive nutrients passing intact into the intestine for absorption. Thus, zein–SPI complex microparticles exhibited features for delivery of hydrophilic nutrients or drugs with significantly improved bioavailability. Moreover, because no organic solvent was involved in this cold gelation method, the zein–SPI microparticles were proposed as a system for delivering hydrophilic nutrients for food applications (Luo and Wang, 2014).

1.3.1.3.4 Zein–omega-3 polyunsaturated fatty acids

Fish oil, flax oil, and, more recently, algae oil are the most commonly used sources of omega-3 polyunsaturated fatty acids (omega-3 PUFAs). Omega-3 PUFAs have been associated with a variety of health benefits, such as reducing the risk of coronary heart disease, hypertension, arthritis, and immune response disorders (Quispe-Condori *et al.*, 2011; Rubio-Rodríguez *et al.*, 2010). However, one of the major drawbacks of oils rich in PUFAs is rapid oxidation of multiple unsaturated carbon–carbon double bonds of PUFAs, which involves the formation of toxic products such as peroxides or undesirable off-flavor compounds (Quispe-Condori *et al.*, 2011).

For encapsulation of fish oil in solid zein particles, a liquid–liquid dispersion process was used that could provide a simple method to produce submicrometer-sized solid particles for incorporating lipophilic bioactive compounds as alternative delivery systems to emulsions (Zhong *et al.*, 2009).

The liquid–liquid dispersion process involved the preparation of stock solutions by dissolving different amounts of zein and fish oil (zein-to-oil ratios of 2:1, 4:1, 6:1, and 8:1) in 90% isopropanol; the stock solution was then sheared into deionized water. The decrease of overall isopropanol concentration resulted in the precipitation of oil-loaded zein particles with diameters of 350 to 450 nm. After freeze-drying, samples of the encapsulated fish oil in solid zein particles (with a zein-to-oil ratio of 4:1 or lower) showed good oxidative stability, as assessed by the development of lipid hydroperoxide values during storage. This result showed that solid zein nanoparticles may be incorporated into food products, such as beverages, snacks, and cereals, to supplement bioactive compounds beneficial to human health (Zhong *et al.*, 2009).

Similarly, flax oil (which is rich in PUFAs and hence has low stability and high susceptibility to oxidation) was stabilized by encapsulation in zein microparticles prepared by spray-drying and freeze-drying (Quispe-Condori *et al.*, 2011).

1.3.2 Inulin

1.3.2.1 Origin and structure

Inulin is a natural polysaccharide belonging to the fructans group. It is a plant-derived compound occurring as storage carbohydrate in many members of the Asteraceae family including chicory, Jerusalem artichoke, and dahlia (Barclay *et al.*, 2010; Beirao-da-Costa *et al.*, 2013). This polysaccharide is also produced by bacteria (*Streptococcus mutans;* Wolff *et al.*, 2000) and fungal species, mainly members of the *Aspergillus* species (Kurakake *et al.*, 2007). Chicory (*Cichorium intybus* L., var. *sativum*) is the main natural source of inulin, which is characterized by a substantial fraction of inulin compounds with a high degree of polymerization (Van Loo *et al.*, 1995; Beirao-da Costa *et al.*, 2013).

Chemically, inulin is a polymer built of linear chains of fructosyl groups bonded by β-2,1 glycosidic linkage, with the reducing end terminated by an α-D-1,2 glucopyranoside ring group. It is described as α-D-glucopyranosyl-[α-D-fructofuranosyl](n-1)-D-fructofuranoside (Figure 1.2) (Dan *et al.*, 2009; Kurakake *et al.*, 2007; Barclay *et al.*, 2010). In general, inulins derived from plants have chains containing from 2 to 100 or more units of fructose. Both origin (the species of plant) and the time of harvest affect inulin's length of chains and

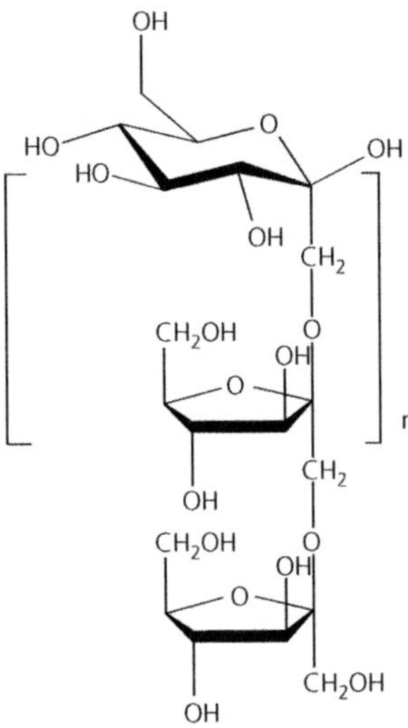

Figure 1.2 Chemical structure of inulin (Dan *et al.*, 2009).

polydispersity (Ronkart *et al.*, 2007; Barclay *et al.*, 2010). The degree of polymerization of inulin produced by microorganisms varies between 10,000 and 100,000 (Franck and De Leenheer, 2002; Barcley *et al.*, 2010).

1.3.2.2 Properties

Multiple application possibilities of inulin are the result of its special physiochemical properties. Inulin is characterized by its biochemical neutrality and nontoxicity (Barclay *et al.*, 2010). In addition, it is described as a substance with a bland neutral taste and without any off flavors or aftertaste. In general, normal inulin has a slightly sweet taste, about one tenth of the sweetness of sugar, but removing from inulin's structure the fraction with polymerization degree below 10 leads to total loss of this flavor (Franck, 2002). Noteworthy is that the presence of β-2,1 glycosidic linkages cause this polymer to be indigestible by humans and higher animals. In the gastrointestinal tract, inulin is digested before it reaches the colon by the activity of inhabiting *Bifidobacterium* species (Lopez-Molina *et al.*, 2005), and hence it acts as dietary fiber and a prebiotic. Its health-promoting effects include improvement of the immune system, increase in calcium and magnesium assimilation, and reduction of cholesterol and serum lipid levels (Coudray *et al.*, 1997; Niness, 1999; Lopez-Molina *et al.*, 2005).

A significant advantage of inulin with respect to its application is its solubility and gelation. Solubility of this polysaccharide is inversely dependent on the chain length, and solubility decreases with increasing chain length. Generally, it is rather poorly water soluble, about 10% at room temperature, creating solutions with quite low viscosity (Franck, 2002). However, inulin with short chains is dissolved in aqueous solution in a concentration up to 80%, whereas longer chain fractions are much less dissolved and even precipitate in the crystalline forms (Kim *et al.*, 2001; Franck and De Leenheer, 2002). Inulin gelation can be performed by cooling a hot solubilized solution or by shearing suspensions of this polymer; the thermal method gives gels that are stronger and smoother and that have smaller particle size. The concentration of inulin to form gels in aqueous solutions, depending on the chain length, is greater than 13% for longer chains and 25% for shorter chains (Kim *et al.*, 2001; Franck and De Leenheer, 2002; Barclay, 2010). This kind of gel consists of a three-dimensional network of insoluble submicrometer crystalline inulin particles in water. Physical gel stability is guaranteed by a high amount of water immobilized in this network (Franck, 2002). Inulin interacts with other gelling agents, including alginate, gellan gum, κ- and ι-carrageenans, gelatin, and maltodextrins, and despite its lack of emulsifying properties, it can be used in encapsulation processes as a stabilizer of matrix (de Barros Fernandes *et al.*, 2014b).

1.3.2.3 Application in the encapsulation process

Inulin is widely used, especially in the food and pharmaceuticals industry. Application of this polysaccharide in food technology is based on its gelation properties. The texture, mouth feel, and even glossy appearance of inulin gels is similar to that of fat, and hence it is mainly used as its replacement. Because of its sweet taste, inulin can also replace sugar. As a result, inulin can be used to produce a low-calorie food (Stevens *et al.*, 2001; Kim *et al.*, 2001; Franck and De Leenheer, 2002; Robertfroid, 2005; Dan *et al.*, 2009; Barclay *et al.*, 2010). In the pharmacy, inulin functions mainly as a stabilizer and excipient (Fuchs, 1987; Dan *et al.*, 2009; Barclay *et al.*, 2010).

A group of scientists has focused on the inulin as an encapsulant agent. They studied the spray-drying encapsulation process of essential oils from oregano and rosemary using inulin separately (Beirao-da-Costa *et al.*, 2012 and 2013) or in complex with other gelling substances (de Barros Fernandes *et al.*, 2014a and 2014b). Researchers noticed that obtained inulin microcapsules were regular, smooth, uninjured, and spherical, with size in the range of 3 to 4.5 μm (Beirao-da-Costa *et al.*, 2013). Those capsules also were more stable in comparison with gelatin–sucrose microparticles (Beirao-da-Costa *et al.*, 2012). Whey protein–inulin mixture in ratios of 1:1 and 3:1 created a good–quality wall matrix of microcapsules with immobilized rosemary essential oil (de Barros Fernandes *et al.*, 2014a). Moreover, in studying the impact of the partial or total replacement of gum arabic by modified starch, maltodextrin, or inulin on properties of microcapsules with rosemary essential oil, it was noticed that the particles containing inulin were characterized by smoother surface. The addition of inulin also had a positive influence on the particles' wettability and decreased the hygroscopicity under high relative humidity. However, the encapsulation process was less efficient (de Barros Fernandes *et al.*, 2014b).

1.3.3 Angum gum

1.3.3.1 Origin and structure

A native biopolymer, Angum gum, is a natural exudate of *Amygdalus scoparia* Spach, which is grown mainly in the southern and western rangelands of Iran. Local people use it as a functional ingredient for nutritional and medicinal purposes (Jafari *et al.*, 2013).

1.3.3.2 Properties and application in the encapsulation process

Angum gum was used as a food flavor encapsulant in spray-drying encapsulation of D-limonene. After gum extraction, gum dispersions with maltodextrin were prepared in water (in 1%–5% concentrations) and emulsified with 5% and 10% D-limonene using high-pressure homogenization. The emulsification properties of this novel biopolymer in comparison with a model Arabic gum (Arg) showed that the increase in the level of Arabic gum leads to a decrease in emulsion droplet size, whereas increasing Angum gum content results in bigger droplet sizes. Gums such as Angum gum have the advantage of being independent of pH and ionic strength of the emulsion, as compared with proteins, which lose their emulsifying abilities in different emulsion environment conditions (Jafari *et al.*, 2013).

Extensive polymer interactions at the interface lead to the formation of an interfacial membrane, which may therefore provide better protection against droplet recoalescence, and this results in more-stable emulsions of Angum gum than Arabic gum. Native and unrecognized biopolymers such as Angum gum can be a good alternative for various applications, such as emulsification and microencapsulation of food flavors and oils, due to their film- and wall matrix–forming properties for covering the active ingredients and producing encapsulated powders (Jafari *et al.*, 2013).

1.3.4 *Opuntia ficus-indica*

1.3.4.1 Origin and structure of mucilage

The cactus pear, *Opuntia ficus-indica* (a member of the Cactaceae family, and colloquially known as prickly pear or nopal), is characterized by the production of a hydrocolloid commonly known as *mucilage* (nopal mucilage), which forms molecular networks that are able to retain large amounts of water (Saag *et al.*, 1975; McGarvie and Parolis, 1981; Medina-Torres *et al.*, 2000; Sepulveda *et al.*, 2007). *O ficus-indica* mucilage is a high-molecular-weight polysaccharide that behaves as a polyelectrolyte and contains a molecular structure of up to 30,000 different sugars. Chemical composition of *O. ficus-indica* mucilage is a complex mixture of polysaccharides, such as L-arabinose, D-galactose, D-xylose, and L-rhamnose, and D-galacturonic acid, which represent up to 10 g per 100 g of total sugars (McGarvie *et al.*, 1981; Medina-Torres *et al.*, 2000; Saenz *et al.*, 2004). In *O. ficus-indica*, the water-soluble polysaccharide fraction with thickening properties, represents less than 10% of the water-soluble material (Majdoub *et al.*, 2001). The mucilage structure is proposed as two distinctive water-soluble fractions, where one is a pectin with gelling properties with Ca^{2+} and the other is a mucilage without gelling properties (Sepulveda *et al.*, 2007).

1.3.4.2 Properties and application of mucilage in the encapsulation process

Nopal mucilage, due to its emulsifying properties and rheological behavior, is an interesting option for use as a carrier of active substances (Medina-Torres *et al.*, 2000). Its use as an edible coating has been reported in strawberry preservation, where it achieved good results in increasing shelf life (Del-Valle *et al.*, 2005) and improving optical properties and water-vapor transport (Espino-Díaz *et al.*, 2010).

This mucilage has also been studied for its capacity for encapsulating bioactive compounds by spray-drying (Medina-Torres *et al.*, 2013; Saenz *et al.*, 2009). An antioxidant compound (gallic acid) was encapsulated using aqueous extracts from *O. ficus-indica* mucilage as wall material. The mucilage presented a macromolecular dispersion that became less agglomerated by the addition of gallic acid. The intermolecular mucilage–gallic acid interactions became favorable and considerably reduced the size of the aggregate, which confirmed the encapsulation properties of nopal mucilage. The results showed that using spray-drying to process nopal mucilage extract produced a stable powder with small particle size and, consequently, higher viscosity, while also exhibiting higher resistance to flow, mainly due to encapsulated structures (Medina-Torres *et al.*, 2013).

The controlled release of microcapsules of mucilage with gallic acid was designed with respect to the conditions of the small intestine, which is where gallic acid is absorbed. The controlled release indicated that 65% of gallic acid was released in 2.47 days, and the microcapsules of mucilage gum showed high efficiency (>60%). The nopal mucilage represents a promising and effective encapsulating agent of bioactive additives for incorporation into functional foods (Medina-Torres *et al.*, 2013).

1.3.5 Shellac

1.3.5.1 Origin and structure

Shellac is a natural biodegradable polymer. It is a resin secreted by the female lac insect *(Laccifer Lacca,* also called *Kerria lacca),* which parasitizes some types of trees in India, Thailand, and China. Shellac is a heterogeneous compound of polar and nonpolar components consisting of polyhydroxy polycarboxylic esters, lactones, and anhydrides, with the main acid components being aleuritic and terpenic acids (Krause and Muller, 2001; Patel *et al.*, 2013a). Its chemical structure is presented in Figure 1.3. Shellac is a nontoxic and harmless substance and GRAS (Okamoto and Ibanez, 1986; Chauhan *et al.*, 2013).

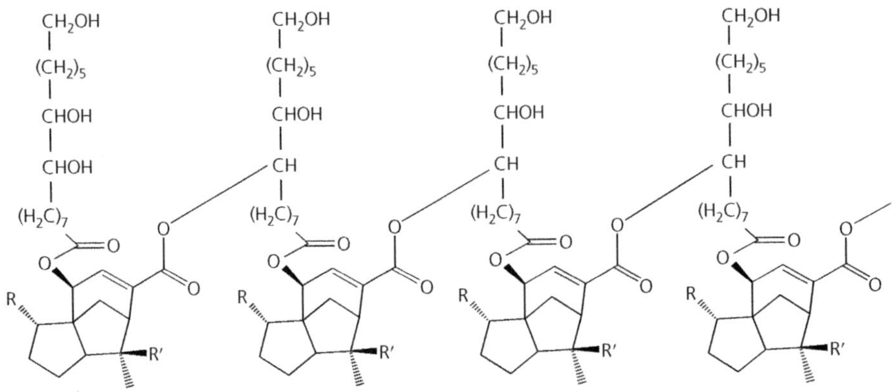

Figure 1.3 Chemical structure of shellac (Limmatvapirat, 2004).

1.3.5.2 Properties

Shellac, as a polymer containing carboxylic groups, is practically insoluble in acidic and pH-neutral aqueous media. Aqueous solutions can be prepared by using alkali salts (Leick *et al.*, 2011). Despite those solubility problems, shellac has some attractive properties, including cohesiveness, thermoplasticity, and insulating and film-forming ability. It is lipophilic and has a tendency to self-assemble into colloidal structures based on its solvent properties (Patel *et al.*, 2013b). Moreover, this resin can interact with some hydrocolloids, including pectin, xanthan gum, and cellulose derivatives (Patel *et al.*, 2011) based on non-covalent interplays, which are attributed to hydroxy aliphatic fatty acid–aleuritic acid, the main component of shellac. Because of the large amounts of carboxylic and hydroxyl groups in the structure of shellac and a strong negative charge, aleuritic acid participates in hydrogen bonding and electrostatic interactions (Coelho *et al.*, 2012; Patel *et al.*, 2013a).

1.3.5.3 Application in the encapsulation process

All of these properties make shellac widely used in industry, especially in pharmaceuticals as an enteric coating material and in the food industry as a glazing agent for confections and nutritional supplements (Boonsongrit *et al.*, 2006; Bouchemal, 2008; Leick *et al.*, 2011). Shellac is applied as an encapsulating agent of active substances (Patent no. 5,164,210; Leick *et al.*, 2011; Patel *et al.*, 2013b).

Patent no. 5,164,210 (1991) discloses the encapsulation of high-intensity sweetener ingredients applied in chewing gum by using as encapsulant mixture of shellac and zein. The encapsulant composition was prepared by dissolving components in ethyl alcohol, mixing them in an appropriate proportion, and then adding sweetener. Finally, the ethyl alcohol was removed from the sweetener–encapsulant mixture by air-drying in a fume hood for 16 hours at room temperature. Obtained capsules had a more positive effect on the shelf life of the chewing gum and sweetener than shellac or zein used separately.

Other researchers have worked on novel all-natural polymeric microcapsules composed of gelatin and shellac. They were obtained using a simple extrusion method without any cross-linkers, which was based on the strong interactions between two oppositely charged polymers and the immediate precipitation of acid-resistant shellac. The mixture of gelatin and shellac was dropped in an acidic medium, causing an instant solidification of liquid drops into solid microcapsules that retained their spherical shape on air-drying. Some possible applications of these novel capsules have been successfully demonstrated for pharmaceuticals (loading and release of bioactives such as silibinin and epigallocatechin gallate), the food industry (encapsulation of colorants and flavors, e.g., curcumin and D-limonene), and biotechnology (immobilization of enzymes) (Patel *et al.*, 2013a).

Leick's group (2010) studied thin-walled, liquid-filled composite capsules where matrix was based on calcium pectinate and shellac. Capsules were also prepared by extrusion. It was shown that the addition of shellac improved mechanical properties of the capsules, which were stronger and showed less deformation than pure pectin capsules. These results are promising for industrial applications in the future.

Acknowledgments

We would like to thank Agnieszka Bednarczyk-Drąg for English-language editing of our chapter.

References

Adhikari, K., Mustapha, A., and Grün, I. U. (2003). Survival and metabolic activity of microencapsulated *Bifidobacterium longum* in stirred yogurt. *Journal of Food Science: Food Microbiology and Safety* 68(1): 275–280.

Aggarwal, B. B., and Sung, B. (2009). Pharmacological basis for the role of curcumin in chronic diseases: An age-old spice with modern targets. *Trends in Pharmacological Sciences* 30: 85–94.

Barclay, T., Ginic-Markovica, M., Cooper, P., and Petrovsky, N. (2010). Inulin - a versatile polysaccharide with multiple pharmaceutical and food chemical uses, *Journal of Excipients and Food Chemicals* 1(3): 27–50.

Beirão da Costa, S., Duarte, C., Bourbon, A. I., Pinheiro, A. C., Serra, A. T., *et al.* (2012). Effect of the matrix system in the delivery and *in vitro* bioactivity of microencapsulated oregano essential oil. *Journal of Food Engineering* 110: 190–199.

Beirão-da-Costa, S., Duarte, C., Bourbon, A. I., Pinheiro, A. C., Januário, M. I. N., *et al.* (2013). Inulin potential for encapsulation and controlled delivery of oregano essential oil. *Food Hydrocolloids* 33: 199–206.

Beristain, C. I., Garcia, H. S., and Vernon-Carter, E. J. (2001). Spray dried encapsulation of cardamom *(Elettaria cardamomum)* essential oil with mesquite *(Prosopis juliflora)* gum. *LWT – Food Science and Technology* 34: 398–401.

Boonsongrit, Y., Mitrevej, A., and Mueller B. W. (2006). Chitosan drug binding by ionic interaction. *European Journal of Pharmaceutics and Biopharmaceutics* 62: 267–274.
Bouchemal, K. (2008). New challenges for pharmaceutical formulations and drug delivery systems characterization using isothermal titration calorimetry. *Drug Discovery Today* 13(21–22): 960–972.
Chauhan, O. P., Nanjappa, C., Ashok, N., Ravi, N. Roopa N., and Raju P. S. (2013). Shellac and aloe vera gel based surface coating for shelf life extension of tomatoes. *Journal of Food Science and Technology* 52(2): 1200–1205.
Chen, L., and Subirade, M. (2009). Elaboration and characterization of soy/zein protein microspheres for controlled nutraceutical delivery. *Biomacromolecules* 10: 3327–3334.
Chen, J., Zheng, J., McClements, D. J., and Xiao, H. (2014). Tangeretin-loaded protein nanoparticles fabricated from zein/β-lactoglobulin: Preparation, characterization, and functional performance. *Food Chemistry* 158: 466–472.
Coelho, C., Nanabala, R., Ménager, M., Commereuc, S., and Verney, V. (2012). Molecular changes during natural biopolymer ageing: The case of shellac. *Polymer Degradation and Stability* 97: 936–940.
Coudray, C., Bellanger, J., Castiglia-Delavaud, C., Remesy, C., Vermorel, M., and Rayssignuier, Y. (1997). Effect of soluble or partly soluble dietary fibres supplementation on absorption and balance of calcium, magnesium, iron and zinc in healthy young men. *European Journal of Clinical Nutrition* 51: 375–380.
Dan, A., Ghosh, S., and Moulik, S. P. (2009). Physicochemical studies on the biopolymer inulin: A critical evaluation of its self aggregation, aggregate-morphology, interaction with water, and thermal stability. *Biopolymers* 91: 687–699.
de Barros Fernandes, R. V., Borges, S. V., Botrel, D. A., and de Oliveira, C. S. (2014a). Physical and chemical properties of encapsulated rosemary essential oil by spray drying using whey protein–inulin blends as carriers. *International Journal of Food Science and Technology*, 49: 1522–1529.
de Barros Fernandesa, R. V., Borgesa, S. V., and Botrel, D. A. (2014b). Gum arabic/starch/maltodextrin/inulin as wall materials on the microencapsulation of rosemary essential oil. *Carbohydrate Polymers* 101: 524–532.
Del-Valle, V., Hernandez-Munoz, P., Guarda, A., and Galotto, M. J. (2005). Development of a cactus-mucilage edible coating *(Opuncia ficus-indica)* and its application to extend strawberry *(Fragaria ananassa)* shelf-life. *Food Chemistry* 91: 751–756.
Espino-Diaz, M., Ornelas-Paz, J. J., Martinez-Tellez, M. A., Santillan, C., Barbosa-Canovas, G. V., *et al.* (2010). Development and characterization of edible films based on mucilage of *Opuntia ficus-indica* (L.). *Journal of Food Science* 75: 347–352.
Fang, X., Shima, M., and Adachi S. (2005). Effects of drying conditions on the oxidation of linoleic acid encapsulated with gum arabic by spray-drying. *Food Science and Technology Research* 11(4): 380–384.
Franck, A., and De Leenheer, L. (2002). Inulin. In: *Polysaccharides II: Polysaccharides from Eukaryotes*, pp. 439–479. A. Steinbüchel and E. J. Vandamme, eds. Berlin: Wiley–VCH Verlag GmbH.
Franck, A. (2002). Technological functionality of inulin and oligofructose. *British Journal of Nutrition* 87(Suppl 2): S287–S291.
Fuchs, A. (1987). Potentials for non-food utilization of fructose and inulin. *Starch-Starke*, 39: 335–343.
Hamakar, B. R, Mohamed, A. A, Habben, J. E, Huang, C. P, and Larkins, B. A. (1995). Efficient procedure for extracting maize and sorghum kernel proteins reveals higher prolamin contents than the conventional method. *Cereal Chemistry* 72: 583–588.
Herrera, E., and Barbas, C. (2001). Vitamin E: Action, metabolism and perspectives. *Journal of Physiology and Biochemistry* 57: 43–56.
Higuera-Ciapara, I., Felix-Valenzuela, L., Goycoolea, F., and Arguelles-Monal W. (2004). Microencapsulation of astaxanthin in a chitosan matrix. *Carbohydrate Polymers* 56: 41–45.

Jafari, S. M., Beheshti, P., and Assadpour, E. (2013). Emulsification properties of a novel hydrocolloid (Angum gum) for D-limonene droplets compared with Arabic gum. *International Journal of Biological Macromolecules* 61: 182–188.

Janiszewska, E., and Włodarczyk, J. (2013). Influence of spray drying conditions on beetroot pigments retention after microencapsulation process. *Acta Agrophysica* 20(2): 343–356.

Jimenez, M., Garcia, H. S., and Beristain, C. I. (2006). Spray-dried encapsulation of conjugated linoleic acid (CLA) with polymeric matrices. *Journal of the Science of Food and Agriculture* 86: 2431–2437.

Kailasapathy, K. (2006). Survival of free and encapsulated probiotic bacteria and their effect on the sensory properties of yoghurt. *LWT – Food Science and Technology* 39: 1221–1227.

Kaushik, V., and Roos, Y. H. (2007). Limonene encapsulation in freeze-drying of gum arabic–sucrose–gelatin systems. *LWT – Food Science and Technology.* 40: 1381–1391.

Kim, Y., Faqih, M. N., and Wang, S. S. (2001). Factors affecting gel formation of inulin. *Carbohydrate Polymers* 46: 135–145.

Klinkesorn, U., Sophanodora, P., Chinachoti, P., Decker, E. A., and McClements, D. J. (2006). Characterization of spray-dried tuna oil emulsified in two-layered interfacial membranes prepared using electrostatic layer-by-layer deposition. *Food Research International* 39(4): 449–457.

Kolanowski, W., Jaworska, D., Weissbrodt, J., and Kunz, B. (2007). Sensory assessment of microencapsulated fish oil powder. *Journal of the American Oil Chemists' Society* 84(1): 37–45.

Krasaekoopt, W., Bhandari, B., and Deeth, H. C. (2006). Survival of probiotics encapsulated in chitosan-coated alginate beads in yoghurt from UHT- and conventionally treated milk during storage. *LWT – Food Science and Technology* 39(2): 177–183.

Krause, K. P., and Muller, R. H. (2001). Production of aqueous shellac dispersions by high pressure homogenization. *International Journal of Pharmaceutics* 223: 89–92.

Kurakake, M., Ogawa, K., Sugie, M., Takemura, A., Sugiura, K., and Komaki, T. (2007). Two types of β-fructofuranosidases from *Aspergillus oryzae* KB. *Journal of Agricultural and Food Chemistry* 56: 591–596.

Lawton, J. W. (2002). Zein: A history of processing and use. *Cereal Chemistry* 79: 1–18.

Leick, S., Kott, M., Degen, P., Henning, S., Pasler, T., *et al.* (2011). Mechanical properties of liquid-filled shellac composite capsules. *Physical Chemistry Chemical Physics,* 13: 2765–2773.

Li, S., Pan, M. H., Lo, C. Y., Tan, D., Wang, Y., *et al.* (2009). Chemistry and health effects of polymethoxyflavones and hydroxylated polymethoxyflavones. *Journal of Functional Foods* 1: 2–12.

López-Molina, D., Navarro-Martinez, M. D., Rojas-Melgarejo, F., Hiner, A. N. P., Chazarra, S., and Rodríguez-López, J. N. (2005). Molecular properties and prebiotic effect of inulin obtained from artichoke (*Cynara scolymus* L.). *Phytochemistry* 66(12): 1476–1484.

Luo, Y., Teng, Z., and Wang, Q. (2012). Development of zein nanoparticles coated with carboxymethyl chitosan for encapsulation and controlled release of vitamin D_3. *Journal of Agricultural and Food Chemistry* 60: 836–843.

Luo, Y., and Wang, Q. (2014). Zein-based micro- and nano-particles for drug and nutrient delivery: A review. *Journal of Applied Polymer Science* 131: 40696.

Luo, Y., Zhang, B., Whent, M., Yo, L., and Wang, Q. (2011). Preparation and characterization of zein/chitosan complex for encapsulation of α-tocopherol, and its *in vitro* controlled release study. *Colloids and Surfaces B: Biointerfaces* 85: 145–152.

Madziva, H., Kailasapathy, K., and Phillips, M. (2006). Evaluation of alginate–pectin capsules in cheddar cheese as a food carrier for the delivery of folic acid. *LWT – Food Science and Technology* 39: 146–151.

Majdoub, H., Roudesli, S., Picton, L., Le Cerf, D., Muller, G., and Grisel, M. (2001). Prickly pear nopal pectin from *Opuntia ficus-indica:* Physico-chemical study in dilute and semi-dilute solutions. *Carbohydrate Polymers* 46: 69–79.

Martins, R., Pereira, S., Siqueira, S., Salomao, W., and Freitas, L. (2013). Curcuminoid content and antioxidant activity in spray dried microparticles containing turmeric extract. *Food Research International* 50: 657–663.

McGarvie, D., and Parolis, H. (1981). Methylation analysis of the mucilage of *Opuntia ficus-indica*. *Carbohydrate Research* 88: 305–314.

McMaster, L. D., Kokott, S. A., and Slatter, P. (2005). Micro-encapsulation of *Bifidobacterium lactis* for incorporation into soft foods. *World J Microbiol Biotechnol* 21:723–728.

Medina-Torres, L., Brito-De La Fuente, E., Torrestiana-Sanchez, B., and Katthain, R. (2000). Rheological properties of the mucilage gum *(Opuntia ficus-indica)*. *Food Hydrocolloids* 14: 417–424.

Medina-Torres, L., García-Cruz, E. E., Calderas, F., González Laredo, R. F., Sánchez-Olivares, G., *et al.* (2013). Microencapsulation by spray drying of gallic acid with nopal mucilage *(Opuntia ficus-indica)*. *LWT – Food Science and Technology* 50: 642–650.

Milani, J., and Maleki, G. (2012). Hydrocolloids in Food Industry. In: *Food Industrial Processes – Methods and Equipment*. B. Valdez, ed. Croatia: InTech.

Miquel, E., Alegria, A., Barbera, R., Farre, R., and Clemente, G. (2004). Stability of tocopherols in adapted milk-based infant formulas during storage. *International Dairy Journal* 14 (11): 1003–1011.

Niness, K. R. (1999). Inulin and oligofructose: What are they? *Journal of Nutrition* 129: 1402S–1406S.

O'Riordan, K., Andrews, D., Buckle, K., and Conway, P. (2001). Evaluation of microencapsulation of a *Bifidobacterium* strain with starch as an approach to prolonging viability during storage. *Journal of Applied Microbiology* 91:1059–1066.

Okamoto, M. Y., and Ibanez, P. S. (1986). Final report on the safety assessment of shellac. *Journal of the American College of Toxicology* 5: 309–327.

Özkan, G., and Bilek, S. F. (2014). Microencapsulation of natural food colourants. *Internationa. Journal of Nutrition and Food Sciences* 3(3): 145–156.

Pan, K., Zhong, Q., and Baek, S. J. (2013). Enhanced dispersibility and bioactivity of curcumin by encapsulation in casein nanocapsules. *Journal of Agricultural and Food Chemistry* 61(25): 6036–6043.

Patel, A. R., Heussen, P. C. M., Hazekamp, J., Drost, E., and Velikov, K. P. (2012). Quercetin loaded biopolymeric colloidal particles prepared by simultaneous precipitation of quercetin with hydrophobic protein in aqueous medium. *Food Chemistry* 133: 423–429.

Patel, A., Heussen, P., Hazekamp, J., and Velikov, K. P. (2011). Stabilisation and controlled release of silibinin from pH responsive shellac colloidal particles. *Soft Matter* 7: 8549–8555.

Patel, A., Hu, Y., Tiwari, J. K., and Velikov, K. P. (2010). Synthesis and characterisation of zein–curcumin colloidal particles. *Soft Matter* 6: 6192–6199.

Patel, A. R., Remijn, C., Mulet Cabero, A.-I., Heussen, P. C. M., Jack, W. M., *et al.* (2013a). Novel all-natural microcapsules from gelatin and shellac for biorelated applications. *Advanced Functional Materials* 23: 4710–4718.

Patel, A. R., Schatteman, D., De Vos, W. H., Lesaffer, A., and Dewettinck, K. (2013b). Preparation and rheological characterization of shellac oleogels and oleogel-based emulsions. *Journal of Colloid and Interface Science* 411: 114–121.

Patel, A. R., and Velikov, K. P. (2014). Zein as a source of functional colloidal nano- and microstructures. *Current Opinion in Colloid & Interface Science* 19: 450–458.

Patent number 5,164,210. (1991). Zein/shellac encapsulation of high intensity sweeteners in chewing gum.

Picciano, M. F. (2010). Vitamin D status and health. *Critical Reviews in Food Science and Nutrition* 50: 24–25.

Picot, A., and Lacroix, C. (2004). Encapsulation of bifidobacteria in whey protein–based microcapsules and survival in simulated gastrointestinal conditions and in yoghurt. *International Dairy Journal* 14(6): 505–515.

Pitalua, E., Jimenez, M., Vernon-Carter, E., and Beristain, C. (2010). Antioxidative activity of microcapsules with beetroot juice using gum arabic as wall material. *Food and Bioprocess Processing* 88(2–3): 253–258.

Pittas, A. G., Chung, M., Trikalinos, T., Mitri, J., Brendel, M., *et al.* (2010). Systematic review: Vitamin D and cardiometabolic outcomes. *Annals of Internal Medicine* 152: 307–314.

Polavarapu, S., Oliver, Ch. M., Ajlouni, S., and Augustin, M. A. (2011). Physicochemical characterisation and oxidative stability of fish oil and fish oil–extra virgin olive oil microencapsulated by sugar beet pectin. *Food Chemistry* 127: 1694–1705.

Porrarud, S., and Pranee, A. (2010). Microencapsulation of Zn–chlorophyll pigment from Pandan leaf by spray drying and its characteristic. *International Food Research Journal* 17: 1031–1042.

Quispe-Condori, S., Saldana, M. D. A., and Temelli F. (2011). Microencapsulation of flax oil with zein using spray and freeze drying, *LWT – Food Science and Technology* 44: 1880–1887.

Roberfroid, M. B. (2005). Introducing inulin-type fructans. *British Journal of Nutrition* 93(Suppl. 1): S13–S25.

Rocha, G., Favaro-Trindade, C., and Ferreira Grosso, C. (2012). Microencapsulation of lycopene by spray drying: Characterization, stability and application of microcapsules. *Food and Bioproducts Processing* 90: 37–42.

Ronkart, S. N., Deroanne, C., Paquot, M., Fougnies, C., Lambrechts, J.-C., and Blecker, C. S. (2007). Characterization of the physical state of spray-dried inulin. *Food Biophysics* 2: 83–92.

Rubio-Rodríguez, N., Beltrán, S., Jaime, I., de Diego, S. M., Sanz, M. T., and Rovira-Carballido, J. (2010) Production of ω-3 polyunsaturated fatty acid concentrates: A review. *Innovative Food Science and Emerging Technologies* 11: 1–12.

Saag, L., Sanderson, G., Moyna, P., and Ramos, G. (1975). Cactaceae mucilage composition. *Journal of the Science of Food and Agriculture*, 26: 993–1000.

Sabliov, C. M., Fronczek, C., Astete, C. E., Khachaturyan, M., Khachatryan, L., and Leonardi, C. (2009). Effect of temperature and UV light degradation of α-tocopherol in free and dissolved form. *Journal of the American Oil Chemists' Society* 86(9): 895–902.

Saenz, C., Sepulveda, E., and Matsuhiro, B. (2004). *Opuntia* spp. mucilages: A functional component with industrial perspectives. *Journal of Arid Environments* 57: 275–290.

Saenz, C., Tapia, S., Chávez, J., and Robert, P. (2009). Microencapsulation by spray drying of bioactive compounds from cactus pear *(Opuntia ficus-indica)*. *Food Chemistry* 114: 616–622.

Sepulveda, E., Saenz, C., Aliaga, E., and Aceituno, C. (2007). Extraction and characterization of mucilage in *Opuntia* spp. *Journal of Arid Environments* 68: 534–545.

Shu, B., Yu, W., Zhao, Y., and Liu, X. (2006). Study on microencapsulation of lycopene by spray-drying. *Journal of Food Engineering* 76: 664–669.

Shukla, R., and Cheryan, M. (2001). Zein: The industrial protein from corn. *Industrial Crops and Products* 13: 171–192.

Silva, D. F., Favaro-Trindade, C. S., Rocha, G. A., and Thomazini, M. (2012). Microencapsulation of lycopene by gelatin–pectin complex coacervation. *Journal of Food Processing and Preservation* 36: 185–190.

Stevens. C. V., Meriggi, A., and Booten, K. (2001). Chemical modification of inulin, a valuable renewable resource, and its industrial applications. *Biomacromolecules* 2: 1–16.

Tan, L. H., Chan, L. W., and Heng, P. W. S. (2005). Effect of oil loading on microspheres produced by spray drying. *Journal of Microencapsulation: Micro and Nano Carriers* 22(3): 253–259.

Torres-Giner, S., Martinez-Abad, A., Ocio, M. J., and Lagaron, J. M. (2010). Stabilization of a nutraceutical omega-3 fatty acid by encapsulation in ultrathin electrosprayed zein prolamine. *Food Science* 75: 69–79.

Tucker, J. M., and Townsend, D. M. (2005). Alpha-tocopherol: Roles in prevention and therapy of human disease. *Biomedicine and Pharmacotherapy* 59: 380–387.

Van Loo, J., Coussement, P., De Leenheer, L., Hoebregs, H., and Smits, G. (1995). On the presence of inulin and oligofrutose as a natural ingredients in the Western diet. *Critical Reviews in Food Science and Nutrition* 35: 525–552.

Wang, Q., Yin, L. L., and Padua, G. W. (2008). Effect of hydrophilic and lipophilic compounds on zein microstructures. *Food Biophysics* 3(2): 174–181.

Wolff, D., Czapla, S., Heyer, A. G., Radosta, S., Mischnick, P., and Springer, J. (2000). Globular shape of high molar mass inulin revealed by static light scattering and viscometry. *Polymer* 41: 8009–8016.

Yáñez-Fernández, J., Ramos-Ramirez, E. G., and Salazar-Montoya, J. A. (2008). Rheological characterization of dispersions and emulsions used in the preparation of microcapsules obtained by interfacial polymerization containing *Lactobacillus* sp. *European Food Research and Technology* 226(5): 957–966.

Zhang, Y., Yang, Y., Tang, K., Hu, X., and Zou, G. (2008). Physicochemical characterization and antioxidant activity of quercetin-loaded chitosan nanoparticles. *Journal of Applied Polymer Science* 107: 891–897.

Zheng, Y., Haworth, I. S., Zuo, Z., Chow, M. S., and Chow, A. H. (2005). Physicochemical and structural characterization of quercetin–beta-cyclodextrin complexes. *Journal of Pharmaceutical Sciences* 94: 1079–1089.

Zhong, Q., and Jin, M. (2009). Zein nanoparticles produced by liquid–liquid dispersion. *Food Hydrocolloids* 23: 2380–2387.

Zhong, Q., Tian, H., and Zivanovic, S. (2009). Encapsulation of fish oil in solid zein particles by liquid–liquid dispersion. *Journal of Food Processing and Preservation* 33: 255–270.

Zhu, F., Kale, A., and Cheryan, M. (2007). Fractionation of zein by size exclusion chromatography. *Journal of Agricultural and Food Chemistry* 55: 3843–3849.

CHAPTER 2

High-pressure-treated corn starch as an alternative carrier of molecules of nutritional interest for food systems

Lorena Deladino[1], Aline Schneider Teixeira[1], Antonio Diego Molina García[2], and Alba Sofia Navarro[1,3]

[1] *Centro de Investigación y Desarrollo en Criotecnología de los Alimentos (CIDCA), CONICET, Facultad de Ciencias Exactas, Universidad Nacional de la Plata, 47 y 116, La Plata, (1900), Argentina*

[2] *Instituto de Ciencia y Tecnología de Alimentos y Nutrición (ICTAN-CSIC), José Antonio Novais 10, 28040, Madrid, Spain*

[3] *Facultad de Ingeniería, Universidad Nacional de la Plata, 1 y 47, La Plata, (1900), Argentina*

2.1 Introduction

Development of novel functional foods includes bioactive compounds such as antioxidants, minerals, vitamins, probiotics, and bioactive peptides, among others, which may have physiological benefits or reduce the risks of diseases. However, all of these materials are sensitive to food processing and storage conditions, as well as to conditions in the gastrointestinal tract after their consumption. Incorporation of nutraceutical compounds into food matrices has led to extensive research on the most appropriate technology to protect them, depending on the active ingredients and the matrix composition.

Encapsulation provides a simple way to protect solid, liquid and gaseous materials in small capsules that release their contents at controlled rates over prolonged periods (Champagne and Fustier, 2007). In addition, encapsulation in food systems can be used to solve formulation problems arising from a limited chemical or physical stability of the active ingredient or an incompatibility between the active ingredient and the food matrix. This technology also allows control of the release of a sensory active compound or the bioavailability of specific nutrients (Deladino *et al.*, 2007).

An understanding of the physical and chemical phenomena of encapsulation process is needed to design the matrix that contains the bioactive compounds, considering their stability, release, perception and digestion. Among the

---

New Polymers for Encapsulation of Nutraceutical Compounds, First Edition.
Edited by Jorge Carlos Ruiz Ruiz and Maira Rubi Segura Campos.

encapsulant materials, polymers such as alginate and pectin have been used to protect active ingredients in capsules (Anbinder *et al.*, 2011; Deladino *et al.*, 2008). Several researchers have focused on starch as a matrix material by modifying this structure (Le Corre *et al.*, 2010; Glenn *et al.*, 2010; Uthumporn *et al.*, 2010; Rodrigues and Emeje, 2012; Elfstrand *et al.*, 2007). Starch is a renewable, natural, low-cost source that can be combined with an advanced technology such as high hydrostatic pressure (HHP) to obtain starch carriers for bioactive compounds. HHP technology allows us to develop new materials with innovative functionalities in common materials such as starches. This chapter describes corn starch as a carrier for bioactive compounds and the modifications in its structure by the HHP technique. The ability of HHP-treated corn starch to bind and carry zinc and magnesium salts and natural antioxidants of yerba mate *(Ilex paraguariensis)* extracts is presented as a case study in section 2.1.

2.2 Trends in nutraceutical foods

Consumer demand for healthy nutritious foods increased the market for nutraceutical products, which are substances that can potentially promote health and wellness and specifically reduce risk of disease (Aryee and Boye, 2015). The global nutraceuticals market was valued at $171.8 billion in 2014 and is expected to reach $241.1 billion by 2019 (BCC Research, 2014).This trend has led food technologists to focus on new ingredients for foods with additional health-promoting functions. Ingredients have to maintain their biological activity during processing and storage. Thus, food technologists are devoted to developing technologies to protect these ingredients from environmental conditions. Controlled release of the bioactive compounds at the target site of the body and compatibility with other components are also important issues for investigation (Ubbink and Krüger, 2006).

Vehiculization of bioactive compounds in food systems is a strategy for delivering micronutrients at suitable levels that provide health benefits. Micronutrient deficiencies still remain a major public health problem in many countries, with more than two billion people suffering from one or more micronutrient deficiencies (Meenakshi, 2009; World Health Organization, 2012). In many areas of the world, poor-quality diet and lack of micronutrients are more widespread problems than low energy intake (Stewart *et al.*, 2010), with devastating consequences: 19 % of all deaths before the age of 5 years can be attributed to deficiency of vitamin A, zinc, iron, and/or iodine (Prentice *et al.*, 2008). Therefore, this problem becomes a major challenge for the entire scientific community. Micronutrient deficiency can be addressed through diversifying the diet or by giving mineral supplements, fortifying food, and/or increasing mineral concentrations in edible crops (biofortification). Food biofortification combined with availability is encouraged as an immediate strategy to spread mineral consumption (Bouis *et al.*, 2003; Genc *et al.*, 2005; White and Broadley, 2005).

Nowadays, natural sources of bioactive compounds are investigated to give an alternative to the use of synthetic additives. Bioactive substances from plant origin, like phytochemicals, have been extensively investigated for their potential functional properties (Shahidi, 2004; Ahmad and Beg, 2001; Heim *et al.*, 2002). Phytochemicals, mainly phenolics, are antioxidant compounds associated with a role in preventing age-related and degenerative diseases, including atherosclerosis, cancer, and diabetes, among others (Shahidi 2004). The antioxidant effect of phenolic compounds in functional foods is produced by different mechanisms, including free-radical scavenging and metal chelation (Heim *et al.*, 2002). However, to achieve this functionality, antioxidants must be protected from the surrounding medium or the processing conditions during food production.

2.2.1 Natural antioxidants from yerba mate extracts

Yerba mate (*Ilex paraguariensis* Saint Hilaire) is a tree originating in South America that grows in a limited zone within Argentina, Brazil, and Paraguay. Their leaves (Figure 2.1) are industrially processed to obtain the yerba mate (Figure 2.2), which can be consumed as an aqueous extract (Figure 2.3). Several authors have extensively studied the composition of yerba mate, and the main bioactive substances reported in the aqueous extracts are phenolic compounds, such as chlorogenic acid and its isomers; gallic, *p*-coumaric, caffeic, and ferulic acids; rutin; epicatechin; gallocatechin; and saponins (Anesini *et al.*, 2012; Dugo *et al.*, 2009; Filip *et al.*, 2001; González de Mejía *et al.*, 2009; Heck *et al.*, 2008).

Some studies have demonstrated that the antioxidant activity of yerba mate increases after enzymatic hydrolysis (Rivelli *et al.*, 2011) and can be higher than that of red wine and green or black tea (Bixby *et al.*, 2005; Campos *et al.*, 1996). Acute or short-term consumption of *I. paraguariensis* infusions can inhibit the lipid peroxidation of plasma and low-density lipoproteins in healthy subjects (Gugliucci, 1996; Silva *et al.*, 2008) and increase plasma antioxidant capacity (Matsumoto *et al.*, 2009; Silva *et al.*, 2008). drinking these infusions can also improve plasma paraoxonase-1 (PON-1) activity (Menini *et al.*, 2007) and increase the gene expression of superoxide dismutase and catalase in peripheral

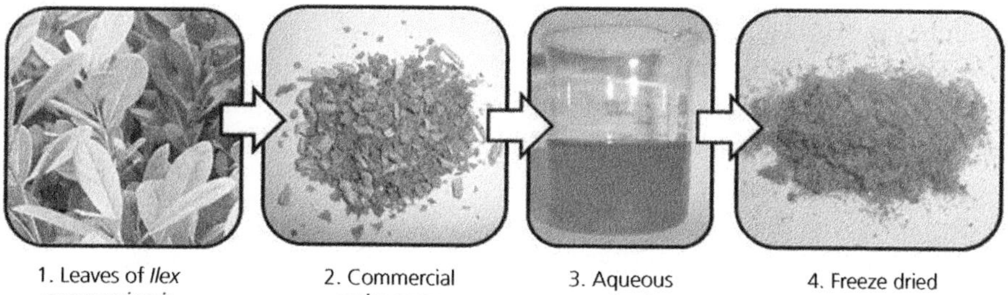

Figure 2.1 Different stages of yerba mate processing.

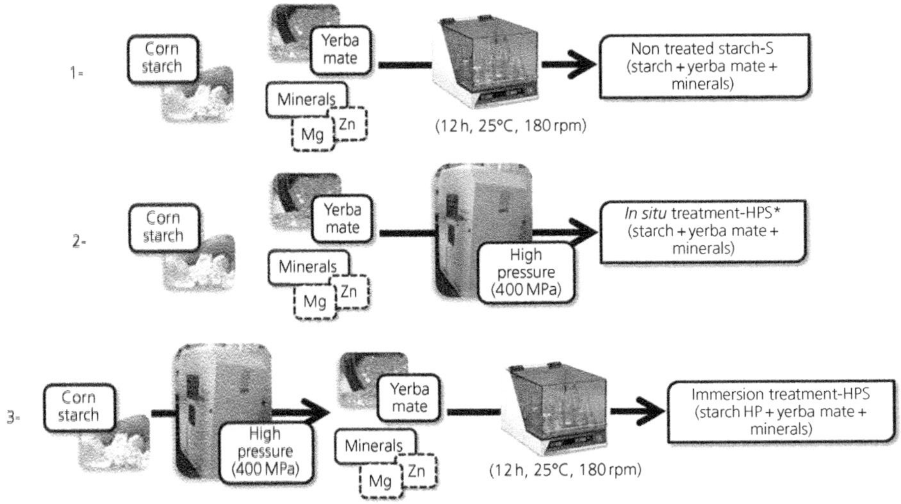

Figure 2.2 Scheme showing the production of bioactive starches. **1,** Nontreated starch (S); **2,** *in situ* treatment (HPS*); **3,** Immersion treatment (HPS).

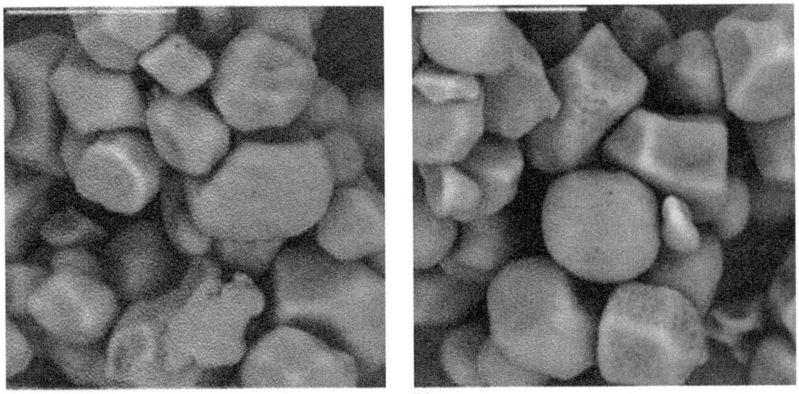

Figure 2.3 SEM photographs showing the external surface of native corn starch granules **(a)** and corn starch after high-pressure treatment **(b).** The *bars* correspond to 20 μm.

blood leukocytes (Matsumoto *et al.*, 2009). These results suggest that yerba mate ameliorates oxidative stress, hyperglycemia, hypercholesterolemia, and endothelial dysfunction, thus potentially acting to prevent atherosclerosis. The effects of *I. paraguariensis* on health have an important role in antioxidant, antiinflammatory, antimutagenic, and lipid-lowering activities, particularly in the prevention of cardiovascular diseases (Bracesco *et al.*, 2011).

Lyophilized yerba mate extract (Figure 2.4) becomes sticky when it is not protected against ambient conditions (Deladino *et al.*, 2007a). Thus, the marked hygroscopic behavior that influences the flowability of this product was minimized through encapsulation technology (Anbinder *et al.*, 2011; Deladino *et al.*, 2007b; Deladino *et al.*, 2008).

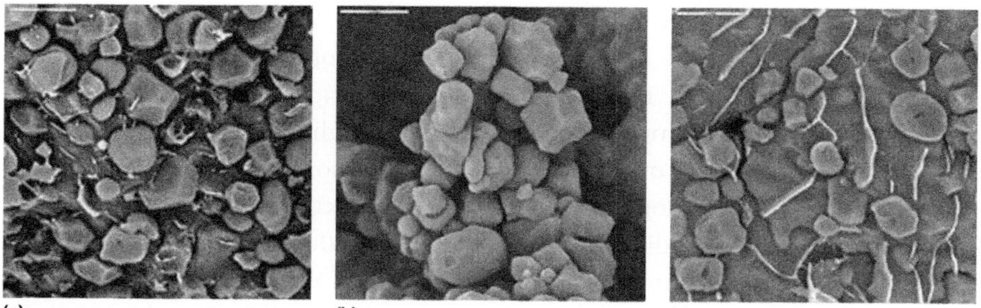

(a) (b) (c)

Figure 2.4 Cryo-SEM micrographs of HPS **(a)**, $HPS_{magnesium}$ **(b)**, and HPS_{zinc} **(c)**. HPS samples showed changes in the surface characteristics of granules influenced for the type of mineral (magnesium or zinc), which indicated alterations in the structure. The *bars* correspond to 10 μm.

2.2.2 Micronutrients: Magnesium and zinc

The human body requires at least 22 mineral elements for its well-being (White and Broadley, 2005). More than 30% of the world's habitants are estimated to have a zinc deficiency, constituting one of the most important nutritional and public health problems affecting developing countries (International Zinc Nutrition Consultative Group, 2004; McLean *et al.*, 2007). Magnesium deficiency is also common in many developed and developing countries (Rude and Gruber, 2004; Thacher *et al.*, 2006). In contrast with macronutrients, which are consumed in large amounts (hundreds of grams daily), micronutrients, such as magnesium and zinc, are ingested in very small amounts (micrograms and milligrams per day). These minerals perform important roles in regulating whole-body metabolism, including energy utilization and work performance.

Magnesium is the second most common intracellular cation, with only 1% of total magnesium found in blood. This mineral has a wide range of functions throughout the body, acting as a cofactor for more than 300 enzymatic reactions, in which food is catabolized and new chemical products are formed, affecting glucose transportation and influencing insulin sensitivity (Shils, 1993). Abundant research focuses on identifying the functions and interactions of magnesium in the body. Examples include glycogen breakdown, fat oxidation, protein synthesis, ATP synthesis, and the second messenger system. Magnesium also serves as a physiologic regulator of membrane stability and is involved in neuromuscular, cardiovascular, immune, and hormonal function (Ebel and Gunther, 1980; Saris *et al.*, 2000). Evidence has shown that low magnesium levels are negatively correlated with the development of insulin resistance and increased risk of the metabolic syndrome and type 2 diabetes mellitus. Hypomagnesemia is present in 10% of patients admitted into hospital and in 65% of patients admitted to intensive care units. Studying the prevention of these diseases is at the forefront of nutrition-focused research (Guerrero-Romero *et al.*, 2015; Takagi *et al.*, 2015). The strong evidence connecting magnesium deficiency with the metabolic syndrome and type 2 diabetes mellitus suggests magnesium supplementation may be an appropriate intervention technique to control the progression of these diseases.

With regard to the zinc, this mineral is located throughout the body, especially as a component of thousands of zinc metalloproteins or zinc-binding proteins and nucleic acids. The ability of zinc to participate in strong but readily exchangeable ligand binding (Williams, 1989) has high biologic value, interacting with a wide range of organic ligands that incorporate zinc into numerous biologic systems. The biologic role of zinc is now recognized in structure and function of proteins, including enzymes (more than 200 enzymes in mammals), transcription factors, hormonal receptor sites, and biological membranes. Zinc has numerous central roles in DNA and RNA metabolism (MacDonald, 2000); it is involved in signal transduction, gene expression, and apoptosis; and it participates in many components of macronutrient metabolism. Zinc metalloenzymes and zinc-dependent enzymes have been identified and are involved in nucleic acid metabolism and cellular proliferation, differentiation, and growth (MacDonald, 2000). In addition, some zinc-containing enzymes, such as carbonic anhydrase and lactate dehydrogenase, are involved in intermediary metabolism during exercise. Another zinc-containing enzyme, superoxide dismutase, protects against free-radical damage (Tapiero and Tew, 2003). More than 3% of all identified human genes contain zinc-finger domains (Maret, 2001). Thus, zinc plays a broad role in gene expression (Truong-Tran *et al.*, 2001).

2.3 Starch as a carrier for bioactive compounds

Starch constitutes the main carbohydrate in the human diet and contributes greatly to the textural properties of many foods. Characteristic properties like thickening, colloidal stabilizing, gelling, bulking, water retention, and adhesion allow several industrial applications of this polysaccharide (Jobling, 2004). Starch exists naturally within the plant cells and is mainly composed of amylose and amylopectin; lipids and minerals are minor components of starch granules. Amylose is a linear polymer of glucopyranose units linked through α-D-(1-4) glycosidic linkages, and amylopectin is a branched polymer containing an average one branch point, which is $1 \rightarrow 4 \rightarrow 6$ linked for every 20 to 25 straight-chain residues. Starch granules are densely packed with semicrystalline structures where the crystalline regions are related to the amylopectin component and the amorphous ones mainly represent amylose.

Distribution of amylose and amylopectin within the starch granules varies among starches from different sources. In the case of corn starch, the amylose-to-amylopectin ratio is 25:75. Extensive research has been carried out into the structure of starch granules using different techniques, among them, x-ray diffraction, differential scanning calorimetry (DSC), scanning electron microscopy (SEM), and confocal scanning laser microscopy (CSLM) (Fredriksson *et al.*, 1998; Huber and BeMiller, 2000; Pérez and Bertoft, 2010; Wu *et al.*, 2014).

Physical and chemical characteristics of the starch granules, such as mean granule size, granule size distribution, amylose-to-amylopectin ratio, and mineral content, influence starch behavior in aqueous systems. When the starch granules are heated in an excess of water, gelatinization takes place. Hydrogen bonds in amorphous regions are disrupted, and water, acting as a plasticizer, is absorbed by the granules, provoking their swelling. The loss of order in the amorphous regions is a nonequilibrium, glass transition process (Slade and Levine, 1993). Melting of the crystallites of amylopectin and leaching of both polymer molecules, mainly amylose, also take place during gelatinization. At the end of the process, an irreversible loss of crystalline order occurs. The gelatinization process takes place over a temperature range that depends on the botanical source of starch, the amount of water present (Parker and Ring, 2000), the perfection of crystallites, and the subpopulations of granules with different physical and chemical properties (Fredriksson *et al.*, 1998; Ji *et al.*, 2004). The temperature range and the enthalpy associated with the gelatinization process can be determined by heating the starch dispersions at different heating rates in a calorimeter (Fredriksson *et al.*, 1998).

Different strategies have been applied to give functionalities to starches through obtaining edible films, porous systems, or encapsulation matrices to hold active compounds. Starch is used to develop edible films due to its capacity to form a continuous matrix that can be used to protect sensitive materials (Bonilla *et al.*, 2013; Mali *et al.*, 2006; Talja *et al.*, 2007). Additives like glycerol, acting as a plasticizer of the starch films, affect crystallinity and glass transition temperature (T_g), the temperature at which the material changes from the glassy to the rubbery state for a given heating rate. This plasticizer seems to limit crystal growth and recrystallization due to the interaction with the polymeric chains (Mali *et al.*, 2006). Starch films can be used to protect bioactive compounds, although the film-forming procedure could affect some antioxidant additives (Bonilla *et al.*, 2013; Corrales *et al.*, 2009; Souza *et al.*, 2011).

Another strategy is to use starch as a holding matrix itself, because starch granules are, themselves, porous systems that can increase their porosity by enzymatic procedures, freezing–solvent exchange techniques, and application of high-pressure treatments, among others (Buckow *et al.*, 2007; Liu *et al.*, Zhou 2008; Qian *et al.*, 2011; Simonin *et al.*, 2011; Uthumporn *et al.*, 2010). The porous structure of starch could be useful to hold and release sensitive materials such as antioxidants, vitamins, and flavors. The product obtained, porous starch, has extensive applications not only in the food industry but also in tissue engineering, agriculture, cosmetics, pulp and paper, and other industries (Chang *et al.*, 2011; Glenn *et al.*, 2010; Nakamatsu *et al.*, 2006).

By the enzymatic procedure, starch structure can be modified by hydrolyzing the amorphous regions with enzymes such as α-amylase and glucoamylase at sub-gelatinization temperature, which generates pores depending on the degree of hydrolysis and the starch type (Uthumporn *et al.*, 2010). Uthumporn and colleagues (2010) showed that corn starch had the highest degree of hydrolysis compared with cassava, mung bean, and sago starches, giving different pore structures. After hydrolysis treatment, corn starch showed pores that penetrated deep into the granules, but enzymatic erosion was observed at the surface for cassava, and isolated pore structures were obtained for mung bean and sago starches. Porous starch can also be obtained by the freezing–solvent exchange technique after ice crystals in the frozen gel are replaced with ethanol. Research of Qian and colleagues (2011) showed that when the concentration of the potato starch paste increased and the ethanol-to-water ratio decreased, the size of the holes in the resulting porous starch gradually decreased (Qian *et al.*, 2011).

An example of the use of starch granules as a holding matrix to protect bioactive compounds is reported by Glenn's team (2010), who encapsulated essential oils in porous microspheres obtained by pumping an aqueous high-amylose starch gelatinous melt through an atomizing nozzle. The atomized starch droplets were air-classified into two fractions (5 and 100 μm mean particle sizes) and collected in ethanol. The essential oils (thymol, clove, origanum, and camphor white oil) were encapsulated within the pore structure, obtaining free-flowing powders, without agglomeration.

Traditionally, starch is used as a common excipient in drug formulations for the pharmaceuticals industry; however, several investigations have been performed about the production of starch microparticles to encapsulate active substances (Le Corre *et al.*, 2010; Rodrigues and Emeje, 2012). Elfstrand and colleagues (2007), based on manufacturing problems of starch microspheres intended for subcutaneous injections, investigated the formation of ordered structure in starch dispersions by DSC. According to these authors, starch microparticles (Biosphere®) were obtained by emulsifying starch in an aqueous two-phase system containing polyethylene glycol and then stabilizing the microspheres by crystallization of the starch matrix. The bioactive compound (protein) was encapsulated into the starch matrix during the manufacturing of the microspheres. Experimental conditions, like incubation time and temperature, were important for the amount of ordered structure and thermal stability of the crystallites. The presence of additives (carbonate buffer, polyethylene glycol, and bovine serum albumin) mainly affected the nucleation phase of the crystallization process. Thus, a specific amount of ordered structure with desired thermal characteristics could be predicted by the optimization procedure (Elfstrand *et al.*, 2007).

Current advances in technology allow us to obtain more novel starches with significantly enhanced functionality. The intended use of this polymer as a carrier for bioactive compounds has led to the application of high hydrostatic pressure to native starches and the evaluation of these carrier systems as vehicles for bioactive compounds.

2.3.1 Starches treated by high-hydrostatic-pressure technology

Pressure, a major thermodynamic variable, is as determining for the stability of chemical compounds and the fate of their reactions as temperature can be, and only the small pressure variation occurring in many natural environments makes us forget it. High-hydrostatic-pressure treatments have become a widespread and growing technology applied in food systems.

The effect of hydrostatic pressure on biological macromolecules derives from the fulfillment of *Le Chatelier's principle* when pressure increases. The classic equation based on this principle

$$d(\Delta G) = (\Delta V)dp + (dS)dT \tag{2.1}$$

specifies the dependence of the free energy (ΔG) of a process with pressure (p) and temperature (T), through the change in volume (ΔV) and entropy (ΔS). At constant temperature, a relation among K (the two-state equilibrium constant), p, and ΔV, can be derived:

$$\ln K = \ln K_0 (p\Delta V) / RT \tag{2.2}$$

ΔV is actually the reaction molar volume increment (Harrington and Kegeles, 1973; Silva *et al.*, 2001). Parallel kinetic equations can be employed to describe the pressure dependence of reaction rate constants (Molina-García, 2003). Consequently, the equilibrium is displaced toward the lower-volume species. For small molecules and moderate increments, pressure changes can be unnoticed because either there is no other conformation available differing in specific volume, or this difference is too small to give rise to a conformational change. In the same way, reactions can be displaced, yielding a combined smaller specific volume, for all the intervening species. This must not be forgotten, because the solvent and its interactions (such as hydrogen bonds) can contribute significantly to the overall volume of the system (Knorr *et al.*, 2006).

Starch can be considered a huge macromolecule where monomers are bound by covalent links into the macromolecular components amylose and amylopectin, and these polysaccharides are linked together by secondary binding forces, mainly by hydrogen bonds, but also by hydrophobic and van der Waals forces (Imberty *et al.*, 1991). The larger size of the molecule allows the existence of smaller volume conformations, but the hydrogen bonds' contributions are determinant for its high-pressure behavior (Knorr *et al.*, 2006). Starch gelatinization can be considered a reaction of starch with water, where many intramolecular hydrogen bonds are replaced by starch–water bonds. Pressure treatments in the absence of water yield unaltered starch granules (Hibi *et al.*, 1993). The special characteristics of water, with its tetrahedral hydrogen bonds network, imply that bulk water has a larger molecular volume than those molecules detached from that network and involved in hydrogen bonds with nonwater molecules, such as starch (Molina-García, 2003).

The effect of thermodynamic changes in equilibrium is intrinsically reversible, and consequently, when pressure is released, displaced reactions would be reversed and the conformational changes induced by pressure increases would be restored (Molina-García, 2003). Nevertheless, the process of starch gelatinization involves a number of irreversible steps, such as the disentangling of the component polysaccharide chains and their exit from the starch granule, when the attaching intracellular hydrogen bonds are dissolved. Thus, starch pressure gelatinization is, like the thermally induced process, irreversible (Knorr *et al.*, 2006).

However, starch gelatinized by pressure is reported to be not completely identical to the thermal product. This may be due to the reduced thermal drift of the released polysaccharide chains, in comparison with the high-temperature product, where higher-energy solvent Brownian movement displaces their chains farther away from the original granular structure. Differences in rheological and microstructural properties have been found, with reduced granular degradation and amylose leaching, as well as smaller swelling index and specific gravity (Douzals *et al.*, 1998; Knorr *et al.*, 2006; Stolt *et al.*, 2000). However, there is no agreement about whether pressure affects the resulting gel retrograde behavior, that is, reordering of the starch structure of gelatinized systems that occurs upon aging.

Temperature and time are synergistically associated with pressure in starch gelatinization. Pressure–temperature phase diagrams have been drawn for several starch types (Rubens and Heremans, 2000; Smeller, 2002). Generally speaking, both pressure and temperature add to the gelatinization of starch, and the process can be completed at higher temperatures, even if pressure is not so elevated (Bauer and Knorr, 2005; Stolt *et al.*,2000). Time has also an effect on the degree of gelatinization achieved. The associated effect of temperature must be carefully taken into consideration in pressure treatments, because there is a considerable (tenths of degrees) rise in temperature associated to the pressure built up at the levels employed to gelatinize starch. This rise could alter experiments and processes if not accounted for, especially as, being fully reversible, the pressure release brings about an equivalent temperature drop (Molina-García, 2003; Otero *et al.*, 2000).

Starches from different biological origins behave differently in high-pressure treatments. Those coming from cereal species are generally less resistant than starches from tuber origin. Potato starch is hardly affected up to pressures of 600 MPa (Błaszczak *et al.*, 2005; Douzals *et al.*, 1996; Oh *et al.*, 2008), whereas wheat, barley, corn, and rice starches are completely gelatinized at lower pressures (500 MPa) (Buckow *et al.*, 2007; Douzals *et al.*, 1996; Hibi *et al.*, 1993; Stolt *et al.*, 2000). Corn starch, as a typical cereal-origin product, can be completely gelatinized in a relatively short time in room-temperature treatments (Hibi *et al.*, 1993; Knorr *et al.*, 2006). Although, as stressed above, pressure gelatinization partially preserves starch granular integrity and independence, these characteristics can be potentiated by applying subgelatinization treatments. Corn starch subjected to 400 MPa at mild temperatures (between room temperature and 40 °C) for 30 to 40 minutes presents a mixed character, preserving many of the native granular properties (granular integrity, reduced intergranular interactions) while acquiring some of those of gelatinized starch (such as the partial substitution of internal hydrogen bridges by water bridges, as derived from the DSC reduction in the enthalpy of gelatinization). This enthalpy is related to the nongelatinized starch fraction, which can be also associated to its digestibility or resistant character.

Starch partially gelatinized under high pressure is easier to obtain than its thermal equivalent, as pressure can be applied homogeneously to the whole of the sample, no matter how large, and from a strict time period, which is not easily achieved in thermal treatments. When observed by cryo-scanning electron microscopy, the resulting partially gelatinized granules present a porous character and a partially open network of chains, which suggest their utility for binding a variety of substances of nutritional and pharmaceutical interest (Molina-García *et al.*, 2007; Deladino *et al.*, 2015; Teixeira *et al.*, 2015). The bioactive starches can be obtained following the procedure shown in Figure 2.2.

Corn starch (S) suspensions (10 g/100 mL) are mixed with freeze-dried yerba mate extracts or/and mineral salts, then the suspensions are submitted to environmental shaking and dried (Figure 2.1). For *in situ* HHP treatment, corn starch suspensions with the active compound were submitted to high pressure (Figure 2.2). Another option is to apply the HHP treatment only to corn starch suspensions, then the resulting treated polymer is immersed with the active compounds in an environmental shaker as mentioned before (Figure 2.3). To obtain the treated starches, the equipment used in our study was a High Pressure Pilot Food Processor (Stansted Fluid Power LTD, Model FP 571000:9/2C, Harlow, UK), operating under 400 MPa, for 35 minutes with 38 °C as the initial vessel temperature and reaching a final process temperature of 40 °C (Deladino *et al.*, 2015; Teixeira *et al.*, 2015).

Thus, the bioactive starches obtained after HHP treatment are easy-handling powders that can be added to different food formulations to protect the functional ingredients from biological or chemical degradation that can occur during processing, storage, and consumption.

2.3.2 Morphology of corn starch carriers

After HHP treatment of starches, granular structure is partially disintegrated, with low quantity of amylose leached out from the granules. When comparing starches with low and high amylose contents submitted to the same HHP treatment, different behavior is observed. Whereas low-amylose starches completely lose the crystalline structure and form a gel-like structure, high-amylose starches retain their granule structure with a lower crystallinity. The amylose present in the granules could have a stabilizing effect to protect starch crystallinity due to the formation of amylose–lipid complexes to restrict the swelling of granules

(Chen *et al.*, 2007; Błaszczak *et al.*, 2007). SEM microscopy allows us to observe the general morphology (Figure 2.3). Once the HHP treatment is applied to native starches, the number of small pores and hollows increases (Figure 2.3b).

According to Błaszczak, Valverde, and Fornal (2005), two different zones can be distinguished: the outer zone of starch granules that remains unchanged after HHP treatment and the inner zone that is completely destroyed and formed gel-like structures. High pressure acts immediately and is independent of the size and the shape of the sample; thus, HHP-treated starches would be more homogeneous than heat-induced gelatinized starches. During the HHP processing, new binding sites are generated and can be exploited to carry and deliver the molecules of interest, such as minerals (Fernández *et al.*, 2008) (Figure 2.4).

Labeling granules with fluorescein isothiocyanate (FITC) allows us to observe fissures cracking the surface and penetrating to the hilum of HHP-treated corn granules (Figure 2.5b, c and d). FITC penetrating behavior reveals a higher

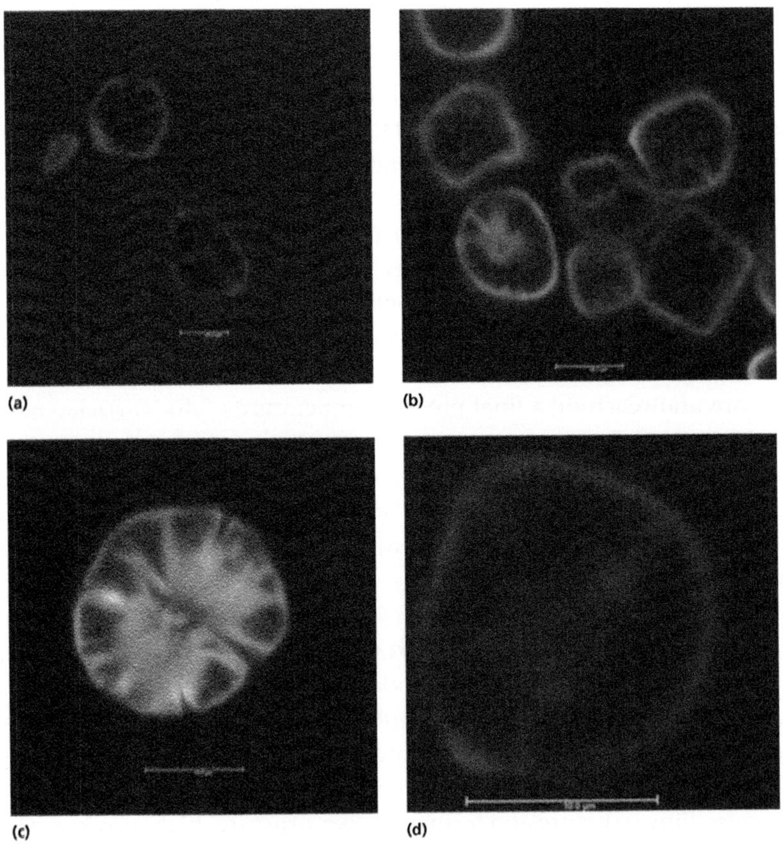

Figure 2.5 Confocal laser scanning micrographs of corn starch granules. **a,** S; **b,** HPS; **c,** HPS_{zinc}, **d,** $HPS_{magnesium}$. HPS_{zinc} showed a higher number of channels, suggesting the presence of more pores. The *bars* correspond to 10 μm.

number of channels, which suggests a presence of more pores, indicating that reagents have access to the granule interior.

2.3.3 Porosity characteristics of treated starch granules

Porosity characteristics of treated starch granules depend on the size, shape, and porosity of the granules. In addition, the specific surface area is proportional to the specific pore volume, and it is inversely related to the pore diameter (Juszczak *et al.*, 2002; Sujka and Jamroz, 2007). The specific surface of starches can be employed as a measure of the surface activity, which, in turn, could help in evaluating the effect of the HHP treatment on the granules. Among many methods of specific surface area examination, the most common are those based on gas or liquid adsorption measurement (Sujka and Jamroz, 2007). The measurements involve determining the isotherms of nitrogen, argon, or krypton adsorption at the temperature of liquid nitrogen and calculating the monolayer capacity basing on BET adsorption isotherm. Specific surface area can be calculated using the formula

$$S_{BET} = V_m S_0 \left(m^2 g^{-1}\right) \tag{2.3}$$

Where S_0 is the surface taken by the adsorbate molecule and V_m is the monolayer volume (Juszczak *et al.*, 2002).

In this way, porosimetric analysis helps researchers understand the effect of the different HHP treatments. Both mercury intrusion and nitrogen adsorption techniques were applied to study the effect of high hydrostatic pressure on the granular structure. Different pore size distribution is obtained by the different encapsulation techniques (Figure 2.6).

Comparing both methods, pore structure analysis by mercury porosimetry is faster than by nitrogen adsorption. In mercury porosimetry and nitrogen adsorption determinations, two different physical interactions take place. Both methods are based on surface tension, capillary forces, and pressure. With mercury porosimetry, large pores at the intrusion phase are determined first, whereas with nitrogen adsorption, the smallest pores are measured at the adsorption phase (Westermarck, 2000). The determination range of high-pressure mercury porosimetry is wider (pore diameter 3 nm to 14 μm) than that of nitrogen adsorption (0.3–300 nm) and detects larger pores that are out of the range of nitrogen adsorption. Thus, the smallest pores that are out of range of mercury porosimetry can be determined with nitrogen adsorption. Results of the two methods can be compared through the following parameters: total pore volume, volume pore size distribution, and specific surface area–to–total pore surface area.

Figure 2.6 shows the pore size distribution of non-treated corn starch and high-pressure-treated starch (HPS). Whereas the prevalent pore size was located between 6 and 14 nm for S and between 4 and 10 nm for HPS, respectively, differences between the pore volumes obtained by each different technique were observed. In addition, nitrogen adsorption allowed detecting a second

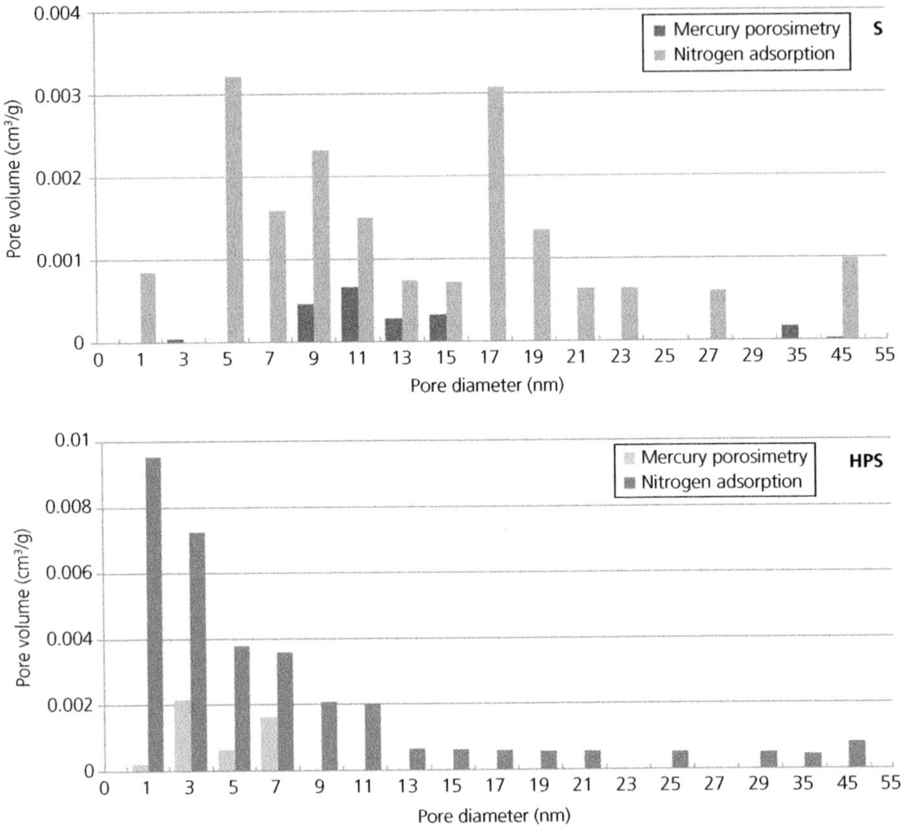

Figure 2.6 Pore size distribution of nontreated and HHP-treated corn starch. Comparison of data obtained by nitrogen gas adsorption and mercury intrusion.

predominant group between 15 and 23 nm with a maximum of 17 nm for native starch and the presence of a lower quantity of pores between 9 and 45 nm for HHP-treated starch.

Juszczak and colleagues (2002) found a group of pores between 10.0 and 14.5 nm to be prevalent in several types of cereal starch granules with nitrogen adsorption. In addition, in corn starch they observed a wide range of pore diameters (from 30 to 10 nm) in the second predominant group of pores. A similar pore size distribution was obtained for waxy maize, with a distinct peak representing the prevalent group of pores 10 to 14.5 nm in diameter. According to Webb and Orr (1997), even if the pore volume values obtained do not agree, surface area values may be similar. This is because small pores have a larger effect on the surface area. However, in our case, surface area values do not agree; total pore area for nontreated starch was 0.989 m^2/g determined by mercury intrusion and 0.2767 m^2/g by nitrogen adsorption; for HHP-treated starch, these values were 3.713 m^2/g and 0.4066 m^2/g, respectively. Similarly, larger surface area values have been obtained with mercury porosimetry than with nitrogen adsorption for other systems like lactose tablets (Dees and Polderman, 1981) and silica samples (Milburn *et al.*, 1991).

2.3.4 Gelatinization properties after high-hydrostatic-pressure treatment

As stated earlier, the degree of gelatinization after the pressure treatment can be determined by differential scanning calorimetry (DSC). Simply, the area under the gelatinization peak is compared before and after the pressure treatment, and the result yields the degree of gelatinization. Another parameter concerning starch gelatinization derived from DSC is the temperature at which the (thermally induced, inside the calorimeter) gelatinization process happens. Actually, several temperatures are observed, a peak temperature and an onset and an end-set temperature. The process spans several degrees, because of both the heterogeneity of starch granules (naturally occurring in a range of sizes and stability) and the different stages of the process.

The effect of pressure treatment in the gelatinization temperature of the remaining nongelatinized starch is controversial: Some authors report a decrease (Błaszczak *et al.*, 2005; Knorr *et al.*, 2006), and others found an increase (Hibi *et al.*, 1993; Muhr *et al.*, 1982; Thevelein *et al.*, 1981) in the gelatinization temperature. The first case could be due to a general destabilization of the granule structure, as is the case in proteins, and the second could work via a preferential gelatinization of the smaller and more unstable granules, leaving the more stable ones unaltered. In our case study, the gelatinization temperature for the HHP-treated corn starch appeared slightly shifted toward lower values as compared to the native one (Figure 2.7). Also, gelatinization enthalpy decreased from 12 J/g to 9 J/g after the treatment. Thus, this 25% of the degree of gelatinization can be attributed to the HHP treatment.

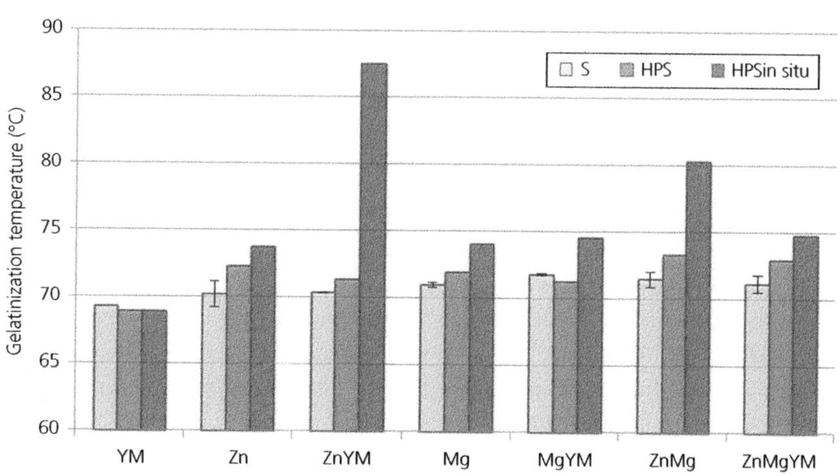

Figure 2.7 Gelatinization temperatures obtained by differential scanning calorimetry for bioactive starches with yerba mate and minerals.

As a general rule, samples containing minerals showed higher peak values due to the presence of zinc and magnesium ions, and the hydroxyl groups of the glucose units would interact with these cations (Teixeira *et al.*, 2015). The starch granule would be stabilized by the presence of the cations, and thus more energy is necessary to reach gelatinization temperatures. As a general trend, peak temperatures increased in the following order: nontreated starch (S) < immersion treatment (HPS) < *in situ* treatment (HPS*) (Figure 2.7); this fact was attributed to the increasing concentration of salts in the HHP-treated samples.

2.3.5 Crystalline structure of starch granules affected by high pressure

The regular packing of amylopectin chains gives rise to a substantial degree of crystallinity on starch granules (from 15% to 45%). Its x-ray patterns are classified as A-type starch (most cereal-origin starches, such as rice, corn, waxy corn, wheat) and B-type starch (tuber origin, such as potato). C-type starch is considered a mixture of A and B types, and retrograded starch shows B-type x-ray diffraction patterns (Imberty *et al.*, 1991; Knorr *et al.*, 2006). B-type starch is found to be more resistant to pressure than A (Katopo *et al.*, 2002). Moreover, pressure has been shown to displace the x-ray pattern from A to B (Hibi *et al.*, 1993; Knorr *et al.*, 2006; Stute *et al.*, 1996). The pressure effects on crystallinity can be considered in terms of the lower density of high-crystallinity granules and accounted for the higher number of water molecules associated to each glucose molecule in the B-type starch, which is consequently more stable and dense. The B-type crystallite has more combined water molecules, which fill up the channel in the cell unit of the crystallite and play a role as a stabilizer, whereas the amylopectin of the A-type starch has a more scattered branching structure (Jane *et al.*, 1997). Hence, the B-type starches are more stable, and the A-type starches with more-flexible scattered branching structures are more active and tend to be rearranged or destroyed by water under high pressure.

In our study, bioactive starches do not show changes in A-type x-ray diffraction patterns after HHP treatment. Characteristic peaks were identified in native and HHP starches (Teixeira *et al.*, 2015). The most interesting parameter that arises from the x-ray diffraction analysis is the determination of the crystalline fraction, which is normally calculated as the ratio between the absorption peaks and the total diffractogram area, expressed as percentage (Teixeira *et al.*, 2015; Mali *et al.*, 2006). In the case of HHP-treated starches carrying minerals, the crystalline fraction can be divided in two portions: The first, common to all samples, is proportion of the starch, which is lower for treated starches (due to a partial gelatinization during the HHP treatment); the second portion is directly related to the amount of mineral loaded in the sample (Figure 2.8).

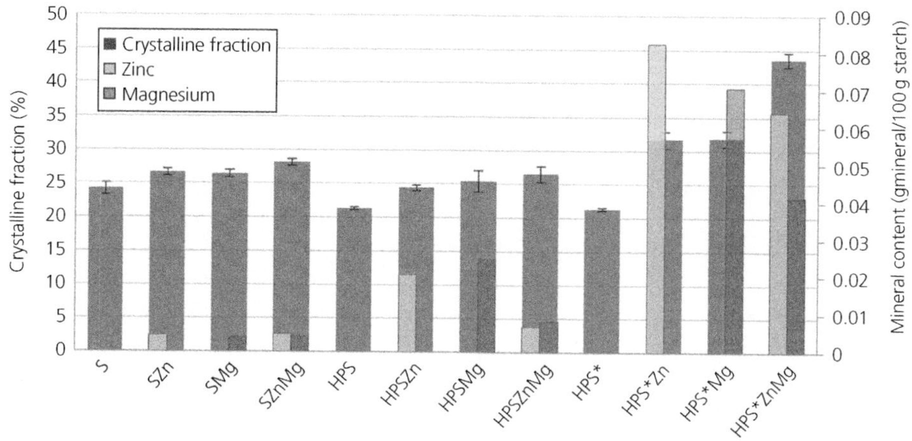

Figure 2.8 Relationship between crystalline fraction of control and bioactive starches and mineral content determined by atomic emission spectrometer. Max sd = 0.0009 for zinc and 0.00004 for magnesium.

2.3.6 Loading of active compounds in bioactive starches

Starch treatment affects mineral content as determined by atomic emission spectrometry following an increasing order of loading: S<HPS<HPS* (Figure 2.8). When two minerals were incorporated into HHP-treated starches, a lower quantity of each mineral alone was loaded. The incorporation of yerba mate extract together with minerals positively affects the zinc load, whereas the opposite effect is reached with magnesium, in both cases, mixing one mineral in turn with yerba mate extracts or the two minerals together and the extract (Teixeira *et al.*, 2015). It has been shown that ions bind to functional groups of starch in different ways (Ciesielski *et al.*, 2003; Łabanowska *et al.*, 2013; Lai *et al.*, 2001). Specifically for the alkali earth metal ions, it is postulated that they can form complexes with starch, but also as for alkali metal ions, there are electrostatic interactions between the cations and anions interacting with –OH groups. Also starch sorption with these metal ions should be taken into account.

The more appropriate methodology to evaluate yerba mate antioxidant loading is HPLC-MS, because it allows us to determine changes in the relative contribution of the different polyphenol compounds generated by HHP treatments and bioactive compound combinations in the sample (Figure 2.9).

Polyphenol composition is preserved when applying HHP-treated starches had the same relative amounts of the main different polyphenols: chlorogenic acid esters (55%), chlorogenic acid isomers (27%), chlorogenic acid (8%), and rutin (10%). This relationship was found for yerba mate lyophilized extracts. Total load of polyphenols is affected by mineral load because the higher amount of minerals loaded in HPS* starches causes a decrease in polyphenol loading. However, when only yerba mate extract is loaded, the highest loading values are obtained by HHP *in situ* treatment (Deladino *et al.*, 2015). Then the hypothesis is

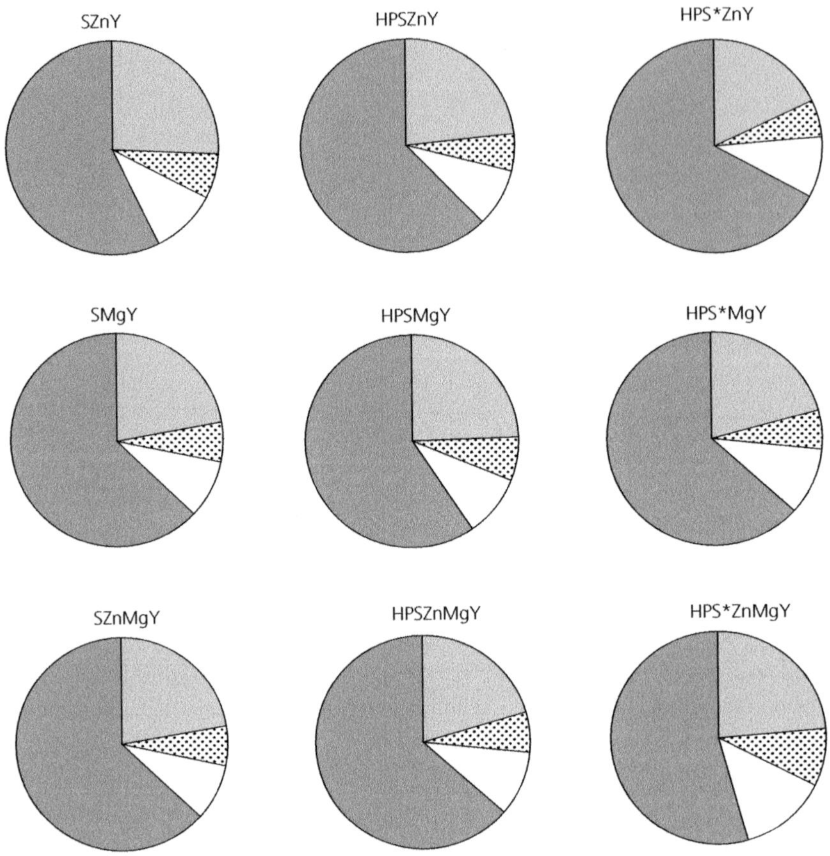

Figure 2.9 Contribution of each polyphenol compound to total polyphenol content of corn starches determined by HPLC-MS. SY, nontreated starch; HPS, HHP-treated starch obtained by immersion; HPS*, HHP-treated starch obtained *in situ*.

that minerals, instead of yerba mate, would occupy free sites of the starch granule when both of these compounds simultaneously undergo the high-pressure treatment.

2.4 Conclusions

The combination of a low-cost and widely available material, such as corn starch, with an advanced technology, such as high-hydrostatic-pressure processing to increase its molecular binding capacity and modify its performance, can yield a very promising wide-use carrier material. The presented approach suggests a new strategy of combining multiple ingredients in a simple carrier such as cornstarch. These bioactive carriers will be suitable additives or ingredients for a wide range of functional foods, such as soups, bakery products, desserts, and other powder formulations.

References

Ahmad, I., and Beg, A. Z. (2001). Antimicrobial and phytochemical studies on 45 Indian medicinal plants against multi-drug resistant human pathogens. *Journal of ethnopharmacology* 74(2): 113–123.

Anbinder, P. S., Deladino, D., Navarro A. S., Amalvy J. I., and Martino, M. N. (2011). Yerba mate extract encapsulation with alginate and chitosan systems: Interactions between active compound encapsulation polymers. *Journal of Encapsulation and Adsorption Sciences* 1: 80–87.

Anesini, C., Turner S., Cogoi L., and and Filip, R. (2012). Study of the participation of caffeine and polyphenols on the overall antioxidant activity of mate *(Ilex paraguariensis). LWT - Food Science and Technology* 45(2): 299–304.

Aryee, A. N. A., and Boye J. I. (2015). Current and Emerging Trends in the Formulation and Manufacture of Nutraceuticals and Functional Food Products. In *Nutraceutical and Functional Food Processing Technology*. J. I. Boye, ed. Hoboken: Wiley-Blackwell.

Bauer, B. A., and Knorr, D. (2005). The impact of pressure, temperature and treatment time on starches: Pressure-induced starch gelatinisation as pressure time temperature indicator for high hydrostatic pressure processing. *Journal of Food Engineering* 68: 329–334.

BCC Research. (2014). *FOD013E Nutraceuticals: Global markets* 2014. http://www.bccresearch.com/market-research/food-and-beverage/nutraceuticals-markets-report-fod013e.html.

Bixby, M., Spieler, L., Menini, T., and Gugliucci, A. (2005). *Ilex paraguariensis* extracts are potent inhibitors of nitrosative stress: A comparative study with green tea and wines using a protein nitration model and mammalian cell cytotoxicity. *Life Sciences* 77: 345–358.

Błaszczak, W., Valverde S., and Fornal, J. (2005). Effect of high pressure on the structure of potato starch. *Carbohydrate Polymers* 59(3): 377–383.

Błaszczak, W., Misharina, T. A., Yuryev, V. P., and Fornal, J. (2007). Effect of high pressure on binding aroma compounds by maize starches with different amylose content. *LWT – Food Science and Technology* 40(10): 1841–1848.

Bonilla, J., Talón E., Atarés, L., Vargas, M., and Chiralt, A. (2013). Effect of the incorporation of antioxidants on physicochemical and antioxidant properties of wheat starch–chitosan films. *Journal of Food Engineering* 118(3): 271–278.

Bouis, H. E., Chassy, B. M., and Ochanda, J. O. (2003). 2. Genetically modified food crops and their contribution to human nutrition and food quality. *Trends in Food Science and Technology* 14(5): 191–209.

Bracesco, N., Sanchez, A. G., Contreras, V., Menini, T., and Gugliucci, A. (2011). Recent advances on *Ilex paraguariensis* research: Minireview. *Journal of Ethnopharmacology* 136(3): 378–384.

Buckow, R., Heinz, V., and Knorr, D. (2007). High pressure phase transition kinetics of maize starch. *Journal of Food Engineering* 81(2): 469–475.

Campos, A. M., Escobar, J., and Lissi, E. A. (1996). The total reactive antioxidant potential (TRAP) and total antioxidant reactivity (TAR) of *Ilex paraguariensis* extracts and red wine. *Journal of the Brazilian Chemical Society* 7: 43–49.

Ciesielski, W., Lii, C., Yen, M.-T., and Tomasik, P. (2003). Interactions of starch with salts of metals from the transition groups. *Carbohydrate Polymers* 51(1): 47–56.

Corrales, M., Han, J. H., and Tauscher, B. (2009). Antimicrobial properties of grape seed extracts and their effectiveness after incorporation into pea starch films. *International Journal of Food Science & Technology* 44(2): 425–433.

Champagne, C. P., and Fustier, P. (2007). Microencapsulation for the improved delivery of bioactive compounds into foods. *Current Opinion in Biotechnology* 18(2): 184–190.

Chang, P. R., Yu, J., and Ma, X. (2011). Preparation of porous starch and its use as a structure-directing agent for production of porous zinc oxide. *Carbohydrate Polymers* 83(2): 1016–1019.

Chen, P., Yu L., Kealy, T., Chen, L., and Li, L. (2007). Phase transition of starch granules observed by microscope under shearless and shear conditions. *Carbohydrate Polymers* 68(3): 495–501.

Dees, P. J., and Polderman, J. (1981). Mercury porosimetry in pharmaceutical technology. *Powder Technology* 29: 187–197.

Deladino, L., Anbinder, P. S., Navarro, A. S., and Martino, M. N. (2008). Encapsulation of natural antioxidants extracted from *Ilex paraguariensis*. *Carbohydrate Polymers* 71(1): 126–134.

Deladino, L., Anbinder, P. S., Navarro, A. S., and Martino, M. N. (2007a). Co-crystallization of yerba mate extract *(Ilex paraguariensis)* and mineral salts within a sucrose matrix. *Journal of Food Engineering* 80(2): 573–580.

Deladino, L., Navarro, A., and Martino, M. N. (2007b). Encapsulation of active compounds: Ionic gelation and cocrystallization as case studies. In *Functional Properties of Food Components*. C. E. Lupano, ed. Trivandrum: Kerala Research Signpost.

Deladino, L., Teixeira, A. S., Navarro, A. S., Alvarez, I., Molina-García, A. D., and Martino, M. (2015). Corn starch systems as carriers for yerba mate *(Ilex paraguariensis)* antioxidants. *Food and Bioproducts Processing* 94: 463–472.

Douzals, J. P., Perrier Cornet, J. M., Gervais, P., and Coquille, J. C. (1996). Hydration and pressure-temperature phase diagram of wheat starch. *Journal of Agriculture and Food Chemistry* 44: 1403–1408.

Douzals, J. P, Perrier Cornet, J. M., Gervais, P., and Coquille, J. C. (1998). High-pressure gelatinization of wheat starch and properties of pressure-induced gels. *Journal of Agriculture and Food Chemistry* 46: 4824–4829.

Dugo, P., Cacciola, F., Donato, P., Assis Jacques, R., Caramao, E. B., and Mondello, L. (2009). High efficiency liquid chromatography techniques coupled to mass spectrometry for the characterization of mate extracts. *Journal of Chromatography A* 1216(43): 7213–7221.

Ebel, H., and Gunther, T. (1980). Magnesium metabolism: A review. *Journal of Clinical Chemistry and Biochemistry* 18: 257–270.

Elfstrand, L., Eliasson, A.-C., Jönsson, M., Larsson, M., Simpraga, A., *et al.* (2007). Recrystallization of waxy maize starch during manufacturing of starch microspheres for drug delivery: Influence of excipients. *Carbohydrate Polymers* 69(4): 732–741.

Fernández, P. P., Sanz, P. D., Martino, M. N., and Molina-García, A. D. (2008). Partially-gelatinised starches by high hydrostatic pressure as oligoelement carriers. *Spanish Journal of Agricultural Research* 6: 129–137.

Filip, R., López, P., Giberti, G., Coussio, J., and Ferraro, G. (2001). Phenolic compounds in seven South American *Ilex* species. *Fitoterapia* 72(7): 774–778.

Fredriksson, H., Silverio, J., Andersson, R., Eliasson, A. C., and Åman, P. (1998). The influence of amylose and amylopectin characteristics on gelatinization and retrogradation properties of different starches. *Carbohydrate Polymers* 35(3–4): 119–134.

Genc, Y., Humphries, J. M., Lyons, G. H., and Graham, R. D. (2005). Exploiting genotypic variation in plant nutrient accumulation to alleviate micronutrient deficiency in populations. *Journal of Trace Elements in Medicine and Biology* 18: 319–324.

Glenn, G. M., Klamczynski, A. P., Woods D. F., Chiou, B. S., Orts, W. J., and Imam, S. H. (2010). Encapsulation of plant oils in porous starch microspheres. *Journal of Agricultural and Food Chemistry* 58(7): 4180–4184.

González de Mejía, E., Song, Y. S., Heck, C. I., and Ramirez-Mares, M. V. (2009). Yerba mate tea *(Ilex paraguariensis):* Phenolics, antioxidant capacity and *in vitro* inhibition of colon cancer cell proliferation. *Journal of Functional Foods* 2(1): 23–34.

Guerrero-Romero, F., Simental-Mendia, L. E., Hernandez-Ronquillo, G., and Rodriguez-Moran, M. (2015). Oral magnesium supplementation improves glycaemic status in subjects with prediabetes and hypomagnesaemia: A double-blind placebo-controlled randomized trial. *Diabetes and Metabolism* 41(3): 202–207.

Gugliucci, A. (1996). Antioxidant effects of *Ilex paraguariensis:* Induction of decreased oxidability of human LDL *in vivo. Biochemical and Biophysical Research Communications* 224: 338–344.

Harrington, W. F., and Kegeles, G. (1973). Pressure effects in ultracentrifugation of interacting systems. *Methods in Enzymology* 27: 306–345.

Heck, C. I., Schmalko, M., and González de Mejía, E. (2008). Effect of growing and drying conditions on the phenolic composition of mate teas *(Ilex paraguariensis). Journal of Agricultural and Food Chemistry* 56(18): 8394–8403.

Heim, K. E., Tagliaferro, A. R., and Bobilya, D. J. (2002). Flavonoid antioxidants: Chemistry, metabolism and structure–activity relationships. *The Journal of nutritional biochemistry* 13(10): 572–584.

Hibi, Y., Matsumoto, T., and Hagiwara, S. (1993). Effect of high pressure on the crystalline structure of various starch granules. *Cereal Chemistry* 70: 671–676.

Huber, K. C., and BeMiller, J. N. (2000). Channels of maize and sorghum starch granules. *Carbohydrate Polymers* 41(3): 269–276.

Imberty, A., Buléon, A., Tran, V., and Pérez, S. (1991). Recent advances in knowledge of starch structure. *Starch-Starke* 43: 375–384.

International Zinc Nutrition Consultative Group. (2004). Assessment of the risk of zinc deficiency in populations and options for its control. In *Food and Nutrition Bulletin.* 25(1 Suppl 2): S99–203.

Jane, J., Wong, K., and McPherson, A. E. (1997). Branch-structure difference in starches of A- and B-type x-ray patterns revealed by their Naegeli dextrins. *Carbohydrate Research* 300(3): 219–227.

Ji, Y., Ao, Z., Han, J. A., Jane, J. L., and BeMiller, J. N. (2004). Waxy maize starch subpopulations with different gelatinization temperatures. *Carbohydrate Polymers* 57(2): 177–190.

Jobling, S. (2004). Improving starch for food and industrial applications. *Current Opinion in Plant Biology* 7(2): 210–218.

Juszczak, L., Fortuna, T., and Wodnicka, K. (2002). Characteristics of cereal starch granules surface using nitrogen adsorption. *Journal of Food Engineering* 54(2): 103–110.

Katopo, H., Song, Y., and Jane, J. (2002). Effect and mechanism of ultrahigh hydrostatic pressure on the structure and properties of starches. *Carbohydrate Polymers* 47(3): 233–244.

Knorr, D., Heinz, V., and Buckow, R. (2006). High pressure application for food biopolymers. *Biochimica et Biophysica Acta* 1764: 619–631.

Łabanowska, M., Kurdziel, M., Bidzińska, E., Pietrzyk, S., *et al.* (2013). Influence of metal ions on thermal generation of carbohydrate radicals in native and modified starch studied by EPR. *Starch-Stärke* 65(5–6): 469–482.

Lai, V. M. F., Tomasik P., Yen, M.-T., Hung, W.-L., and Lii, C. (2001). Re-examination of the interactions between starch and salts of metals from the non-transition groups. *International Journal of Food Science & Technology* 36(3): 321–330.

Le Corre, D., Bras, J., and Dufresne, A. (2010). Starch nanoparticles: A review. *Biomacromolecules* 11(5): 1139–1153.

Liu, Y., Selomulyo, V. O., and Zhou, W. (2008). Effect of high pressure on some physicochemical properties of several native starches. *Journal of Food Engineering* 88(1): 126–136.

MacDonald, R. S. (2000). The role of zinc in growth and cell proliferation. *Journal of Nutrition* 130(5): 1500S–1508S.

Mali, S., Grossmann, M. V. E., García, M. A., Martino, M. N., and Zaritzky, N. E. (2006). Effects of controlled storage on thermal, mechanical and barrier properties of plasticized films from different starch sources. *Journal of Food Engineering* 75(4): 453–460.

Maret, W. (2001). Zinc biochemistry, physiology, and homeostasis – recent insights and current trends. *Biometals* 14: 187–90.

Matsumoto, R. L. T., Bastos, D. H. M., Mendonça, S., Nunes V. S., Bartchewsky, W., *et al.* (2009). Effects of mate tea *(Ilex paraguariensis)* ingestion on mRNA expression of antioxidant enzymes, lipid peroxidation, and total antioxidant status in healthy young women. *Journal of Agricultural and Food Chemistry* 57(5): 1775–1780.

McLean, E., Egli, I., Cogswell, M., de Benoist, B., and Wojdyla, D. (2007). *Worldwide prevalence of anemia in preschool aged children, pregnant women and non-pregnant women of reproductive age.* Geneva: World Health Organization.

Meenakshi, J. V. (2009). *Biofortification. Best practice paper: New advice from CC08.* Copenhagen: Copenhagen Consensus Center.

Menini, T., Heck, C., Schulze, J., De Mejia, E., and Gugliucci, A. (2007). Protective action of *Ilex paraguariensis* extract against free radical inactivation of paraoxonase-1 in high-density lipoprotein *Planta Medica* 73: 1141–1147.

Milburn, M. V., Prive, G. G., Milligan, D. L., Scott, W. G., Yeh, J., *et al.* (1991). Three-dimensional structures of the ligand-binding domain of the bacterial aspartate receptor with and without a ligand. *Science* 254(5036): 1342–1347.

Molina-García, A. D., Horridge, E., Sanz, P. D., and Martino, M. N. (2007). Nanostructure of starch high-pressure treated granules discovered by low temperature scanning electron microscopy. In: *Modern Research and Educational Topics in Microscopy, Microscopy Series 3. Applications in Physical/Chemical Sciences.* D. J. Méndez-Vilas, ed. Badajoz, Spain: Formatex Research Center.

Molina-García, A. D. (2003). The effect of hydrostatic pressure on biological systems. In: *Biotechnology & Genetic Engineering Reviews.* S. E. Harding, ed. Andover, UK: Intercept Ltd.

Muhr, A. H., Wetton, R. E., and Blanshard, J. M. V. (1982). Effect of hydrostatic pressure on starch gelatinisation, as determined by DTA. *Carbohydrate Polymers* 2: 91–102.

Nakamatsu, J., Torres, F. G., Troncoso, O. P., Yuan, M.-L., and Boccaccini, A. R. (2006). Processing and characterization of porous structures from chitosan and starch for tissue engineering scaffolds. *Biomacromolecules* 7(12): 3345–3355.

Oh, H. E., Pinder, D. N., Hemar Y., Anema, S. G., and Wong, M. (2008). Effect of high-pressure treatment on various starch-in-water suspensions. *Food Hydrocolloids* 22: 150–155.

Otero, L., Molina-García, A. D., and Sanz, P. D. (2000). The thermal effect of food quasi-adiabatic high pressure treatments. *Innovative Food Science and Emerging Technologies* 1: 119–226.

Parker, R., and Ring, S. (2000). Macromolecular aspects of bread staling. In: *Bread Staling.* P. Chinachoti, and Y. Vodovotz, eds. Boca Raton, FL: CRC Press.

Pérez, S., and Bertoft, E. (2010). The molecular structures of starch components and their contribution to the architecture of starch granules: A comprehensive review. *Starch-Stärke* 62(8): 389–420.

Prentice, A. M., Gershwin, M. E., Schaible, U. E., Keusch, G. T., Victoria, L. G., and Gordon, J. I. (2008). New challenges in studying nutrition disease interactions in the developing world. *Journal of Clinical Investigation* 118: 1322–1329.

Qian, D., Chang, P. R., and Ma, X. (2011). Preparation of controllable porous starch with different starch concentrations by the single or dual freezing process. *Carbohydrate Polymers* 86(3): 1181–1186.

Rivelli, D. P., Almeida, R. L., Ropke, C. D., and Barros, S. B. (2011). Hydrolysis influence on phytochemical composition, antioxidant activity, plasma concentration, and tissue distribution of hydroethanolic Ilex paraguariensis extract components. *Journal of Agricultural and Food Chemistry* 59(890): 1–7.

Rodrigues, A., and Emeje, M. (2012). Recent applications of starch derivatives in nanodrug delivery. *Carbohydrate Polymers* 87(2): 987–994.

Rubens, P., and Heremans, K. (2000). Pressure-temperature gelatinization phase diagram of starch: An *in situ* Fourier transform infrared study. *Biopolymers* 54: 524–530.

Rude, R. K., and Gruber, H. E. (2004). Magnesium deficiency and osteoporosis: Animal and human observations. *Journal of Nutritional Biochemistry* 15(12): 710–716.

Saris, N. E., Mervaala, E., Karppanen, H., Khawaja, J. A., and Lewenstam, A. (2000). Magnesium. An update on physiological, clinical and analytical aspects. *Clinica Chimica Acta* 294(1–2): 1–26.

Shahidi, F. (2004). Functional foods: Their role in health promotion and disease prevention. *Journal of Food Science* 69(5): R146–R149.

Shils, M. E. (1993). Magnesium. In *Modern Nutrition in Health and Disease*, 8th ed. M. E. Shils, J. A. Olson, and M. Shike, eds. Philadelphia: Lea & Febiger.

Silva, E. L., Neiva, T. J. C., Shirai, M., Terao, J., and Abdalla, D. S. P. (2008). Acute ingestion of yerba mate infusion *(Ilex paraguariensis)* inhibits plasma and lipoprotein oxidation. *Food Research International* 41: 973–979.

Silva, J. L., Foguel, D., and Royer, C. A. (2001). Pressure provides new insights into protein folding, dynamics and structure. *Trends in Bochemical Siences* 6: 612–618.

Simonin, H., Guyon, C., Orlowska, M., de Lamballerie, M., and Le-Bail, A. (2011). Gelatinization of waxy starches under high pressure as influenced by pH and osmolarity: Gelatinization kinetics, final structure and pasting properties. *LWT – Food Science and Technology* 44(3): 779–786.

Slade, L., and Levine, H. (1993). Water relationships in starch transitions. *Carbohydrate Polymers* 21(2–3): 105–131.

Smeller, L. (2002). Pressure–temperature phase diagrams of biomolecules. *Biochimica et Biophysica Acta (BBA) – Protein Structure and Molecular Enzymology* 1595: 11–29.

Souza, C. O., Silva, L. T., Silva, J. R., López, J. A., Veiga-Santos, P., and Druzian, J. I. (2011). Mango and acerola pulps as antioxidant additives in cassava starch bio-based film. *Journal of Agricultural and Food Chemistry* 59(6): 2248–2254.

Stewart, C. P., Dewey, K. G., and Ashorn, P. (2010). The undernutrition epidemic: An urgent health priority. *Lancet* 375(9711): 282.

Stolt, M., Oinonen, S., and Autio, K. (2000). Effect of high pressure on the physical properties of barley starch. *Innovative Food Science & Emerging Technologies* 1: 167–175.

Stute, R., Klingler, R. W., Boguslawski, S., Eshtiaghi, M. N., and Knorr, D. 1996. Effects of high pressures treatment on starches. *Starch* 48: 399–408.

Sujka, M., and Jamroz, J. 2007. Starch granule porosity and its changes by means of amylolysis. *International Agrophysics* 21: 107–113.

Takagi, H., Kobayashi, Y., Taguchi, O., Takei, Y., and Sumida, Y. (2015). Influence of dietary intake of fish oil, magnesium, and zinc on metabolic parameters among individuals tested for diabetes. *Nutrition* 31(7–8): 988–993.

Talja, R. A., Helén, H., Roos, Y. H., and Jouppila, K. (2007). Effect of various polyols and polyol contents on physical and mechanical properties of potato starch–based films. *Carbohydrate Polymers* 67(3): 288–295.

Tapiero, H., and Tew, K. D. (2003). Trace elements in human physiology and pathology: Zinc and metallothioneins. *Biomedicine & Pharmacotherapy* 57(9): 399–411.

Teixeira, A. S., Navarro, A. S., Molina-García, A. D., Martino, M., and Deladino, L. (2015). Corn starch systems as carriers for yerba mate *(Ilex paraguariensis)* antioxidants: Effect of mineral addition. *Food and Bioproducts Processing* 94: 39–49.

Thacher, T. D., Fischer, P. R. Strand, M. A., and Pettifor, J. M. (2006). Nutritional rickets around the world: Causes and future directions. *Annals of Tropical Paediatrics* 26(1): 1–16.

Thevelein, J. M., Van Assche, J. A., Heremans, K., and Gerlsma, S. Y. (1981). Gelatinisation temperature of starch, as influenced by high pressure. *Carbohydrate Research* 93: 304–307.

Truong-Tran, A. Q., Carter, J., Ruffin, R. E., and Zalewski, P. D. (2001). The role of zinc in caspase activation and apoptotic cell death. *Biometals* 14(3–4): 315–330.

Ubbink, J., and Krüger, J. (2006). Physical approaches for the delivery of active ingredients in foods. *Trends in Food Science & Technology* 17(5): 244–254.

Uthumporn, U., Zaidul, I. S. M., and Karim, A. A. (2010). Hydrolysis of granular starch at sub-gelatinization temperature using a mixture of amylolytic enzymes. *Food and Bioproducts Processing* 88(1): 47–54.

Webb, P. A., and Orr, C. (1997). *Analytical methods in fine particle technology*. Norcross, GA: Micromeritics Instrument Corp.

Westermarck, S. (2000). Use of mercury porosimetry and nitrogen adsorption in characterisation of the pore structure of mannitol and microcrystalline cellulose powders, granules and tablets. PhD dissertation, Pharmaceutical Technology Division, University of Helsinki.

White, P. J., and Broadley, M. R. (2005). Biofortifying crops with essential mineral elements. *Trends in Plant Science* 10(12): 586–593.

World Health Organization (2012). *World Health Statistics* 2012. http://www.who.int/gho/publications/world_health_statistics.

Williams, R. J. P. (1989). An introduction to the biochemistry of zinc. In: *Zinc in Human Biology*. C. Mills, ed. London: Springer-Verlag.

Wu, A. C., Li, E., and Gilbert, R. G. (2014). Exploring extraction/dissolution procedures for analysis of starch chain-length distributions. *Carbohydrate Polymers* 114: 36–42.

CHAPTER 3

Protein-based nanoparticles as matrices for encapsulation of lipophilic nutraceuticals

Adrián A. Perez, Osvaldo E. Sponton, and Liliana G. Santiago
Grupo de Biocoloides, Instituto de Tecnología de Alimentos (ITA), Facultad de Ingeniería Química (FIQ), Universidad Nacional del Litoral (UNL), 1 de Mayo 3250, Santa Fe, (3000), Argentina

3.1 General aspects of encapsulating lipophilic nutraceuticals

The most interesting lipophilic nutraceuticals to be incorporated into different products are extracted from animal and vegetable resources. For example, some polyphenols have important actions as antioxidants due to their ability to capture free radicals (Mulder *et al.*, 2008; Saladino *et al.*, 2008). Carotenoids are other kind of natural antioxidants that protect cells against oxidative stress (Sies and Stahl, 1995). Polyunsatured fatty acids (PUFAs) are relevant for immunity regulation and for preventing cardiovascular diseases, among other benefits (Hsieh *et al.*, 2007). Finally, several amino acids, peptides, vitamins, and phytochemicals are usually used in the development of delivery systems in order to induce different healthy effects (McClements and Li, 2010). In spite of their recognized bioactive actions, the simple addition of lipophilic nutraceuticals into different products usually it is not enough for reaching the desired objectives. The main reason is that lipophilic nutraceuticals show poor solubilization in aqueous systems, which strongly affects their physicochemical stability and bioavailability (Zimet and Livney, 2009). To solve these problems, different lipophilic nutraceutical encapsulation strategies were developed, taking into account the physicochemical properties and environmental susceptibility of lipophilic nutraceuticals (Matalanis *et al.*, 2011).

In general, encapsulation of lipophilic nutraceuticals could be defined as a process in which lipophilic nutraceuticals are covered or incorporated into a matrix (homogeneous or heterogeneous) in order to create capsules or functional structures that promote their vehiculization. The main objectives of encapsulating lipophilic nutraceuticals are solubilization or vehiculization into

---

New Polymers for Encapsulation of Nutraceutical Compounds, First Edition.
Edited by Jorge Carlos Ruiz Ruiz and Maira Rubi Segura Campos.

aqueous matrices; protection against environmental physicochemical changes, such as oxidation, UV radiation, and temperature (Gouin, 2004; McClements, 2007); and controlled delivery in desired conditions (Matalanis *et al.*, 2011).

In this chapter, some examples about innovative systems to encapsulate lipophilic nutraceuticals are shown. Special emphasis is placed in the development of encapsulation systems based on lipophilic nutraceuticals' binding ability with some globular proteins. As examples, PUFAs were chosen because of their increasing use in the formulation of different nutraceutical products. There are some studies in the literature about the biological actions of complexes formed by assembly of proteins and PUFAs. Information about formation of nanocomplexes with biological action could be exploited in formulating new functional foods that contribute to the prevention and/or treatment of certain pathologies.

3.2 Polyunsaturated fatty acid encapsulation systems

PUFAs constitute one of the most interesting lipophilic nutraceuticals to be incorporated into foods, pharmaceuticals, and cosmetic formulations. Examples of important PUFAs are α-linolenic acid (ALA, 18:3n-3), γ-linolenic acid (GLA, 18:3n-6), linoleic acid (LA, 18:2n-6), and conjugated linoleic acid (CLA, 18:2n-6, 18:2n-7). From a nutritional point of view, some of these PUFAs are considered essential fatty acids because they cannot be synthesized by the human organism, so they must be incorporated in diet. The most common form of consumption of these PUFAs is through the intake of vegetable oils (e.g., olive, sunflower, soybean, flaxseed, rapeseed, chia seed), fish oils (e.g., cod, salmon) and crustacean (e.g., krill, crayfish, lobster) oils, which vary in composition and physicochemical properties. The intake is usually conditioned by factors such as dietary patterns, cultural factors, and consumer preferences (Ilyasoglu and El, 2014; Zimet and Livney, 2009). ALA consumption is important due to its participation as a precursor in the synthesis of eicosapentaenoic acid (EPA, 20:5n-3) and docosapentaenoic acid (DHA, 22:6n-3) (Plourde and Cunnane, 2007). Biological implications of PUFAs have been clinically demonstrated in a number of scientific reports (Al *et al.*, 2000; Boelsma, *et al.*, 2001; Calder and Zurier, 2001; Freeman, 2000; Gogos, *et al.*, 2000; Roche and Gibney, 2000; von Schacky, 2003).

PUFAs are very sensitive to oxidation (McClements *et al.*, 2007). Moreover, it is well known that high temperatures enhance lipid oxidation kinetics (Farhoosh *et al.*, 2008). The addition of antioxidants to PUFA-rich oils was proposed as a strategy for retarding the effects of lipid oxidation (Becker and Knorr, 1996; Sherwin, 1976). However, this strategy does not solve the problem of incorporating PUFAs into aqueous media, which is the main requisite for increasing their bioavailability (McClements and Li, 2010).

Hence, in order to increase solubilization of PUFAs, different encapsulation systems have been developed. Some examples are systems based on conventional emulsions (McClements, 2005a), multiple emulsions (Garti and Bisperink, 1998), and multilayer emulsions (Fioramonti *et al.*, 2015; McClements, 2005b); solid lipid particles (Wissing *et al.*, 2004); hydrogel beads (Chen *et al.*, 2006); and biopolymer nanoparticles (Zimet and Livney, 2009). Each of these strategies has advantages and disadvantages. For example, microcapsules of PUFA-rich oils based in conventional emulsions are relatively easy to produce, but they have stability problems because physicochemical properties of protective cover are not easy to control. PUFA-rich oils encapsulated through multiple emulsion systems could lose stability during processing or storage of foods due to mechanical forces, heating, freezing, or dehydration.

Systems based on multilayer emulsions could resolve these problems mainly because protective biopolymer cover is easier to control (Fioramonti *et al.*, 2015a,b; McClements *et al.*, 2007). For each of these strategies, the final size of the system allows us to distinguish between nano- and microencapsulation which can determine their potential applications (Chen *et al.*, 2006; McClements and Li, 2010). It is important to take into account the physicochemical aspects involved in the digestive process in order to rationally design PUFA-encapsulation systems. In the literature, there is some information showing that the uptake of different microencapsulated oils can produce changes in the oil's bioaccessibility (Cummings and Overduin, 2007; Maljaars *et al.*, 2009; McClements and Li, 2010). However, the effect of gastrointestinal digestion on the bioaccessibility of microencapsulated oils is not yet known.

In this chapter, special emphasis is on the design of protein-based systems for encapsulating lipophilic nutraceuticals. The systems described in the following sections are based on native globular protein, protein aggregates, and biopolymer particles, all obtained at the nanoscale.

3.2.1 Native globular proteins as carriers of polyunsaturated fatty acids

Some globular proteins show interesting properties for the development of PUFA-delivery systems because, in general, they are nontoxic, nonimmunogenic, biocompatible, and biodegradable materials. The formation of protein–PUFA nanocomplexes exploits the binding properties that show some globular proteins. In the case of PUFAs, binding ability is driven by hydrophobic forces involving certain protein domains. Although there are some controversies about the real binding site of globular proteins, most authors agree that binding requires special structural conditions, mainly when native globular proteins are considered. This is evident in some protein families that present a great conservation pattern in their amino acid sequences. However, it is important to keep in mind that structural conditions do not always suggest molecular specificity, mainly due to the promiscuous nature of protein–ligand interactions; that is, one protein is able to bind many different ligands.

One of the most-studied globular proteins showing ligand binding properties is β-lactoglobulin. β-Lactoglobulin is the main protein fraction of milk whey proteins, which are widely used in food industry due to their good nutritional and functional properties (Essemine *et al.*, 2011; Perez *et al.*, 2012a,b). β-Lactoglobulin is a globular protein with 162 amino acid residues, an atomic mass of 18.3 kDa, and a pI of about 5.1 (Bhattacharjee and Das, 2000; Bolder *et al.*, 2007). At pH higher than 7.5 or lower than 2.0, β-lactoglobulin shows a monomeric structure. At pH between 2.0–3.7 and 5.1–7.5, β-lactoglobulin forms dimers, whereas at pH between 3.7 and 5.1, it forms octamers. Two disulfide bounds (Cys106–Cys119, Cys66–Cys160) stabilize β-lactoglobulin's globular structure (Cheison *et al.*, 2011). In this conformation, hydrophobic domains are mainly buried into the protein, minimizing free energy, while hydrophilic domains are located at protein–water interface (Kato and Nakai, 1980). The biological role of β-lactoglobulin remains unknown, although one possibility is its contribution to lipid metabolism during the neonatal period. Moreover, because of its homology with retinol-binding proteins, it was suggested β-lactoglobulin could play an important role in retinol vehiculization (Perez and Calvo, 1995).

The acquired knowledge about β-lactoglobulin's molecular characteristics has allowed researchers to develop new technologies and products (Matalanis *et al.*, 2011; McClements and Li, 2010). In this sense, β-lactoglobulin's binding properties have received considerable attention due to their potential uses in PUFA-delivery strategies (Livney, 2010; Sponton, *et al.*, 2014; Zimet and Livney, 2009). β-Lactoglobulin has two lipophilic ligand-binding sites: a central hydrophobic β-barrel (or *calyx*) and a superficial *pocket* (Cheison *et al.*, 2011; Wang *et al.*, 1998, 1999). The superficial *pocket* is located close to the dimer contact region, between an α-helix (sited laterally to the *calyx*) and the *calyx* surface (Cheison *et al.*, 2011; Frapin *et al.*, 1993; Wang et al., 1998, 1999). Thus, β-lactoglobulin could simultaneously link two lipophilic molecules (Frapin *et al.*, 1993; Wang *et al.*, 1999).

The PUFA-binding properties of β-lactoglobulin are generally characterized by two parameters: stoichiometry or number of ligand molecules bound (n) and association constant (K_a), which could be evaluated by means of fluorescence, equilibrium dialysis, or isothermal titration calorimetry (ITC). For PUFAs, and fatty acids in general, it was reported that affinity constant increases with the length of the hydrocarbon chain, which could be explained by considering an increment in hydrophobic interactions. Moreover, it was established that the number and position of double bonds within a PUFA only weakly affect its interaction with β-lactoglobulin (Frapin *et al.*, 1993). Regarding stoichiometry, there is an agreement that one PUFA molecule is bound at the β-lactoglobulin calyx. However, because of diversity of techniques employed, there are discrepancies among values of binding parameters. The existence of impurities in the β-lactoglobulin sample could also strongly affect the parameters' magnitude.

Regarding biological properties of β-lactoglobulin–PUFA complexes, a modification of PUFA bioaccessibility after complexation has been reported. Jiang and Liu (2010) have demonstrated that CLA–β-lactoglobulin complexes were more active on Caco-2 cells after 48 hours of exposure as compared with free CLA. A similar cytotoxic effect was reported for β-lactoglobulin–oleic acid (Lisková *et al.*, 2011).

3.2.2 Protein aggregates as carriers of polyunsaturated fatty acids

It is well known that globular functional properties are easily modified by different processes, including heating (Foegeding *et al.*, 2002, 2006), high pressure, and enzymatic hydrolysis (Perez *et al.*, 2012a,b). The structure of β-lactoglobulin is highly sensitive to the processing conditions used in food manufacturing, especially heat treatments, which are routinely used to change food textures or reduce microbial load. Such treatments denature the protein, leading to the formation of aggregates. Hence, with the exception of raw milk, β-lactoglobulin is often found in a nonnative conformations in food products.

These changes in protein structure can have a strong impact on lipophilic nutraceuticals' binding properties of β-lactoglobulin. Fioramonti and colleagues (2014) have shown that a controlled heat treatment could promote conformational changes in the tertiary structure of milk whey proteins, affecting their functional properties and interactions with other molecules. Structural modifications were attributed to exposition of reactive and hydrophobic amino acid residues buried in the protein (Cairoli *et al.*, 1994). Therefore, the induction of a suitable structural modification could be used in the development of delivery systems with improved encapsulation efficiency, changes in binding affinity, and/or repercussions in the release of lipophilic nutraceuticals (Fioramonti *et al.*, 2014; Sponton *et al.*, 2014).

The use of aggregate proteins for encapsulation strategies for lipophilic nutraceuticals involves the knowledge of the principles that govern protein denaturation and aggregation. In the case of β-lactoglobulin, different mechanisms of aggregate formation have described. In respect to this, the kinetic model proposed by de Jong and colleagues (1992) could be more suitable for describing the heat-induced β-lactoglobulin aggregation process. The denaturation stage is considered an equilibrium first–order reaction between native and partially unfolded protein. At this stage, β-lactoglobulin dimers dissociate to monomers, and free sulfhydryl groups are exposed onto the protein surface (Hoffman *et al.*, 1997).

The second step consists in several aggregation reactions. These are bimolecular second-order reactions driving to irreversible formation of protein aggregates via thiol–disulfide interchange reactions and disulfide bounds (Verheul *et al.*, 1998). In addition to covalent bonds, other noncovalent interactions (ionic, hydrophobic, and van der Waals) could be involved in a heat-induced β-lactoglobulin aggregation process (Hoffman *et al.*, 1997). According to literature, formation and characteristics of β-lactoglobulin aggregates strongly depend on heating temperature and on bulk conditions, such as pH, ionic strength, salt type, concentration (Hoffman *et al.*, 1997; Nicolai *et al.*, 2011; Verheul *et al.*, 1998) and the presence of co-solutes, such as sorbitol and glycerol (Chanasatru *et al.*, 2009). β-Lactoglobulin aggregates would be more hydrophobic than native β-lactoglobulin due to the greater exposition of buried hydrophobic domains as a consequence of heat treatment (Bhattacharjee and Das, 2000). These characteristics support the idea that β-lactoglobulin aggregates can be used as carriers of lipophilic nutraceuticals. Moreover, as a consequence of a highly exposed hydrophobic surface, the amount of loaded lipophilic nutraceuticals could be greater in comparison with native β-lactoglobulin.

The hypothesis that heat-induced β-lactoglobulin aggregates, with improved hydrophobic properties, could have a greater ability to bind PUFAs onto their hydrophobic surfaces than native β-lactoglobulin was tested in a study using linoleic acid as a PUFA model (Perez *et al.*, 2014). It was concluded that pH in the range of 6.5 to 7.5 had a greater effect on formation of heat-induced β-lactoglobulin aggregate formation. β-Lactoglobulin aggregates formed at pH 6.5 were the most hydrophobic and could be applied as carriers of bioactive lipophilic molecules. However, the mechanism of linoleic acid binding to β-lactoglobulin aggregates was characterized by complex behavior that depends on aggregate formation conditions (pH, heating time, or combination of both). However, under similar experimental conditions, Le Maux and colleagues (2012, 2013) observed an increasing amount of linoleic acid (linoleate form) bound per protein monomer when β-lactoglobulin was heated. The obtained heat-induced aggregates did not corroborate the hypothesis that the greater the surface hydrophobicity, the greater the ability to bind linoleic acid. This finding could suggest that complexation should require the preservation of the linoleic acid binding site. Nevertheless, information derived from this study called attention to the impact of heat treatment (temperature and time) and pH on the development of PUFA-encapsulation strategies using β-lactoglobulin as carrier.

Linoleic acid's binding properties with ovalbumin heat induced aggregates that have been studied. Ovalbumin is a globular protein of 43 kDa molecular weight and is composed of 385 amino acids, half of which are hydrophobic and mainly buried in the protein structure. Charged amino acids (a third of the total amino acids) are mainly located on protein surface in contact with aqueous medium (Croguennec *et al.*, 2007). Ovalbumin has one disulfide bond and four free sulfhydryl groups. The effect of heat treatment on ovalbumin's molecular structure has been extensively studied (Galazka *et al.*, 1999). Heating promotes protein unfolding and aggregation, conferring an increase in protein surface hydrophobicity (Croguennec *et al.*, 2007). This phenomenon depends on environmental conditions, and it is normally driven by molecular interactions between exposed hydrophobic patches and formation of disulfide bonds. Therefore, the systematic study of heating and environment variables is very important in order to control the ovalbumin's aggregate physicochemical properties required to enhance PUFAs' binding ability.

In relation to this, the influence of heat treatment (temperature and time) and environmental conditions (pH and protein concentration) on the physicochemical properties of ovalbumin aggregates (particle size and surface characteristics) has been determined (Sponton *et al.*, 2015a). Interactions between PUFA and ovalbumin aggregates were explained in the following way. PUFA molecules are formed by a hydrophilic head, composed of carboxylic groups, and a hydrophobic tail, which correspond to the aliphatic chains. PUFAs' low solubility in aqueous solution is conferred by hydrophobic tails (Fontana *et al.*, 2013). When PUFA concentration in aqueous medium exceeds the critical micelle concentration, around 60 μM at pH 7.6, fatty acid molecules assemble, forming micelles and vesicles (Fontana *et al.*, 2013; Zimet and Livney, 2009). These supramolecular assemblies are mainly formed by hydrophobic interaction between aliphatic chains. In the resulting configuration, polar heads are located in the outside of the supramolecular structure in contact with water molecules. Formation of micelles and vesicles confers appreciable turbidity to the PUFA aqueous solution. Nevertheless, a turbid PUFA aqueous solution becomes clear when ovalbumin aggregate solution is added.

Following this approach, it was demonstrated that nanometric ovalbumin aggregates had greater ability to bind linoleic acid than native ovalbumin. Differences in linoleic acid's binding ability were attributed not only to differences in surface hydrophobicity but also to differences in their size and so their specific surface area. In general, the highest binding ability was for ovalbumin aggregates with the lowest size. The fact that linoleic acid was bound to ovalbumin aggregates in a more effective way than native ovalbumin may suggest that they could be applied as carriers of PUFAs favoring its incorporation in aqueous systems (Sponton *et al.*, 2015b). Information derived from this study provides some practical data about requirements of particle size and surface properties of ovalbumin nanoparticles with improved binding ability.

3.2.3 Biopolymer nanoparticles as carriers of polyunsaturated fatty acids

Biopolymer nanoparticles (BNPs) are the subjects of increasing interest in the development of lipophilic nutraceutical encapsulation systems with applications in several industrial sectors. In general, BNPs could protect lipophilic nutraceuticals from degradation and enhance their bioavailability. BNPs can be designed to obtain improved load capacity and lower opsonization. Moreover, BNPs show interesting physicochemical properties associated with their small size, such as great surface-to-volume ratio and the possibility to modulate their characteristics in response to different environmental conditions (Desai *et al.*, 1997; Panyam *et al.*, 2003). Small size could also prevent the alteration of textural, optical, and rheological properties of the products (Lesmes and McClements, 2009, Matalanis *et al.*, 2011; McClements ανδ Li, 2010).

In the literature, systems are described that are based on gelatin, collagen, casein, albumin, and milk whey proteins. In general, BNPs can be easily prepared under soft process conditions yielding a smaller size (50–300 nm) compared to microparticles and, in general, better controlled-release properties than other delivery systems, such as liposomes. Production methods for BNPs can be classified into several techniques: desolvation, emulsification, thermal gelation, nano-spray-drying, nab-technology, and self-assembly. For more details, an interesting review of different methods of obtaining BNPs is available (Elzoghby *et al.*, 2012).

Currently, using BNPs to encapsulate PUFAs by applying self-assembly approaches have gained great interest for the following reasons: great colloidal stability (Zimet and Livney, 2009), increased bioavailability (Ilyasoglu and El, 2014), and potential beneficial biological actions, in particular, potential antitumor activity (Fontana *et al.*, 2013). However, the production of BNPs to encapsulate PUFAs requires an exhaustive knowledge about principles of molecular self-assembly, which is strongly dependent on the molecular characteristics and physicochemical properties of the involved biopolymers (proteins and polysaccharides) and lipophilic nutraceuticals (Zimet and Livney, 2009). Usually, these BNPs are obtained by applying two self-assembly principles: lipophilic nutraceuticals binding at a particular protein domain in order to form protein–lipophilic nutraceuticals complexes, and electrostatic deposition of a polysaccharide onto the surface of the preformed protein–lipophilic nutraceutical complexes. In general, the term *electrostatic deposition* should be interpreted as simple biopolymer interaction between protein and polysaccharide. Usually, these interactions take place under aqueous medium conditions that favor attraction between polysaccharide anionic groups and protein cationic groups. Considering these interactions, designing BNPs should involve the systematic study of the individual biopolymer's functional properties, molecular interactions between biopolymers and bioactive compounds, and the effect of the process variables that govern such interactions.

The most important process variables in BNP design are aqueous medium pH, ionic strength, biopolymer charge density (i.e., the number of charges per monomeric unit), biopolymer relative concentration, and biopolymer total concentration in the system. In general, the adequate magnitudes for these variables depend on the particular biopolymer systems and their potential applications. It is desirable to achieve the highest colloidal stability so that BNPs remain in solution as long as possible. Regarding this, it is well established that lower particle size and higher electrical potential are requirements for high colloidal stability in aqueous media (Lesmes and McClements, 2009).

Experimental information about the design of BNPs as PUFA carriers was provided by Perez and colleagues (2015). Linoleic acid and high-methoxyl pectin were employed as models of PUFA and anionic polysaccharide, respectively. The applied strategy consisted of obtaining β-lactoglobulin–linoleic acid complexes via β-lactoglobulin binding to linoleic acid, and producing BNPs via electrostatic deposition of high-methoxyl pectin onto the surface of preformed β-lactoglobulin–linoleic acid complexes. The experimental work provides a systematic study of the process variables, such as pH and protein–polysaccharide concentration ratio ($R_{Prot:HMP}$), in order to obtain BNPs to carry PUFA, with special emphasis on their phase behavior and colloidal stability. In summary, results show that at pH 4.0, stable BNPs are obtained at 1:1 and 2:1 $R_{Prot:HMP}$, exhibiting sizes around 337 to 364 nm and ζ potential between −25 and −28 mV. These characteristics allow the application of BNPs for linoleic acid encapsulation systems in liquid acidic media. Regarding high-methoxyl pectin's protective role at the linoleic acid binding site, it was noted that an 2:1 $R_{Prot:HMP}$ could favor linoleic acid's protective effect, turning this condition into the most suitable for the design of the encapsulation system. This strategy was previously reported by Zimet and Livney (2009), supporting the idea that a cover of polysaccharide onto the surface of protein–PUFA complexes could favor the protection of PUFA molecules mainly against oxidation.

3.3 Conclusions

Molecular structures of some globular proteins suitable for encapsulating lipophilic nutraceuticals has been extensively researched. The most important feature of these proteins is the special protein conformation that promotes the spontaneous binding of lipophilic nutraceuticals. The formation of protein–PUFA complexs modifies the bioaccessibility of the PUFA and, in some cases, promotes a cytotoxic effect. These findings highlight potential applications of β-lactoglobulin–PUFA complexes in cancer therapies. Unfortunately, the binding parameters for characterizing the development of these encapsulation systems are difficult to measure, which leads to a great discrepancy of the results. Although the real biological actions of some native globular proteins remains unknown, this property may enhance the design of PUFA delivery systems. Protein-based nanoparticles could have a bright future in the controlled delivery of PUFAs. In particular, protein aggregates and biopolymer nanoparticles have shown high PUFA-loading capacity in combination with biodegradability and biocompatibility features. However, a better understanding of the properties of these carriers will provide a basis for their optimization, thus opening new challenges in the area of lipophilic nutraceuticals encapsulation.

Acknowledgments

Authors acknowledge the financial support of the following projects: CAI+D PI – 2011 501 201 101 00 171 LI (UNL, Santa Fe, Argentina), PICT 2014-2636 (ANPCyT, Argentina), and Consejo Nacional de Investigaciones Científicas y Técnicas de la República Argentina (CONICET).

References

Al, M. D., van Houwelingen, A. C., and Hornstra, G. (2000). Long-chain polyunsaturated fatty acids, pregnancy, and pregnancy outcome. *American Journal of Clinical Nutrition* 71(1): 285–291.

Becker, R., and Knorr, A. (1996). An evaluation of antioxidants for vegetable oils at elevated temperatures. *Lubrication Science* 8(2): 95–117.

Bhattacharjee, C., and Das, K. P. (2000). Thermal unfolding and refolding of β-lactoglobulin: An intrinsic and extrinsic fluorescence study. *European Journal of Biochemistry* 267: 3957–3964.

Boelsma, E., Hendriks, H. F., and Roza, L., (2001). Nutritional skin care: Health effects of micronutrients and fatty acids. *American Journal of Clinical Nutrition* 73(5): 853–864.

Bolder, S., Vasbinder, A., Sagis, L., and van der Linden, E. (2007). Heat-induced whey protein isolate fibrils: Conversion, hydrolysis, and disulphide bond formation. *International Dairy Journal* 17: 846–853.

Cairoli, S., Iametti, S., and Bonomi, F. (1994). Reversible and irreversible modifications of β-lactoglobulin upon exposure to heat. *Journal of Protein Chemistry* 13(3): 347–354.

Calder, P. C., and Zurier, R. B. (2001). Polyunsaturated fatty acids and rheumatoid arthritis. *Current Opinion in Clinical Nutrition & Metabolic Care* 4(2): 115–121.

Chanasattru, W., Jones, O. G., Decker, E. A., and McClements, D. J. (2009). Impact of cosolvents on formation and properties of biopolymer nanoparticles formed by heat treatment of β-lactoglobulin–pectin complexes. *Food Hydrocolloids* 23(8): 2450–2457.

Cheison, S., Lai, M., Leeb, E., and Kulozik, U. (2011). Hydrolysis of β-lactoglobulin by trypsin under acidic pH and analysis of the hydrolysates with MALDI–TOF–MS/MS. *Food Chemistry* 125: 1241–1248.

Chen, L., Remondetto, G. E., and Subirade, M. (2006). Food protein–based materials as nutraceutical delivery systems. *Trends in Food Science & Technology* 17(5): 272–283.

Cummings, D. E., and Overduin, J. (2007). Gastrointestinal regulation of food intake. *Journal of Clinical Investigation* 117(1): 13–23.

de Jong, P., Bouwman, S., and van der Linden, H. J. L. J. (1992). Fouling of heat treatment equipment in relation to the denaturation of β-lactoglobulin. *Journal of the Society of Dairy Technology* 45: 3–8.

Desai, M. P., Labhasetwar, V., Walter, E., Levy, R. J., and Amidon, G. L. (1997). The mechanism of uptake of biodegradable microparticles in Caco-2 cells is size dependent. *Pharmaceutical Research* 14(11): 1568–1573.

Elzoghby, A. O., Samy, W. M., and Elgindy, N. A. (2012). Albumin-based nanoparticles as potential controlled release drug delivery systems. *Journal of Controlled Release,* 157(2): 168-182.

Essemine, J., Hasnia, I., Carpentiera, R., Thomas, T. J., and Tajmir-Riahia, H. A. (2011). Binding of biogenic and synthetic polyamines to β-lactoglobulin. *International Journal of Biological Macromolecules* 49: 201–209.

Farhoosh, R., Niazmand, R., Rezaei, M., and Sarabi, M. (2008). Kinetic parameter determination of vegetable oil oxidation under Rancimat test conditions. *European Journal of Lipid Science and Technology* 110(6): 587–592.

Fioramonti, S. A., Perez, A. A., Aringoli, E., Rubiolo, A. C., and Santiago, L. G. (2014). Design and characterization of soluble biopolymer complexes produced by electrostatic self-assembly of a whey protein isolate and sodium alginate. *Food Hydrocolloids* 35: 129–136.

Fioramonti, S. A., Martinez, M. J., Pilosof, A. M. R. Rubiolo, A. C., and Santiago, L. G. (2015a). Multilayer emulsions as a strategy for linseed oil microencapsulation: Effect of pH and alginate concentration. *Food Hydrocolloids* 43: 8–17.

Fioramonti, S. A., Martinez, M. J., Pilosof, A. M. R., Rubiolo, A. C., and Santiago, L. G. (2015b). Influence of freezing temperature and maltodextrin concentration on stability of linseed oil-in-water multilayer emulsions. *Journal of Food Engineering* 156: 31–38.

Foegeding, E. A., Luck, P. J., and Davis, J. P. (2006). Factors determining the physical properties of a protein foams. *Food Hydrocolloids* 20: 284–292.

Foegeding, E. A., Davis, J. P., Doucet, D., and McGuffey, M. K. (2002). Advances in modifying and understanding whey protein functionality. *Trends in Food Science & Technology* 13: 151–159.

Fontana, A., Spolaore, B., and Polverino de Laureto, P. (2013). The biological activities of protein/oleic acid complexes reside in the fatty acid. *Biochimica et Biophysica Acta* 1834: 1125–1143.

Frapin, D., Dufour, E., and Haertle, T. (1993). Probing the fatty acid binding site of β-lactoglobulins. *Journal of Protein Chemistry* 12(4): 443–449.

Freeman, M.P. (2000). Omega-3 fatty acids in psychiatry: A review. *Annals of Clinical Psychiatry* 12(3): 159–165.

Galazka, V., Smith, D., Ledward, D., and Dickinson, E. (1999). Interactions of ovalbumin with sulphated polysaccharides: Effects of pH, ionic strength, heat and high pressure treatment. *Food Hydrocolloids* 13: 81–88

Garti, N., and Bisperink, C. (1998). Double emulsions: Progress and applications. *Current Opinion in Colloid & Interface Science* 3(6): 657–667.

Gogos, C.A., Skoutelis, A., and Kalfarentzos, F. (2000). The effects of lipids on the immune response of patients with cancer. *Journal of Nutrition, Health, and Aging* 4(3): 172–175.

Gouin, S. (2004) Microencapsulation: Industrial appraisal of existing technologies and trends. *Trends in Food Science & Technology* 15: 330–347.

Hoffmann, M. A., and van Mil, P. J. (1997). Heat-induced aggregation of β-lactoglobulin: Role of the free thiol group and disulfide bonds. *Journal of Agricultural and Food Chemistry* 45: 2942–2948.

Hsieh, A. T., Anthony, J. C., Diersen-Schade, D. A., Rumsey, S. C., Lawrence, P., and Li, C. (2007). The influence of moderate and high dietary long chain polyunsaturated fatty acids (LCPUFA) on baboon neonate tissue fatty acids. Pediatric Research, 61: 537–545.

Ilyasoglu, H., and El, S. N. (2014) Nanoencapsulation of EPA/DHA with sodium caseinate–gum arabic complex and its usage in the enrichment of fruit juice. *Food Science and Technology* 56: 461–468.

Jiang, H. R., and Liu, N. (2010). Self-assembled β-lactoglobulin–conjugated linoleic acid complex for colon cancer–targeted substance. *Journal of Dairy Science* 93(9): 3931–3939.

Kato, A., and Nakai, S. (1980). Hydrophobicity determined by a fluorescence probe method and its correlation with surface properties of proteins. *Biochimica et Biophysica Acta* 624: 13–20.

Le Maux, S., Giblin, L., Croguennec, T., Bouhallab, S., and Brodkorb, A. (2012). Beta-lactoglobulin as a molecular carrier of linoleate: Characterisation and effects on intestinal epithelial cells *in vitro*. *Journal of Agricultural and Food Chemistry* 60(37): 9476–9483.

Le Maux, S., Bouhallab, S., Giblin, L., Brodkorb, A., and Croguennec, T. (2013). Complexes between linoleate and native or aggregated β-lactoglobulin: Interaction parameters and *in vitro* cytotoxic effect. *Food Chemistry* 141: 2305–2313.

Lesmes, U., and McClements, D. J. (2009). Structure–function relationships to guide rational design and fabrication of particulate food delivery systems. *Trends in Food Science & Technology* 20(10): 448–457.

Lisková, K., Auty, M. A. E., Chaurin, V., Min, S., Mok, K. H., *et al.* (2011). Cytotoxic complexes of sodium oleate with β-lactoglobulin. *European Journal of Lipid Science and Technology* 113(10): 1207–1218.

Maljaars, J., Peters, H. P. F., Haddeman, E., and Masclee, A. (2009). Distribution of small intestinal fat delivery influences satiety and food intake. *European Journal of Gastroenterology and Hepatology* 21(3): A86–A87.

Matalanis, A., Jones, O. G., and McClements, D. J. (2011). Structured biopolymer-based delivery systems for encapsulation, protection, and release of lipophilic compounds. *Food Hydrocolloids* 25(8): 1865–1880.

McClements, D. J. (2005a). *Food Emulsions: Principles, Practice, and Techniques*, 2nd ed. Boca Raton, FL: CRC Press.

McClements, D. J. (2005b). Theoretical analysis of factors affecting the formation and stability of multilayered colloidal dispersions. *Langmuir* 21(21): 9777–9785.

McClements, D. J., Decker, E. A., and Weiss, J. (2007). Emulsion-based delivery systems for lipophilic bioactive components. *Journal of Food Science* 72(8): 109–124.

McClements, D. J., and Li, Y. (2010). Structured emulsion-based delivery systems: Controlling the digestion and release of lipophilic food components. *Advances in Colloid and Interface Science* 159(2): 213–228.

Mulder, A. M., Connellan, P. A., Oliver, C. J., Morris, C. A, and Stevenson, L. M. (2008) Bovine lactoferrin supplementation supports immune and antioxidant status in healthy human males. *Nutrition Research* 28: 583–589.

Nicolai, T., Britten, M., and Schmitt, C. (2011). β-Lactoglobulin and WPI aggregates: Formation, structure and applications. *Food Hydrocolloids* 30: 1–18.

Panyam, J., and Labhasetwar, V. (2003). Biodegradable nanoparticles for drug and gene delivery to cells and tissue. *Advances in Drug Delivery Reviews* 55(3): 329–347.

Perez, A. A., Carrera Sánchez, C., Rodríguez Patino, J., Rubiolo, A., and Santiago, L. (2012a). Effect of enzymatic hydrolysis and polysaccharide addition on the β-lactoglobulin adsorption at the air–water interface. *Journal of Food Engineering* 109(4): 712–720.

Perez, A. A., Carrera Sánchez, C., Rodríguez Patino, J., Rubiolo, A., and Santiago, L. (2012b). Foaming characteristics of β-lactoglobulin as affected by enzymatic hydrolysis and polysaccharide addition: Relationships with the bulk and interfacial properties. *Journal of Food Engineering* 113(1): 53-60.

Perez, A. A., Andermatten, R. B., Rubiolo, A. C., and Santiago, L. G. (2014). Beta-lactoglobulin heat-induced aggregates as carriers of polyunsaturated fatty acids. *Food Chemistry* 158(1): 66–72.

Perez, A. A., Andermatten, R. B., Rubiolo, A. C. and Santiago, L. G. (2015). Biopolymer nanoparticles designed for polyunsaturated fatty acid vehiculization: Protein–polysaccharide ratio study. *Food Chemistry* 188: 543–550.

Perez, M. D., and Calvo, M. (1995). Interaction of β-lactoglobulin with retinol and fatty acids and its role as a possible biological function for this protein: A review. *Journal of Dairy Science* 78: 978–988.

Plourde, M., and Cunnane, S. C. (2007). Extremely limited synthesis of long chain polyunsaturates in adults: Implications for their dietary essentiality and use as supplements. *Applied Physiology, Nutrition and Metabolism* 32: 619–634.

Roche, H. M., and Gibney, M. J. (2000). Effect of long-chain n-3 polyunsaturated fatty acids on fasting and postprandial triacylglycerol metabolism. *American Journal of Clinical Nutrition* 71(1): 232–237.

Sherwin, E. R. (1976). Antioxidants for vegetable oils. *Journal of the American Oil Chemists' Society* 53(6): 430–436.

Sies, H., and Stahl, W. (1995) Beta-carotene, and other carotenoids as antioxidants. *American Journal of Clinical Nutrition* 62: 1315–1321.

Sponton, O. E., Perez, A. A., Carrara, C. R., and Santiago, L. G. (2014). Effect of limited enzymatic hydrolysis on linoleic acid binding properties of β-lactoglobulin. *Food Chemistry* 146: 577–582.

Sponton, O. E., Perez, A. A., Carrara, C. R., Santiago, L. G. (2015a). Impact of environment conditions on physicochemical characteristics of ovalbumin heat-induced nanoparticles and on their ability to bind PUFAs. *Food Hydrocolloids* 48: 165–173.

Sponton, O. E., Perez, A. A., Carrara, C. R., Santiago, L. G. (2015b). Linoleic acid binding properties of ovalbumin nanoparticles. *Colloids and Surfaces, B: Biointerfaces* 128: 219–226.

Verheul, M., and Roefs, S. P. F. M. (1998). Structure of particulate whey protein gels: Effect of NaCl concentration, pH, heating temperature and protein composition. *Journal of Agricultural and Food Chemistry* 46: 4909–4916.

von Schacky, C. (2003). The role of omega-3 fatty acids in cardiovascular disease. *Current Atherosclerosis Reports* 5(2): 139–145.

Wang, Q., Allen, J. C., and Swaisgood, H. E. (1998). Protein concentration dependence of palmitate binding to β-lactoglobulin. *Journal of Dairy Science* 81: 76–81.

Wang, Q., Allen, J. C., and Swaisgood, H. E. (1999). Binding of lipophilic nutrients to β-lactoglobulin prepared by bioselective adsorption. *Journal of Dairy Science* 82: 257–264.

Wissing, S.A., Kayser, O., Müller, R. H. (2004). Solid lipid nanoparticles for parenteral drug delivery. *Advanced Drug Delivery Reviews* 56(9): 1257–1272.

Zimet, P., and Livney, Y. D. (2009) Beta-lactoglobulin and its nanocomplexes with pectin as vehicles for ω-3 polyunsaturated fatty acids. *Food Hydrocolloids* 23(4): 1120–1126.

CHAPTER 4

Surface modifications that benefit protein-based nanoparticles as vehicles for oral delivery of phenolic phytochemicals

Zheng Li

Food Science and Human Nutrition Department, Institute of Agricultural and Food Sciences, University of Florida, Gainesville, FL, 32611, USA

4.1 Overview

Phenolic phytochemicals are defined as secondary metabolites synthesized in fruits and vegetables during their growth and development stages (Li *et al.*, 2015a; Li *et al.*, 2011a; Xing *et al.*, 2015; Zhang *et al.*, 2014). Phenolic phytochemicals basically consist of aromatic rings attached with multiple hydroxyl groups. Phenolic phytochemicals show multiple nutritional and pharmaceutical benefits. For example, phenolic phytochemicals have been confirmed to prevent chronic diseases, improve human longevity, delay the human aging process, and reduce incidences of cancers and other diseases (; Castañeda-Ovando *et al.*, 2009Haslam, 1996; Li *et al.*, 2015a).

Phenolic phytochemicals are not well absorbed in the gastrointestinal tract, leading to low bioactivity (Acosta, 2009; Li *et al.*, 2015a; Li *et al.*, 2015b). Firstly, the gastrointestinal tract contains numerous reactive oxygen species (Figure 4.1). These species can easily oxidize and degrade phenolic phytochemicals, lowering the presence of phenolic phytochemicals (Gao and Hu, 2010; Nagle *et al.*, 2006; Wang *et al.*, 2008). Secondly, phenolic phytochemicals have poor aqueous solubility, which lowers their residences with epithelial cells and reduces their transport through epithelium in the small intestine (Holt *et al.*, 2002). More importantly, no specific receptors on epithelial cells can recognize phenolic phytochemicals, making phenolic phytochemical transport through epithelial cells by passive diffusion (Gao and Hu, 2010; Li *et al.*, 2015a). Moreover, metabolism in epithelial cells metabolizes phenolic phytochemicals into phase II metabolites.

New Polymers for Encapsulation of Nutraceutical Compounds, First Edition.
Edited by Jorge Carlos Ruiz Ruiz and Maira Rubi Segura Campos.

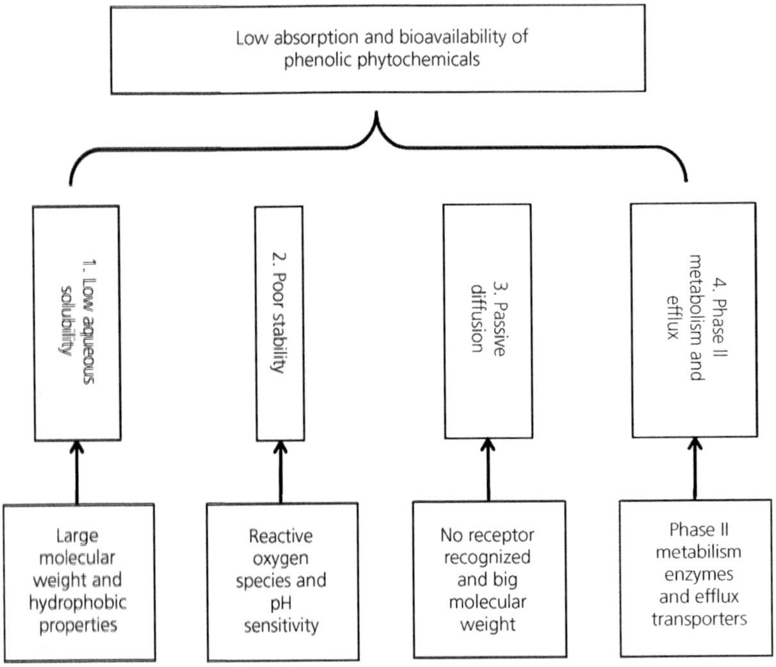

Figure 4.1 Factors for extremely low bioavailability of phenolic phytochemicals.

Both phenolic phytochemicals and phase II metabolites can be captured by efflux transporters on the surface of epithelial cells and pumped back to lumen (Day *et al.*, 2001 Walgren *et al.*, 1998; Yang *et al.*, 1998).

Nanoparticles have been extensively studied as delivery systems in the field of pharmaceutical science because their unique physicochemical properties provide them with cellular uptake features compared to bulk materials (Roger *et al.*, 2010). Particles are defined using particle diameter; nanoparticles have particle diameters between 1 and 100 nm. However, pharmaceutical science also classifies particles with size below 1,000 nm as nanoparticles because the unique properties can also be observed from these particles in a biological aspect (Li *et al.*, 2015a). For example, it has been observed that nanoparticles can be directly taken up by cells, and cellular uptake essentially depends on particle size. Particles with size around 1,000 to 2,000 nm can be engulfed into cells via macropinocytosis although the efficacy of uptake is relatively limited. Nanoparticles with size around 200 nm can stabilize clathrin-coated pits and thus are easily internalized via clathrin-mediated endocytosis into cells, whereas the smaller nanoparticles (60 nm and below) are more likely to be transported into cells via caveolae-mediated endocytosis (Li *et al.*, 2015a). These direct cellular uptakes help to increase bioactivity of encapsulated phenolic phytochemicals.

Protein has been extensively designed into delivery systems for phenolic phytochemicals because the affinity between protein and phenolic phytochemicals results in the encapsulation of phenolic phytochemicals into protein-based nanoparticles. In the meantime, protein-based nanoparticles have more biocompatible and biodegradable features compared to synthesized nanoparticles (Jahanshahi and Babaei, 2008). Therefore, this chapter introduces methods of fabricating protein-based nanoparticles for delivering phenolic phytochemicals. The obstacles to protein-based nanoparticles as oral delivery systems are highlighted and discussed regarding their instability and digestion risk in the gastrointestinal tract. Surface modifications of protein-based nanoparticles are emphasized in terms of modification mechanisms and oral delivery improvement. Coating applications and covalent coupling for protein-based nanoparticles are specifically discussed.

4.2 Fabrication of protein-based nanoparticles

Protein is an attractive macromolecule that possesses biodegradable, biocompatible, and nontoxic or low-toxic properties (Hawkins *et al.*, 2008). The primary structure of protein consists of amino acids via peptide bonds, whereas intermolecular interactions result in the secondary structure of protein. The spatial interactions, mainly including hydrophobic interactions, salt bridges, hydrogen bonds, and disulfide bonds, establish the tertiary structure of protein, and the subproteins/polypeptides further interact to form the quaternary structure (Schulz and Schirmer, 1979). The common proteins that are used for nanoparticle fabrication include albumin, zein, casein, collagen, gelatin, and whey protein (El-Samaligy and Rohdewald, 1983; Li *et al.*, 2014; Li *et al.*, 2011b; Zhang and Zhong, 2010; Zimet *et al.*, 2011). Protein-based nanoparticles have hydrophobic sites inside and hydrophilic groups (hydrophilic amino and carboxyl groups) on the surface, which provides interaction potentials with hydrophobic phenolic phytochemicals. Phenolic phytochemicals possess multiple hydroxyl groups on their structure, which can interact with protein hydrophobic sites via hydrogen bonds and hydrophobic interactions, and these interactions result in their encapsulation into protein-based nanoparticles (Chen *et al.*, 2010; Shutava *et al.*, 2009). Protein-based nanoparticles can be fabricated by several approaches, including desolvation, heating gelation, and self-assembly (Figure 4.2).

4.2.1 Desolvation method

The desolvation approach has been extensively applied to fabricate protein-based nanoparticles. During the desolvation process, antisolvent is normally used to reduce the solubility of protein molecules in a solution system under continuous stirring. When protein molecules lose their solubility in the solution, they start to be separated from the phase and result in turbidity in the system, causing the formation of protein-based nanoparticles (Weber *et al.*, 2000; Zhong and Jin, 2009). Phenolic phytochemicals due to multiple hydroxyl groups tend to interact with protein molecules via hydrogen bonds and hydrophobic

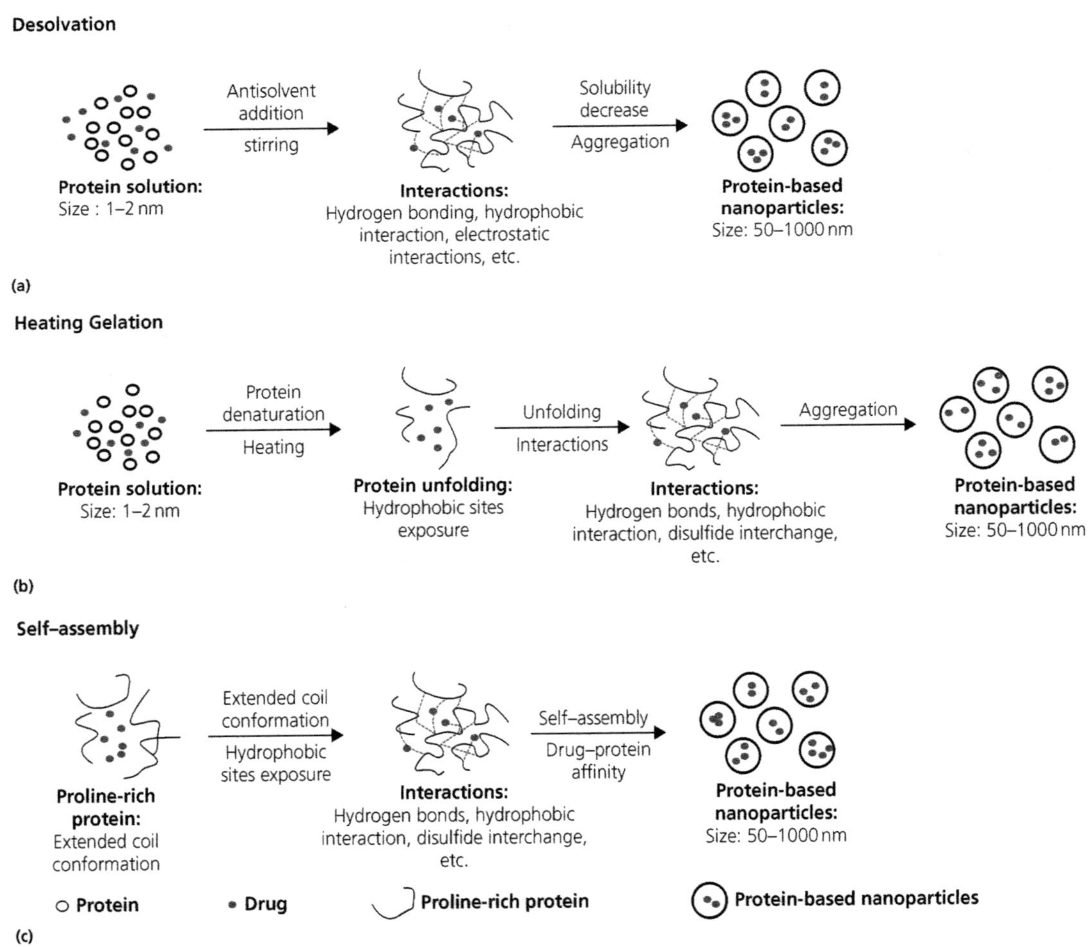

Figure 4.2 Protein-based nanoparticle fabrication approaches via desolvation **(a)**, heating gelation **(b)**, and self-assembly **(c)**.

interactions during the desolvation process, which leads to their encapsulation into protein-based nanoparticles. A crosslinking reagent is normally added to the resultant suspension to further stabilize protein-based nanoparticles by crosslinking amino residues. Afterward, the protein-based nanoparticle suspension is centrifuged to remove solvent and free cross-linker, and the pellet is resuspended into water to yield the nanoparticle suspension.

Water-soluble proteins, like albumin and gelatin, are initially dissolved in water to form protein aqueous solution. Afterward, ethanol is normally used as a desolvation reagent and is added dropwise to the protein aqueous solution. The ethanol-to-water ratio plays an important role in determining the solubility of proteins in the system, and it directly affects the characteristics of the resultant protein nanoparticles. For example, bovine serum albumin was used to form nanoparticles to carry epigallocatechin gallate (EGCG), a kind of tea catechin (Li *et al.*, 2014). The fabrication process started with addition of ethanol to bovine serum albumin aqueous solution under stirring until a milk-white suspension was observed. Afterward, glutaraldehyde was added dropwise to the suspension for further solidification of the nanoparticles. The suspension was centrifuged to remove the supernatant containing free glutaraldehyde and the solids were re-suspended to water. The resultant suspension was mixed with EGCG solution for EGCG encapsulation due to EGCG–bovine serum albumin's nanoparticle affinity.

Acetone is also used as an antisolvent to fabricate protein-based nanoparticles. For example, gelatin nanoparticles were prepared through a two-step desolvation process to encapsulate natural polyphenols, including EGCG, tannic acid, curcumin, and theaflavin (Shutava *et al.*, 2009). Initially, gelatin was dissolved in water by gentle heating and followed by adding acetone white gently shaking for 2 minutes. The precipitate was redissolved in water with gentle heating and the pH was adjusted to range from 1.5 to 5. Afterward, acetone was slowly added to the solution at 40 °C under stirring till a milk-like suspension was observed. Finally, glutaraldehyde was mixed with suspension, the gelatin nanoparticles were washed out several times using deionized water, and then polyphenols were loaded to gelatin nanoparticles.

Zein is a storage protein derived from corn and has a water-insoluble but alcohol-soluble property. This water-insoluble feature makes zein a good candidate for nanoparticle fabrication using the desolvation approach, with water as a desolvation reagent (Zou *et al.*, 2012a). For example, purified cranberry procyanidins and zein protein with different mass ratios were dissolved together in a ethanol–water (4:1, vol/vol) solution. Then water was added to the solution under vigorous stirring to reduce the solubility of both zein and procyanidins. As a result, procyanidins and zein were separated from solution and interacted with each other to form the nanoparticle suspension. The resultant suspension was centrifuged, and the collected sediments were resuspended to water to form a procyanidin–zein nanoparticle suspension.

4.2.2 Heating gelation

Heating can induce the denaturation of protein. During the controlled heating process, protein molecules start to unfold to expose hydrophobic groups. This process helps to enhance protein–protein and protein–phenolic phytochemical interactions by hydrogen bonding, hydrophobic interactions, electrostatic interactions, and disulfide bond interchanges. After a cooling step, refolding protein molecules results in the formation of protein-based nanoparticles that encapsulate phenolic phytochemicals (Chen *et al.*, 2006; Elzoghby *et al.*, 2012; Shimada and Cheftel, 1989).

For example, β-lactoglobulin-EGCG nanovehicles were prepared using the heating approach (Shpigelman *et al.*, 2012). β-Lactoglobulin, a major whey protein in cow's milk, was dissolved in a phosphate buffer (pH 7) containing 0.02% sodium azide and stirred overnight at room temperature. β-Lactoglobulin was heated at 70 °C for 20 min to expose hydrophobic groups. Subsequently, EGCG phosphate buffer solution (pH 2.5) was added to the β-lactoglobulin solution and then vertexed for 20 seconds to allow EGCG to interact with β-lactoglobulin. Finally, the mixture was cooled to room temperature, and β-lactoglobulin-EGCG nanovehicles were fabricated with particle sizes around 20 nm and high EGCG loading capacity.

4.2.3 Self-assembly

Proteins with compact tertiary structure normally show coil conformation in aqueous solution. The limited hydrophobic sites significantly restrict their interactions with phenolic phytochemicals, resulting in less affinity with phenolic phytochemicals (Langer *et al.*, 2003). However, some proteins, such as gelatin, are proline-rich proteins, which display extended random coil conformations in aqueous solution with more exposures of hydrophobic sites. These features enhance the affinity between protein and phenolic phytochemicals and thus assist in self-assembly of these molecules. Of course, the structure of phenolic phytochemicals also affects the fabrication performance. Higher-molecular-weight phenolic phytochemicals possess more hydroxyl groups and advanced spatial structure. These improve interactions between protein and phenolic phytochemicals during self-assembly (Li and Gu, 2011; Yi *et al.*, 2006).

Self-assembled pomegranate ellagitannin–gelatin nanoparticles were fabricated under different reaction conditions (Li and Gu, 2011). It was observed that a higher-molecular-weight ellagitannin, punicalagin, in pomegranate was encapsulated into the nanoparticles with higher loading content, whereas ellagic acid and ellagic acid–hexoside did not bind with gelatin. These demonstrated that the larger structure and more hydroxyl groups of punicalagin significantly increased the affinity toward gelatin. Additionally, the ellagitannin-to-gelatin mass ratio affected the interaction of the molecules, and the higher mass ratio exceeded the saturation point of gelatin, leading to precipitation. pH affected conformations of gelatin and ellagitannins. Acidic and neutral pH conditions caused the degradation of punicalagin, which did not lead to formation of self-assembled nanoparticles. Temperatures between 25 °C and 50 °C resulted in self-assembled nanoparticles with a size of 500 nm, whereas lower temperature caused the aggregation. The self-assembly process was complete after 12 hours, and the suspension remained stable for 4 days.

In another study, tea catechins were encapsulated into gelatin nanoparticles using self-assembly (Chen *et al.*, 2010). Gelatin solution was mixed with different concentrations of tea catechin under magnetic stirring at room temperature. The mixed solution continued to be stirred until the suspension was observed. These self-assembled nanoparticles had a size between 100 and 300 nm, negative zeta-potentials, and spherical morphology. The interaction mechanism was claimed to be hydrogen bonding and hydrophobic interactions due to the hydroxyl groups on tea catechins and hydrophobic sites of gelatin molecules.

4.3 Obstacles to protein-based nanoparticles as oral delivery vehicles

Protein-based nanoparticles after oral administration experience a complicated gastrointestinal condition before they reach the small intestinal epithelial cells for cellular uptake. Because protein-based nanoparticles are made of protein, one of the major macronutrients, they havea high risk of precipitation and digestion, which would make protein-based nanoparticles lose their unique properties, limiting their delivery efficacy for phenolic phytochemicals.

4.3.1 Physiology of the gastrointestinal tract

The gastrointestinal tract mainly consists of mouth, esophagus, stomach, small intestine, large intestine, rectum, and anus (Schneeman, 2002). The mouth takes care of grinding foods to release nutrients (Figure 4.3). This process improves the digestion process of nutrients by increasing the total surface of foods. The esophagus transports food from the mouth to the stomach (Tandler *et al.*, 2001). The stomach is an important organ in the gastrointestinal tract; in the stomach, food is further converted into chyme for better digestion. Two tubular glands in the stomach secrete gastric juices containing pepsinogen and hydrochloric acid. Pepsinogen is further activated to pepsin in the presence of hydrochloric acid, and pepsin splits protein into polypeptides from at pH 1.8 to 3.5 (Rothman *et al.*, 2000; Schneeman, 2002). In the small intestine, large quantities of alkaline mucus are secreted to neutralize acidic juices from the stomach. The mucus also contains a large excess of bicarbonate ions to provide optimal conditions for food digestion by pancreatic juices. The pancreatic juices are secreted by the pancreas, and they contain multiple digestive enzymes. Trypsin, chymotrypsin, and carboxypolypeptidase digest protein to polypeptides and amino acids, whereas pancreatic amylase takes in charge of splitting carbohydrates.

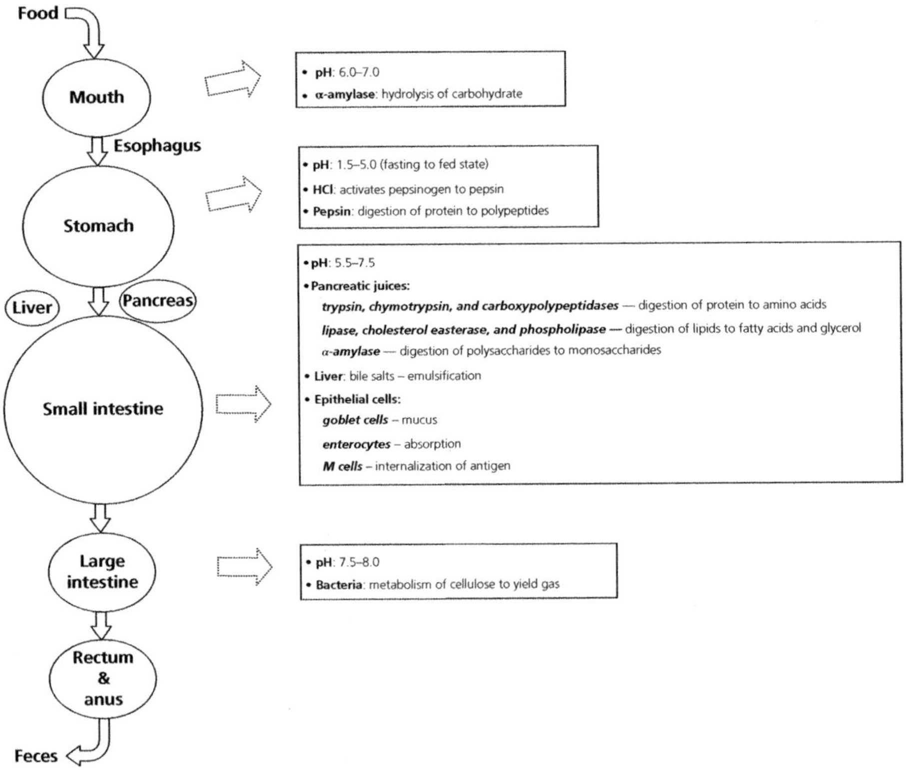

Figure 4.3 Digestive system in the gastrointestinal tract.

Fat digestion in the small intestine is conducted by pancreatic lipase, cholesterol esterase, and phospholipase (Flemström and Isenberg, 2001; Pácha, 2001; Schneeman, 2002). These digested nutrients then pass through the small intestinal epithelium into the circulation. The large intestine only absorbs water and electrolytes. Numerous bacteria in the large intestine metabolize cellulose and other materials to produce gas (Macfarlane and Gibson, 1997).

4.3.2 pH effect

Different pH segments exist in the gastrointestinal tract. The pH in the mouth and esophagus is around 6.0 to 7.0, which allows optimal amylase activity of digestive juices secreted from saliva (Tandler *et al.*, 2001). Parietal cells in the gastric gland secrete hydrochloric acid, which activates pepsinogen for protein digestion. The gastric juices have a pH ranging from 1.5 to 5.0 based on the fasting and fed states, respectively (Schneeman, 2002). In the small intestine, Brunner's glands have the capacity to release large quantities of alkaline bicarbonate to neutralize juices from the stomach, and these bicarbonate ions keep the small intestine at a pH from 5.5 to 7.0. The mucous cells in the large intestine also excrete large amounts of bicarbonate to maintain the pH of the large intestine around 7.5 to 8.0 (Ensign *et al.*, 2012; Schneeman, 2002).

Protein molecules possess carboxyl groups and charged amino groups on the surface, and these residues are sensitive to different pH conditions. The nature of protein molecules causes protein-based nanoparticles to be sensitive to conditions in the gastrointestinal tract. The stability of protein-based nanoparticles is determined by their interparticle repulsions. These interparticle repulsions are essentially affected by the surface charges of proteins. It has been known that the weakest stability of protein-based nanoparticles occurs when the pH condition of the nanoparticle suspension is near the isoelectric point of the corresponding protein (Kantardjieff and Rupp, 2004). This is because protein molecules at or near its isoelectric point significantly reduce surface charges.

This dramatic reduction of surface charges immediately enhances the hydrophobic interactions among protein molecules. As a result, protein-based nanoparticles start to aggregate to yield precipitates. For example, bovine serum albumin nanoparticles were fabricated to encapsulate EGCG as an oral delivery system. The stability of bovine serum albumin–EGCG nanoparticles was investigated under different pH conditions ranging from 1.5 to 7.0 (Li *et al.*, 2014). It was observed that bovine serum albumin–EGCG nanoparticles became turbid at pH 4.5 to 5.0, and precipitates were observed with significant increase of particle sizes. This observation was also accompanied by the dramatic reduction of zeta-potential of bovine serum albumin–EGCG nanoparticles. The zeta-potential was reduced because the isoelectric point of bovine serum albumin is around 4.7, and bovine serum albumin nanoparticles significantly reduced their surface charges around the isoelectric point, increasing hydrophobic interaction among particles and thus leading to precipitation.

Gelatin, a protein hydrolyzed from collagen, has an isoelectric point around 6 to 7. Thus, gelatin nanoparticles are not stable at pH 6 to 7. For example, pomegranate ellagitannin–gelatin self-assembled nanoparticles showed good particle stability at pH from 3 to 5, and the particle sizes were smaller than 200 nm. However, increasing pH condition to 6 and 7 dramatically elevated the size of ellagitannin–gelatin nanoparticles to micrometer scale and accompanied by precipitation and turbidity. Zeta-potentials of the nanoparticles were significantly reduced to around 0, demonstrating the elimination of interparticle repulsions determined by particle surface charges (Li and Gu, 2011).

4.3.3 Ionic strength effect

Large quantities of ions are secreted in the gastrointestinal tract to provide protective and lubrication functions. Also, numerous ions exist in the gastrointestinal tract to balance the pH conditions for optimal activity of digestive enzymes. Some ions in the small intestine are responsible for transportation of digested nutrients through epithelial cells. Moreover, digestive enzymes need to be activated in the presence of several key ions for digestion to occur (Schneeman, 2002). Saliva in the mouth secretes large amounts of potassium and bicarbonate ions to maintain the pH between 6.0 and 7.0. This also helps amylase release from saliva to split polysaccharides. Gastric juices contain hydrochloric acid, which is present to activate pepsin to digest protein in the stomach. Large volumes of bicarbonates are secreted from small ductules and large ducts of the pancreas and Brunner's glands in the small intestine. These ions in the small intestine provide an alkali condition to neutralize hydrochloric acid from the stomach and induce optimal activity of pancreatic enzymes. Sodium ions in the small intestine enhance the transport of amino acids and monosaccharides on epithelial cells via a cotransport pathway.

Ions also affect the stability of protein-based nanoparticles (Melander and Horváth, 1977). Protein-based nanoparticles can be stable due to the carboxyl and hydrophilic amino groups on the surface. These groups need to have enough hydration to make the nanoparticles stable in suspension. Appropriate amounts of ions in the nanoparticle suspension can favor the hydration of nanoparticles with water molecules by ionic attraction, and as a result, particle sizes tend to be increased somewhat (Arakawa and Timasheff, 1984). This can be explained in part because nanoparticles visualized by electron miscroscopy showed smaller sizes than those in aqueous suspension. However, excessive ions provide a strong ionic strength, which dramatically interacts with water molecules via attractions. This could decrease the hydration performance of protein-based nanoparticles with water, and as a result particles are no longer stable and start to aggregate and form precipitates (Bootz *et al.*, 2004; Kuehner *et al.*, 1996; Sanguansri and Augustin, 2006; Stone *et al.*, 2007).

4.3.4 Digestive enzyme effect

Before nutrients are absorbed from the gastrointestinal tract to the systemic circulation, macronutrients need to be fully digested to pass through epithelial cells in the small intestine. Protein digestion mainly occurs in the stomach and small intestine. Pepsinogen, secreted from peptic cells in the gastric gland of the stomach, is activated and converted into pepsin with the presence of hydrochloric acid with pH of 1.5 to 3.5. The activity of pepsin is significantly reduced when the stomach pH reaches 4.0. The pancreas secretes pancreatic juices and mixes with the chyme at the upper portion of the small intestine. The digestive enzymes, released from pancreatic acini, contain multiple enzymes that split macronutrients, including protein, polysaccharides, and lipids, into small molecules for absorption.

Trypsin, chymotrypsin, and carboxypolypeptidase are the main digestive enzymes that split proteins. These enzymes are activated from their inactive forms. Initially, enterokinase in the small intestine initiates activation of trypsin from trypsinogen under neutral pH conditions, and then trypsin continues to activate trypsinogen, chymotrpsinogen, and procarboxypolypeptidase to trypsin, chymotrypsin, and carboxypolypeptidase. Trypsin and chymotrypsin digest proteins to polypeptides, and polypeptides are further digested into amino acids with the activity of carboxypolypeptidase (Schneeman, 2002).

Protein-based nanoparticles, after oral administration, expose themselves to digestive enzymes in the gastrointestinal tract. Therefore, they have an extremely high risk of being digested and collapsed. The collapse and degradation of protein-based nanoparticles causes release of encapsulated phenolic phytochemicals. These compounds can be easily oxidized with reactive oxygen species and only absorbed into circulation system by passive diffusion. More importantly, the collapsed protein-based nanoparticles cannot be taken up by epithelial cells because they lose their features as nanoparticles (Livney, 2010).

For example, bovine serum albumin–EGCG nanoparticles were incubated at 37 °C with simulated gastric and intestinal fluids with and without digestive enzymes for 0.5 and 2 hours, respectively, and the release profiles of EGCG were investigated. Higher release of EGCG was observed in these simulated fluids with the presence of digestive enzymes compared to that without these enzymes, indicating that the integrity of protein nanoparticles was significantly destroyed by enzymes and the nanoparticle collapse dramatically increased the release of EGCG (Li *et al.*, 2014).

The release of β-carotene encapsulated in β-lactoglobulin nanoparticles was studied in simulated gastrointestinal juices with pepsin and trypsin, respectively (Yi *et al.*, 2014). They reported that the limited release of β-carotene was observed from β-lactoglobulin nanoparticles in simulated gastric juice with pepsin for 2 hours. However, this nanoparticle delivery system released β-carotene much faster in simulated intestinal juice with trypsin for 2 hours, which was explained by the collapse of β-lactoglobulin protein by trypsin. It was also noted that only trypsin, instead of trypsin and chymotrypsin, was used in the study. Therefore, a much higher release profile of β-carotene was speculated with pancreatic enzymes in the small intestinal environment.

4.3.5 Mucus barriers

Mucus in the gastrointestinal tract plays an important role in lubricating and protecting epithelial cells (Lai *et al.*, 2009). Mucus is a complex hydrogel consisting of protein, carbohydrates, lipids, salts, antibodies, bacteria, and cellular debris. It clears pathogens and foreign particulates by entrapping these molecules (Atuma *et al.*, 2001). The submandibular gland can secrete mucus in saliva in the mouth, whereas mucous neck cells in the gastric gland release large quantities of mucus to protect the stomach from excoriation. In the small intestine, Brunner's glands also excrete alkaline mucus to protect the duodenum by neutralizing acidic juices from the stomach. Goblet cells on the surface of crypts and villi also release mucus to protect the small intestine lumen. The mucous layer has a negative charge due to mucin, the major protein in mucus (Corfield *et al.*, 2000). Thus, positively charged nanoparticles can interact with mucus via electrostatic interactions by which nanoparticles can rapidly penetrate the mucus layer and attach to the surface of epithelial cells for better cellular uptake. On the other hand, the electrostatic interaction as well as other weak interactions (hydrophobic interaction and hydrogen bonds) can entrap nanoparticles in the mucus layer, reducing the contact between nanoparticles and epithelial cells in the small intestine and lowering the uptake efficacy. For negative charged nanoparticles, the charge repulsion restricts the transport of nanoparticles through the mucus layer, which directly lowers the uptake performance (Li *et al.*, 2015a; Roger *et al.*, 2010).

Albumin, gelatin, zein, and whey protein are the major proteins for fabricating nanoparticles. These proteins possess negative charges around pH conditions in the small intestine, so that the protein-based nanoparticles have negative charges. Therefore, these nanoparticles have difficulty penetrating through mucous layer due to the charge repulsion, which affects absorption of phenolic phytochemicals in the small intestine.

4.4 Surface modifications of protein-based nanoparticles for better delivery

There are certain obstacles to protein serving as an oral-delivery vehicle for phenolic phytochemicals. Therefore, surface modification is extensively studied and designed for protein-based nanoparticles, aiming to improve their stability in the gastrointestinal tract, enhance their mucus-penetrating ability, and/or improve their targeting properties on cells. According to conjugation mechanisms, surface modification of protein-based nanoparticles can be divided into noncovalent coating and covalent conjugation.

4.4.1 Noncovalent coating

Regarding noncovalent coating, biomaterials are generally adsorbed on the surface of particles via weak molecular interactions, such as electrostatic interaction, hydrogen bonds, and hydrophobic interactions (Figure 4.4). Protein-based nanoparticles possess carboxyl groups and charged amino groups that provide particle surface charges, whereas hydrophobic groups sit in the core of protein-based nanoparticles. Therefore, electrostatic interaction can be applied between protein nanoparticles by coating their surface with oppositely charged biomaterials. On the other hand, emulsifier with a hydrophobic site at one end and at the other a hydrophilic site can noncovalently adsorb with hydrophobic groups of protein-based nanoparticles via hydrogen bonds and hydrophobic interactions. As a result, the hydrophilic groups can be exposed on the surface of protein-based nanoparticles. These noncovalent coatings can alter physic and chemical properties of protein-based nanoparticles, which would stabilize nanoparticles in the gastrointestinal tract and improve their uptake efficacy for better absorption of encapsulated phenolic phytochemicals.

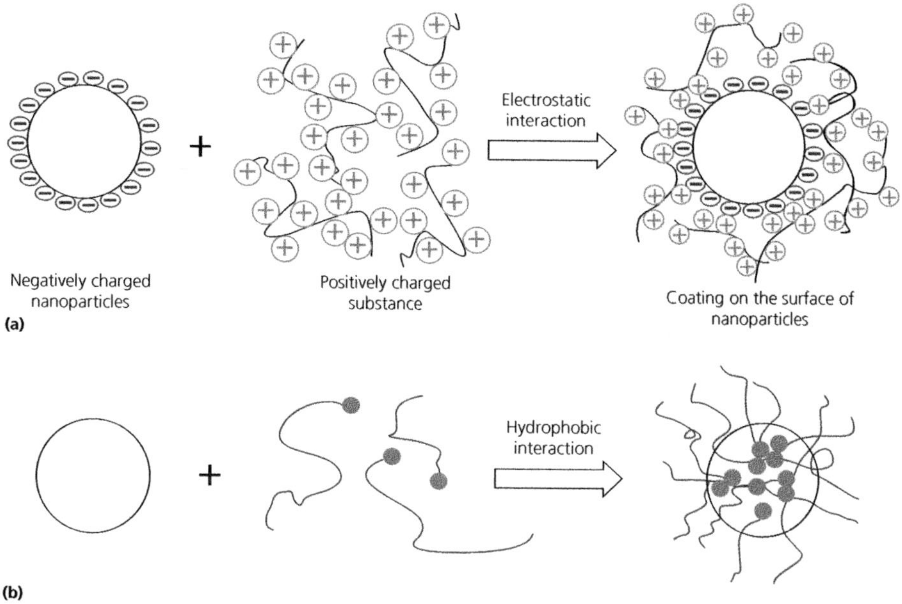

Figure 4.4 Noncovalent coating application on protein-based nanoparticles via electrostatic interactions **(a)** and hydrogen bonding and hydrophobic interactions **(b)**.

4.4.1.1 Chitosan

Chitosan, a linear polysaccharide consisting of D-glucosamine and *N*-acetyl-D-glucosamine via random β-1,4 linkage, is yielded by deacetylation of chitin under concentrated alkaline conditions (Ravi Kumar, 2000). Chitosan is a cationic polysaccharide that is water soluble in acidic solution due to the protonation of amine groups, but it is water insoluble in neutral and basic solutions (Ravi Kumar, 2000). Chitosan has biocompatible, mucoadhesive, and biodegradable properties, and it does not cause toxicity and allergic reactions. Chitosan also serves as a cellular absorption enhancer to increase bioavailability of bioactive compounds via reversible disruption of tight junctions among epithelial cells and/or improving cellular uptake by endocytosis (Ilium, 1998; Smith *et al.*, 2004). Due to its cationic properties, chitosan can be adsorbed on the surface of protein-based nanoparticles to form the coating via electrostatic interactions, and chitosan-coated protein-based nanoparticles exhibit better oral delivery performance for phenolic phytochemicals (Li *et al.*, 2014,; Mei *et al.*, 2008).

For example, bovine serum albumin–EGCG nanoparticles were initially prepared and then coated with chitosan (Li *et al.*, 2014). The chitosan-coated bovine serum albumin–EGCG nanoparticles were investigated in terms of pH stability, digestion stability, and permeability of EGCG on Caco-2 monolayers. The results showed that chitosan coating significantly stabilized bovine serum albumin–EGCG nanoparticles at pH of 4.5 to 5.0, and it induced the delay of

EGCG release from the nanoparticles in the simulated gastric and intestinal fluids with digestive enzymes. More importantly, chitosan coating significantly improved the apparent permeability coefficient of 357 EGCG on Caco-2 monolayers, suggesting that chitosan might benefit EGCG delivery of bovine serum albumin nanoparticles.

In another study, procyanidins purified from cocoa were encapsulated into gelatin nanoparticles using desolvation approach and then adsorbed to chitosan for better stability and improved bioactivity (Zou *et al.*, 2012b). The driving forces between procyanidins and gelatin were hydrogen bonds and hydrophobic interactions, whereas chitosan was attached on the procyanidin–gelatin nanoparticles by electrostatic interactions. The nanoparticles significantly prevented procyanidins from degradading in a harsh condition, and it dramatically induced more THP-1 cancer cells into an early apoptotic stage due to the enhanced cellular uptake.

4.4.1.2 Polylysine

Polylysine is a cationic polymer that results from polymerization of amino acid lysines. Polylysine is positively charged in aqueous solution due to hydrophilic lysine residues and can be used commercially as a food preservative due to its antimicrobial properties on yeast, fungi, and gram-positive and gram-negative bacteria in foods (Shih *et al.*, 2004). Polylysine's structure is similar to that of cell-penetrating peptides that have been demonstrated to translocate across cells under an energy-independent pathway. Therefore, polylysine has been extensively studied as an enhancer for drug delivery (Gupta *et al.*, 2005; Vivès *et al.*, 2008). Similar to chitosan, the polycationic properties of polylysines enable them to be coated on the surface of protein-based nanoparticles due to electrostatic interactions (Singh *et al.*, 2010). This noncovalent conjugation provides a surface barrier to delay the degradation of protein-based nanoparticles in the gastrointestinal tract, which favors encapsulated phenolic phytochemical delivery. In the meantime, cationic lysine residues from polylysines can efficiently attach to epithelial cells via electrostatic interactions, prolonging the residence of protein-based nanoparticles in epithelial cells and thus potentially increasing cellular uptake efficacy for improved absorption of encapsulated phenolic phytochemicals (Vivès *et al.*, 2008).

For example, polylysine was successfully adsorbed on the surface of bovine serum albumin–EGCG nanoparticles, and resulting coated nanoparticles were larger (Li *et al.*, 2014). The coated nanoparticles remained at nano-scale sizes at a pH of 4.5 to 5.0 due to the high positively charged surface. Polylysine delayed the contact between bovine serum albumin and digestive enzymes in simulated gastrointestinal fluids, delaying the release of EGCG. A Caco-2 monolayer study indicated that polylysine might increase absorption of EGCG in bovine serum albumin nanoparticles.

4.4.1.3 D-α-Tocopheryl polyethylene glycol succinate

D-α-Tocopheryl polyethylene glycol succinate (TPGS) is a water-soluble biomaterial that is produced by esterification of vitamin E succinate and polyethylene glycol. TPGS possesses multiple beneficial properties for drug delivery and delivery systems and is classed as generally recognized as safe (GRAS) (Varma and Panchagnula, 2005). For example, TPGS has been reported to enhance drug absorption and stabilize delivery systems in the gastrointestinal tract. Also, it has been reported as an inhibitor of P-glycoprotein, a type of multidrug-resistance protein located on the surface of cells, to reduce efflux behavior. This helps to improve the oral bioavailability of low absorbed phenolic phytochemicals and drugs (Zhang *et al.*, 2012).

TPGS exhibits amphiphilic properties, with a lipophilic alkyl tail and a hydrophilic polar head. This structural feature makes TPGS a good emulsifier for preparing protein-based nanoparticles. Its lipophilic alkyl tail can interact with hydrophobic sites of protein by hydrogen bonds and hydrophobic interactions, whereas the hydrophilic polar head remains on the surface to increase the hydrophilic properties of protein-based nanoparticles (Zou and Gu, 2013). These altered surface physicochemical properties can reduce the collapse of protein-based nanoparticles in the gastrointestinal tract and maintain particle sizes in different pH segments. The properties of TPGS also increase protein nanoparticle delivery performance by inhibiting active efflux of phenolic phytochemicals driven by P-glycoprotein on the surface of epithelial cells.

For example, TPGS-emulsified zein nanoparticles were designed using the desolvation method to improve the oral bioavailability of daidzin, an isoflavone glycoside (Zou and Gu, 2013). The resultant TPGS-emulsified zein nanoparticles showed average sizes around 200 nm and a low polydispersity. TPGS addition increased the encapsulation efficiency compared to zein nanoparticles and showed a slower daidzin release in a simulated gastrointestinal digestion model due to TPGS on the surface of zein nanoparticles. A Caco-2 permeation study showed a higher permeability of daidzin in TPGS-emulsified nanoparticles due to the enhanced cellular uptake confirmed by the confocal study. TPGS-emulsified zein nanoparticles significantly increased the absorption of daidzin in a pharmacokinetic study.

4.4.2 Covalent conjugation

Covalent conjugation refers to coupling of substances to protein-based nanoparticles via covalent binding (Figure 4.5). Protein-based nanoparticles have amino acid groups and they can provide reactive sites to covalent links with other molecules to alter their physicochemical properties (Choi *et al.*, 2005). Compared to noncovalent coating via weak interactions, covalent attachment can show much greater advantages for protein-based nanoparticles. Due to covalent conjugation, surface-modified protein-based nanoparticles may significantly improve their pH and ionic stability (Li and Yao, 2009; Yi *et al.*, 2014).

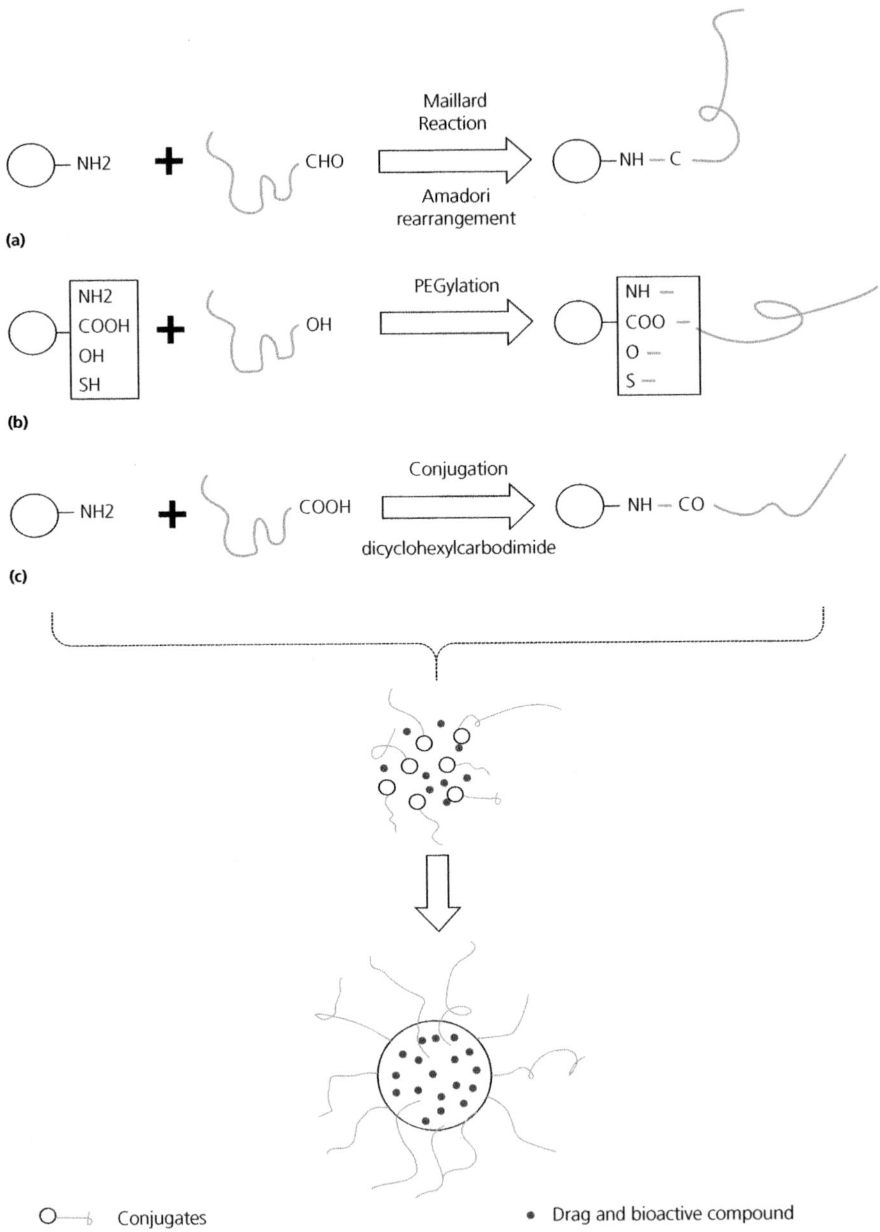

Figure 4.5 Covalent conjugation application on the surface of protein-based nanoparticles via Maillard reaction **(a)**, PEGylation **(b)**, and folic acid conjugation **(c)**.

Covalent conjugated biomaterials cannot be easily detached from protein-based nanoparticles, making them good barriers to prevent protein from degrading in the presence of digestive enzymes (Li and Gu, 2014). What is more, some of the coatings can be recognized by cells, which increases the targeting properties for protein-based nanoparticles (Kouchakzadeh *et al.*, 2010).

These beneficial features would help to promote bioavailability and bioactivity of phenolic phytochemicals encapsulated in protein-based nanoparticles.

4.4.2.1 Dextran

Dextran is a branched polysaccharide that consists of a number of glucose molecules. Its straight chain is composed of glucose molecules via α-1,6 glycosidic linkage, whereas α-1,3 linkage of glucose molecules results in its branch chains. Dextran has the potential to reduce vascular thrombosis, improve colloidal effects, and prevent coagulation (Moncrief *et al.*, 1963). Dextran has been used to conjugate protein molecules to enhance protein stability in the gastrointestinal tract because dextran is resistant to digestion by α-amylase in the gastrointestinal environment (Sery and Hehre, 1956).

The Maillard reaction is a natural chemical reaction that results in foods with brown color and unique flavor without any catalysts. The reactive carbonyl groups in polysaccharides and nucleophilic amino groups of amino acids in protein result in conjugation under high temperature to produce Schiff's based glycosylamines. These glycosylamines further undergo structure rearrangements to form Amadori products. These open-chain Amadori products after Amadori arrangement are then dehydrated and deaminated to yield dicarbonyls. Strecker degradation makes dicarbonyls and amines to yield Strecker aldehydes, which provides colors and flavors for foods (Ledl and Schleicher, 1990; Martins *et al.*, 2000). Dextran has a reducing carbonyl group in its molecular structure, and thus it is able to conjugate on protein molecules under the Maillard reaction. The covalent conjugation is controlled at the Amadori rearrangement stage of the Maillard reaction for better properties of protein–dextran conjugates (Zhou *et al.*, 2012).

After conjugation, the hydrophilic property and hydration behavior of protein-based nanoparticles can be significantly enhanced. Protein-based nanoparticles have a hydrophobic core with a hydrophilic surface. Dextran can remain on the surface of protein-based nanoparticles, restricting the particles' attractions under or near the isoelectric point of the proteins. Secondly, dextran conjugated on the surface of protein-based nanoparticles significantly increases the hydration ability of the nanoparticles, preventing the precipitation that ionic strength effect causes. Thirdly, dextran can work as a protective barrier of protein-based nanoparticles, which effectively delays the contact between protein nanoparticles and digestive enzymes in the gastrointestinal tract. This helps to delay the collapse of protein-based nanoparticles.

For example, gelatin has been reported to be modified with dextran via the Maillard reaction, and the resultant gelatin–dextran conjugate biopolymer was used to self-assemble tea polyphenol to form tea polyphenol gelatin–dextran conjugate nanoparticles (Zhou *et al.*, 2012). The fabricated nanoparticles were claimed to have a hydrophobic core with a dextran hydrophilic shell. These nanoparticles remained particle sizes between 100 and 150 nm in a pH range from 3.0 to 8.0. This result revealed that the conjugated dextran prevented gelatin nanoparticles from aggregation/precipitation whether the pH was near or far from gelatin's isoelectric points (Zhou *et al.*, 2012). The resultant tea polyphenol gelatin–dextran conjugated nanoparticles significantly induced more MCF-7 cells into early stage of apoptosis, indicating the nanoparticles improved the bioactivity of tea polyphenols.

Ovalbumin has also been investigated on its surface modification using dextran (Li and Gu, 2014). The conjugates were yielded after 2-day incubation at 60 °C. The formed ovalbumin--dextran conjugates were further used to encapsulate EGCG via self-assembly. The resultant EGCG ovalbumin–dextran conjugate nanoparticles retained its particle characteristics in simulated gastric and intestinal fluids, indicating the hydration behavior of nanoparticles was enhanced. The release study of the nanoparticles in simulated gastric and intestinal fluids with digestive enzymes revealed that the conjugated dextran helped to result in a small release of EGCG from nanoparticles. These improvements that dextran provided to ovalbumin also increased the permeation of EGCG on Caco-2 monolayers, indicating a potential enhancement of EGCG absorption (Li and Gu, 2014).

Bovine serum albumin was also conjugated with dextran to form conjugates using the Maillard reaction, and doxorubicin was used as a model drug for self-assembled nanoparticles (Deng *et al.*, 2010). These resultant nanoparticles significantly prolonged the life of murine ascites hepatoma H22 tumor-bearing mice compared to free doxorubicin, which might result from the enhanced stability of doxorubicin bovine serum albumin–dextran conjugated nanoparticles (Deng *et al.*, 2010).

4.4.2.2 Polyethylene glycol

Polyethylene glycol (PEG) is a hydrophilic polymer prepared by polymerization of ethylene oxide. Depending on different molecular weights from ethylene oxide polymerization, PEG is also known as polyethylene oxide and polyoxyethlene, and its molecular weights range from 300 to 10,000,000 g/mol (Zalipsky, 1995). PEG has a low toxicity, and it has been reported to be a mucoadhesive compound. PEG can promote enhanced retention effect of drugs and reduce their toxicity by prolonging their circulation half-life. PEG has been widely studied and proposed to improve the penetration of nanoparticles through the mucus layer network (Lai *et al.*, 2009; Mert *et al.*, 2012; Zalipsky, 1995).

The covalent coupling between protein and PEG is achieved by PEGylation, a chemical reaction in which PEG polymer chains are attached to another molecule. At the beginning of PEGylation, PEG is activated and functionalized by activating one or both terminals. These activated PEGs can further react with reactive groups of amino acids in protein, such as $-NH_2-$, -NH-, -COOH, -OH, -SH, and -S-S- bonds. The resultant polymers can be separated and purified using size exclusion, ion exchange, hydrophobic interaction chromatography technologies (Veronese and Pasut, 2005; Zalipsky, 1995).

After PEGylation, protein molecules are expected to increase their hydrophilicity, which can improve their stability in the gastrointestinal tract with different pH segments and large quantities of ions. More importantly, conjugation of PEG on the surface of protein-based nanoparticles significantly enhances the mucus-penetrating properties of nanoparticles, increasing contact of nanoparticles with cells (Mert *et al.*, 2012; Zhang *et al.*, 2012).

For example, bovine serum albumin protein was prepared initially and then covalently conjugated with PEG through PEGylation (Kouchakzadeh *et al.*, 2010). The PEGylation process was optimized using response surface methodology, and the optimized PEGylation resulted in a significant reduction of surface charges of bovine serum albumin nanoparticles from −31.7 mV to −14 mV. The PEG surface–modified bovine serum albumin nanoparticles significantly slowed the release process of 5-fluorouracil, suggesting that the PEG layer on the bovine serum albumin nanoparticles made extra resistance in opposition to drug diffusion (Kouchakzadeh *et al.*, 2010).

Gelatin was also conjugated with PEG to show better delivery performance (Kaul and Amiji, 2002). Type-B gelatin and PEG-epoxide were reacted to synthesize PEG-modified gelatin by pH and temperature-controlled ethanol–water solvent displacement technique. Then, tetramethylrhodamine-labeled dextran was used as a model drug to investigate release performance of PEG modified gelatin nanoparticles with protease. The PEG-modified gelatin nanoparticles had mean sizes between 200 and 500 nm and spherical morphology. The conjugation of PEG significantly decreased the percentage release of labeled dextran from gelatin nanoparticles in the presence of protease due to enhanced steric repulsion. PEGylated gelatin nanoparticles did not show cytotoxicity to BT-20 human breast cancer cells, and they were mainly found in perinuclear regions of these cells after 12 hours of incubation due to endocytosis (Kaul and Amiji, 2002).

4.4.2.3 Folate

Folic acid is a B vitamin with molecular weight of 441 g/moL. It is extensively applied in pharmaceutical sciences for drug delivery because it possesses cancer cell targeting properties. Normally, the surfaces of human cancer cells overexpress folate-receptor proteins, whereas normal human cells do not. These folate-receptor proteins show much higher affinity with folic acid, which can induce cellular uptakes of folate–drug conjugates (Butterworth and Tamura, 1989; Sudimack and Lee, 2000).

The covalent conjugation can be achieved between carboxyl group in folic acid and amino groups of protein-based nanoparticles. Before conjugation with amino groups, the reactive carboxyl groups are activated from folic acid with the presence of dicyclohexylcarbodiimide. Subsequently, the reaction between amino groups and activated folate results in the formation of amide bonds (Ren *et al.*, 2007; Sudimack and Lee, 2000). The folic acid conjugated protein–based nanoparticles significantly improve targeting properties, which benefits anticancer features of phenolic phytochemicals.

For example, bovine serum albumin was used to fabricate nanoparticles and then cross-linked by glutaraldehyde. Afterward, these nanoparticles were further reacted with the activated folic acid to couple folate to the nanoparticles. The folate conjugated bovine serum albumin was investigated regarding the cellular uptake efficacy on human ovarian cancer SKOV3 cells. These conjugated nanoparticles showed a much higher uptake percentage on SKOV3 cells. However, the association of these particles with SKOV3 cells was inhibited by excessive amounts of folic acid. This suggested that the uptake was mediated by folate receptors, and folate conjugated bovine serum albumin nanoparticles increased targeting properties of cancer cells due to folic acid binding with folate receptors on cancer cells (Zhang *et al.*, 2004).

4.5 Summary

Protein-based nanoparticles are good candidates for delivering drugs and bioactive compounds. However, their poor gastrointestinal tract stability restricts their applications as oral delivery systems. Surface modifications include nonconjugation coatings and covalent coupling on the surface of protein-based nanoparticles, and they can alter physicochemical properties of protein-based nanoparticles, which can improve the stability and delivery performance of protein-based nanoparticles in the gastrointestinal tract.

References

Acosta, E. (2009). Bioavailability of nanoparticles in nutrient and nutraceutical delivery. *Current Opinion in Colloid Interface Science* 14: 3–15.

Arakawa, T., and Timasheff, S. N. (1984). Mechanism of protein salting in and salting out by divalent cation salts: Balance between hydration and salt binding. *Biochemistry* 23: 5912–5923.

Atuma, C., Strugala, V., Allen, A., and Holm, L. (2001). The adherent gastrointestinal mucus gel layer: thickness and physical state *in vivo*. *American Journal of Physiology. Gastrointestinal and Liver Physiology* 280(5): G922–G929.

Bootz, A., Vogel, V., Schubert, D., and Kreuter, J. (2004). Comparison of scanning electron microscopy, dynamic light scattering and analytical ultracentrifugation for the sizing of poly(butyl cyanoacrylate) nanoparticles. *European Journal of Pharmaceutics and Biopharmaceutics* 57: 369–375.

Butterworth, C. E., and Tamura, T. (1989). Folic acid safety and toxicity: a brief review. *American Journal of Clinical Nutrition* 50: 353–358.

Castañeda-Ovando, A., Pacheco-Hernández, M. d. L., Páez-Hernández, M. E., Rodríguez, J. A., and Galán-Vidal, C. A. (2009). Chemical studies of anthocyanins: A review. *Food Chemistry* 113: 859–871.

Chen, L., Remondetto, G. E., and Subirade, M. (2006). Food protein–based materials as nutraceutical delivery systems. *Trends in Food Science & Technology* 17: 272–283.

Chen, Y.-C., Yu, S.-H., Tsai, G.-J., Tang, D.-W., Mi, F.-L., and Peng, Y.-P. (2010). Novel technology for the preparation of self-assembled catechin/gelatin nanoparticles and their characterization. *Journal of Agricultural and Food Chemistry* 58: 6728–6734.

Choi, S. J., Kim, H. J., Park, K. H., and Moon, T. W. (2005). Molecular characteristics of ovalbumin–dextran conjugates formed through the Maillard reaction. *Food Chemistry* 92: 93–99.

Corfield, A. P., Myerscough, N., Longman, R., Sylvester, P., Arul, S., and Pignatelli, M. (2000). Mucins and mucosal protection in the gastrointestinal tract: New prospects for mucins in the pathology of gastrointestinal disease. *Gut* 47: 589–594.

Day, A. J., Mellon, F., Barron, D., Sarrazin, G., Morgan, M. R. A., and Williamson, G. (2001). Human metabolism of dietary flavonoids: Identification of plasma metabolites of quercetin. *Free Radical Research* 35: 941–952.

Deng, W., Li, J., Yao, P., He, F., and Huang, C. (2010). Green preparation process, characterization and antitumor effects of doxorubicin–BSA–dextran nanoparticles. *Macromolecular Bioscience* 10: 1224–1234.

El-Samaligy, M. S., and Rohdewald, P. (1983). Reconstituted collagen nanoparticles, a novel drug carrier delivery system. *Journal of Pharmacy and Pharmacology* 35: 537–539.

Elzoghby, A. O., Samy, W. M., and Elgindy, N. A. (2012). Albumin-based nanoparticles as potential controlled release drug delivery systems. *Journal of Controlled Release* 157: 168–182.

Ensign, L. M., Cone, R., and Hanes, J. (2012). Oral drug delivery with polymeric nanoparticles: The gastrointestinal mucus barriers. *Advanced Drug Delivery Reviews* 64: 557–570.

Flemström, G., and Isenberg, J. I. (2001). Gastroduodenal mucosal alkaline secretion and mucosal protection. *News in Physiological Sciences* 16: 23–28.

Gao, S., and Hu, M. (2010). Bioavailability challenges associated with development of anti-cancer phenolics. Mini Reviews in Medicinal Chemistry 10: 550–567.

Gupta, B., Levchenko, T. S., and Torchilin, V. P. (2005). Intracellular delivery of large molecules and small particles by cell-penetrating proteins and peptides. *Advanced Drug Delivery Reviews* 57: 637–651.

Haslam, E. (1996). Natural polyphenols (vegetable tannins) as drugs: Possible modes of action. *Journal of Natural Products* 59: 205–215.

Hawkins, M. J., Soon-Shiong, P., and Desai, N. (2008). Protein nanoparticles as drug carriers in clinical medicine. *Advanced Drug Delivery Reviews* 60: 876–885.

Holt, R. R., Lazarus, S. A., Sullards, M. C., Zhu, Q. Y., Schramm, D. D. *et al.* (2002). Procyanidin dimer B2 [epicatechin-(4β-8)-epicatechin] in human plasma after the consumption of a flavanol-rich cocoa. *American Journal of Clinical Nutrition* 76: 798–804.

Ilium, L. (1998). Chitosan and its use as a pharmaceutical excipient. *Pharmaceutical Research* 15: 1326–1331.

Jahanshahi, M., and Babaei, Z. (2008). Protein nanoparticle: A unique system as drug delivery vehicles. *African Journal of Biotechnology* 7: 4926–4934.

Kantardjieff, K. A., and Rupp, B. (2004). Protein isoelectric point as a predictor for increased crystallization screening efficiency. *Bioinformatics* 20: 2162–2168.

Kaul, G., and Amiji, M. (2002). Long-circulating poly(ethylene glycol)-modified gelatin nanoparticles for intracellular delivery. *Pharmacological Research* 19: 1061–1067.

Kouchakzadeh, H., Shojaosadati, S., Maghsoudi, A., and Vasheghani Farahani, E. (2010). Optimization of PEGylation conditions for BSA nanoparticles using response surface methodology. *AAPS PharmSciTech* 11: 1206–1211.

Kuehner, D. E., Blanch, H. W., and Prausnitz, J. M. (1996). Salt-induced protein precipitation: Phase equilibria from an equation of state. *Fluid Phase Equilibria* 116: 140–147.

Lai, S. K., Wang, Y.-Y., and Hanes, J. (2009). Mucus-penetrating nanoparticles for drug and gene delivery to mucosal tissues. *Advanced Drug Delivery Reviews* 61: 158–171.

Langer, K., Balthasar, S., Vogel, V., Dinauer, N., von Briesen, H., and Schubert, D. (2003). Optimization of the preparation process for human serum albumin (HSA) nanoparticles. *International Journal of Pharmaceutics* 257: 169–180.

Ledl, F., and Schleicher, E. (1990). New aspects of the Maillard reaction in foods and in the human body. *Angewandte Chemie* International Edition in English 29: 565–594.

Li, J., and Yao, P. (2009). Self-assembly of ibuprofen and bovine serum albumin–dextran conjugates leading to effective loading of the drug. *Langmuir* 25: 6385_6391.

Li, Z., and Gu, L. (2014). Fabrication of self-assembled (−)-epigallocatechin gallate (EGCG) ovalbumin–dextran conjugate nanoparticles and their transport across monolayers of human intestinal epithelial Caco-2 cells. *Journal of Agricultural and Food Chemistry* 62: 1301–1309.

Li, Z., and Gu, L. (2011). Effects of mass ratio, pH, temperature, and reaction time on fabrication of partially purified pomegranate ellagitannin – gelatin nanoparticles. *Journal of Agricultural and Food Chemistry* 59: 4225–4231.

Li, Z., Ha, J.-H., Zou, T., and Gu, L. (2014). Fabrication of coated bovine serum albumin (BSA)–epigallocatechin gallate (EGCG) nanoparticles and their transport across monolayers of human intestinal epithelial Caco-2 cells. *Food & Function* 5: 1278–1285.

Li, Z., Jiang, H., Xu, C., and Gu, L. (2015a). A review: Using nanoparticles to enhance absorption and bioavailability of phenolic phytochemicals. *Food Hydrocolloids* 43: 153–164.

Li, Z., Pan, Q., Jin, Z., Mu, L., and Duan, C. (2011a). Comparison on phenolic compounds in *Vitis vinifera* cv. Cabernet Sauvignon wines from five wine-growing regions in China. *Food Chemistry* 125: 77–83.

Li, Z., Percival, S. S., Bonard, S., and Gu, L. (2011b). Fabrication of nanoparticles using partially purified pomegranate ellagitannins and gelatin and their apoptotic effects. *Molecular Nutrition & Food Research* 55: 1096–1103.

Li, Z., Zeng, J., Tong, Z., Qi, Y., and Gu, L. (2015b). Hydrogenolytic depolymerization of procyanidin polymers from hi-tannin sorghum bran. *Food Chemistry* 188: 337–342.

Livney, Y. D. (2010). Milk proteins as vehicles for bioactives. *Current Opinion in Colloid & Interface Science* 15: 73–83.

Macfarlane, G., and Gibson, G. (1997). Carbohydrate Fermentation, Energy Transduction, and Gas Metabolism in the Human Large Intestine. In: *Gastrointestinal Microbiology*, pp. 269–318. R. Mackie and B. White, eds. New York: Springer.

Martins, S. I. F. S., Jongen, W. M. F., and van Boekel, M. A. J. S. (2000). A review of Maillard reaction in food and implications to kinetic modelling. *Trends in Food Science & Technology* 11: 364–373.

Mei, D., Mao, S., Sun, W., Wang, Y., and Kissel, T. (2008). Effect of chitosan structure properties and molecular weight on the intranasal absorption of tetramethylpyrazine phosphate in rats. *European Journal of Pharmaceutics and Biopharmaceutics* 70: 874–881.

Melander, W., and Horváth, C. (1977). Salt effects on hydrophobic interactions in precipitation and chromatography of proteins: An interpretation of the lyotropic series. *Archives of Biochemistry and Biophysics* 183: 200–215.

Mert, O., Lai, S. K., Ensign, L., Yang, M., Wang, Y.-Y., *et al.* (2012). A poly(ethylene glycol)-based surfactant for formulation of drug-loaded mucus penetrating particles. *Journal of Controlled Release* 157: 455–460.

Moncrief, J. A., Darin, J. C., Canizaro, P. C., and Sawyer, R. B. (1963). Use of dextran to prevent arterial and venous thrombosis. *Annals of Surgery* 158: 553–559.

Nagle, D. G., Ferreira, D., and Zhou, Y.-D. (2006). Epigallocatechin-3-gallate (EGCG): Chemical and biomedical perspectives. *Phytochemistry* 67: 1849–1855.

Pácha, J. (2001). Development of intestinal transport function in mammals. *Physiological Reviews* 80(4): 1633–1667.

Ravi Kumar, M. N. V. (2000). A review of chitin and chitosan applications. *Reactive and Functional Polymers* 46: 1–27.

Ren, Y., Wong, S. M., and Lim, L.-Y. (2007). Folic acid–conjugated protein cages of a plant virus: A novel delivery platform for doxorubicin. *Bioconjugate Chemistry* 18: 836–843.

Roger, E., Lagarce, F., Garcion, E., and Benoit, J.-P. (2010). Biopharmaceutical parameters to consider in order to alter the fate of nanocarriers after oral delivery. *Nanomedicine* 5: 287–306.

Rothman, S., Liebow, C., and Isenman, L. (2000). Conservation of digestive enzymes. *Physiological Reviews* 82: 1–18.

Sanguansri, P., and Augustin, M. A. (2006). Nanoscale materials development – a food industry perspective. *Trends in Food Science & Technology* 17: 547–556.

Schneeman, B. O. (2002). Gastrointestinal physiology and functions. *British Journal of Nutrition* 88: S159–S163.

Schulz, G. E., and Schirmer, R. H. (1979). *Principles of Protein Structure*. Berlin: Springer-Verlag.

Sery, T. W., and Hehre, E. J. (1956). Degradation of dextrans by enzymes of intestinal bacteria. *Journal of Bacteriology* 71(3): 373–380.

Shih, I. L., Van, Y. T., and Shen, M. H. (2004). Biomedical applications of chemically and microbiologically synthesized poly(glutamic acid) and poly(lysine). *Mini Reviews in Medicinal Chemistry* 4: 179–188.

Shimada, K., and Cheftel, J. C. (1989). Sulfhydryl group/disulfide bond interchange reactions during heat-induced gelation of whey protein isolate. *Journal of Agricultural and Food Chemistry* 37: 161–168.

Shpigelman, A., Cohen, Y., and Livney, Y. D. (2012). Thermally-induced β-lactoglobulin–EGCG nanovehicles: Loading, stability, sensory and digestive-release study. *Food Hydrocolloids* 29: 57–67.

Shutava, T. G., Balkundi, S. S., Vangala, P., Steffan, J. J., Bigelow, R. L., *et al.* (2009). Layer-by-layer-coated gelatin nanoparticles as a vehicle for delivery of natural polyphenols. *ACS Nano* 3: 1877–1885.

Singh, H. D., Wang, G., Uludag, H., and Unsworth, L. D. (2010). Poly-L-lysine–coated albumin nanoparticles: Stability, mechanism for increasing *in vitro* enzymatic resilience, and siRNA release characteristics. *Acta Biomaterialia* 6: 4277–4284.

Smith, J., Wood, E., Dornish, M. (2004). Effect of chitosan on epithelial cell tight junctions. *Pharmacological Research* 21: 43–49.

Stone, V., Johnston, H., and Clift, M. J. D. (2007). Air pollution, ultrafine and nanoparticle toxicology: Cellular and molecular interactions. *IEEE Transactions on Nanobioscience* 6: 331–340.

Sudimack, J., and Lee, R. J. (2000). Targeted drug delivery via the folate receptor. *Advanced Drug Delivery Reviews* 41: 147–162.

Tandler, B., Gresik, E. W., Nagato, T., and Phillips, C. J. (2001). Secretion by striated ducts of mammalian major salivary glands: Review from an ultrastructural, functional, and evolutionary perspective. *Anatomical Record* 264: 121–145.

Varma, M. V. S., and Panchagnula, R. (2005). Enhanced oral paclitaxel absorption with vitamin E-TPGS: Effect on solubility and permeability *in vitro, in situ* and *in vivo*. *European Journal of Pharmaceutical Sciences* 25: 445–453.

Veronese, F. M., and Pasut, G. (2005). PEGylation, successful approach to drug delivery. *Drug Discovery Today* 10: 1451–1458.

Vivès, E., Schmidt, J., and Pèlegrin, A. (2008). Cell-penetrating and cell-targeting peptides in drug delivery. *Biochimica et Biophysica Acta – Reviews on Cancer* 1786: 126–138.

Walgren, R. A., Walle, U. K., and Walle, T. (1998). Transport of quercetin and its glucosides across human intestinal epithelial Caco-2 cells. *Biochemical Pharmacology* 55: 1721–1727.

Wang, R., Zhou, W., Jiang, X. (2008). Reaction kinetics of degradation and epimerization of epigallocatechin gallate (EGCG) in aqueous system over a wide temperature range. *Journal of Agricultural and Food Chemistry* 56: 2694–2701.

Weber, C., Coester, C., Kreuter, J., and Langer, K. (2000). Desolvation process and surface characterisation of protein nanoparticles. *International Journal of Pharmaceutics* 194: 91–102.

Xing, R.-R., Li, S.-Y., He, F., Yang, Z., Duan, C.-Q., *et al.* (2015). Mass spectrometric and enzymatic evidence confirm the existence of anthocyanidin 3,5-*O*-diglucosides in cabernet sauvignon (*Vitis vinifera* L.) grape berries. *Journal of Agricultural and Food Chemistry* 63(12): 3251–360.

Yang, C. S., Chen, L., Lee, M. J., Balentine, D., Kuo, M. C., and Schantz, S. P. (1998). Blood and urine levels of tea catechins after ingestion of different amounts of green tea by human volunteers. *Cancer Epidemiology Biomarkers & Prevention* 7: 351–354.

Yi, J., Lam, T. I., Yokoyama, W., Cheng, L. W., and Zhong, F. (2014). Controlled release of β-carotene in β-lactoglobulin–dextran-conjugated nanoparticles' *in vitro* digestion and transport with Caco-2 monolayers. *Journal of Agricultural and Food Chemistry* 62: 8900–8907.

Yi, K., Cheng, G., and Xing, F. (2006). Gelatin/tannin complex nanospheres via molecular assembly. *Journal of Applied Polymer Science* 101: 3125–3130.

Zalipsky, S. (1995). Chemistry of polyethylene glycol conjugates with biologically active molecules. *Advanced Drug Delivery Reviews* 16: 157–182.

Zhang, L., Hou, S., Mao, S., Wei, D., Song, X., and Lu, Y. (2004). Uptake of folate-conjugated albumin nanoparticles to the SKOV3 cells. *International Journal of Pharmaceutics* 287: 155–162.

Zhang, M., Nan, H., Wang, Y., Jiang, X., and Li, Z. (2014). Comparison of flavonoid compounds in the flavedo and juice of two pummelo cultivars (*Citrus grandis* L. Osbeck) from different cultivation regions in China. *Molecules* 19: 17314–17328.

Zhang, W., and Zhong, Q. (2010). Microemulsions as nanoreactors to produce whey protein nanoparticles with enhanced heat stability by thermal pretreatment. *Food Chemistry* 119: 1318–1325.

Zhang, Z., Tan, S., and Feng, S.-S. (2012). Vitamin E TPGS as a molecular biomaterial for drug delivery. *Biomaterials* 33: 4889–4906.

Zhong, Q., and Jin, M. (2009). Zein nanoparticles produced by liquid–liquid dispersion. *Food Hydrocolloids* 23: 2380–2387.

Zhou, H., Sun, X., Zhang, L., Zhang, P., Li, J., and Liu, Y.-N. (2012). Fabrication of biopolymeric complex coacervation core micelles for efficient tea polyphenol delivery via a green process. *Langmuir* 28: 14553–14561.

Zimet, P., Rosenberg, D., and Livney, Y. D. (2011). Re-assembled casein micelles and casein nanoparticles as nano-vehicles for ω-3 polyunsaturated fatty acids. *Food Hydrocolloids* 25: 1270–1276.

Zou, T., and Gu, L. (2013). TPGS emulsified zein nanoparticles enhanced oral bioavailability of daidzin: *In vitro* characteristics and *in vivo* performance. *Molecular Pharmaceutics* 10: 2062–2070.

Zou, T., Li, Z., Percival, S. S., Bonard, S., and Gu, L. (2012a). Fabrication, characterization, and cytotoxicity evaluation of cranberry procyanidins–zein nanoparticles. *Food Hydrocolloids* 27: 293–300.

Zou, T., Percival, S. S., Cheng, Q., Li, Z., Rowe, C. A., and Gu, L. (2012b). Preparation, characterization, and induction of cell apoptosis of cocoa procyanidins–gelatin–chitosan nanoparticles. *European Journal of Pharmaceutics and Biopharmaceutics* 82: 36–42.

TOPIC 2

Stability of nutraceutical compounds encapsulated with modified polymers

CHAPTER 5

Novel polymer systems and additives to protect bioactive substances applied in spray-drying

Artur Bartkowiak, Wioletta Krawczyńska, and Alicja Federowicz
Center of Bioimmobilisation and Innovative Packaging Materials, Faculty of Food Sciences and Fisheries, West Pomeranian University of Technology, Szczecin, Poland, Ul. Klemensa Janickiego 35 71-270 Szczecin, Poland

5.1 Introduction

Research on and application of nutraceutical compounds, including fatty acids, polyphenols, probiotics, and prebiotics, have attracted significant attention in the functional foods, nutraceuticals, and pharmaceuticals industries due to their potential health benefits. The stability of bioactive substances is important and desirable to preserve healthy properties during the production process and storage. For this purpose, immobilization processes are used in which utilized substances create carriers. The most commonly used biopolymers, such as polysaccharides or proteins, have high biocompatibility, but scientists are still looking for a better solution and create novel polymers based on the existing ones.

Novel polymers can include hydrocolloids obtained from trees and bushes; extracts from plants or seaweeds, seeds, or grains; gummy slimes from fermentation processes; and modified hydrocolloids and complexes of different compounds.

The spray-drying process has found many applications in the food industry. This process is used to protect bioactive molecules (e.g., antioxidants, vitamins, fatty acids, phytosterols, flavors, colorants, oils) and living cells (e.g., probiotics) (Gharsallaoui, *et al.*, 2007; Dziezak, 1988). In general, bioactive compounds are characterized by their quick inactivation in adverse conditions. Thus, these components must be kept fully functional during processing. Carrier substances used in spray-drying may provide a barrier between bioactive molecules and the environment during processing, during storage under various

New Polymers for Encapsulation of Nutraceutical Compounds, First Edition.
Edited by Jorge Carlos Ruiz Ruiz and Maira Rubi Segura Campos.

conditions, and during passage through the gastrointestinal system (Desai and Park, 2005). Powder product is easier to transport than the liquid form because the weight and volume of powder are smaller than those of liquid (Cal and Sollohub, 2010).

Encapsulation may be defined as a process to entrap one substance (active agent) within another substance (carrier material) (Fang and Bhandari, 2010). This process is also defined as a "technology of packaging solids, liquids, or gaseous materials in small capsules that release their contents at controlled rates over prolonged periods and under specific conditions" (Desai and Park, 2005).

The substance that is immobilized may be called the core material, internal phase, active agent, fill, or payload phase. The substance that immobilizes the core material may be called the membrane, carrier or wall material, coating, shell, external phase, or matrix (Zuidam and Shimoni, 2010).

In this chapter, we focus on well-known polymers and novel polymers that can be used in the spray-drying processes most commonly applied in the food industry.

5.2 Spray-drying process

Spray-drying consists of four main stages, which include atomization, spray contact with drying medium, evaporation, and separation of product from airflow (Cal and Sollohub, 2010). Spray-drying is commonly achieved by dissolving, dispersing, or emulsifying the sensitive ingredients in an aqueous solution of coating material, followed by atomization and spraying of the mixture into a drying chamber. The droplet and drying medium (typically hot air) is contacted and the solvent is evaporated; then the dried particles are separated in a cyclone from the humid air and collected in powder form (Gharsallaoui *et al.*, 2007; Zuidam and Shimoni, 2010).

A liquid feed to be dried is pumped through an atomizer and sprayed into the chamber with hot gas flow (air or other gases) (Bajsic and Kranjcevic, 2001). During atomization, a film is formed at the droplet surface, and water is rapidly evaporated (Gharsallaoui i 2007). As a result, the raw material is transformed from a fluid state into a powder form. The product can be a single particle or agglomerates (Mujumdar, 2000).

Efficiency of encapsulation of bioactive substances by spray-drying is affected by a number of factors, including outlet and inlet air temperatures, type of wall material, and drying time (Table 5.1). Spray-drying has often been described as a harsh drying method because high temperatures are used. Under high temperatures, thermolabile ingredients can be damaged or inactivated (Yoshii *et al.*, 2008). Therefore, a very important step of microencapsulation of active ingredients by spray-drying is the choice of a carrier material.

Table 5.1 Factors affecting encapsulation by spray-drying.

Type of factors	Type of Bioactive Substances						References
	Probiotics	Food Flavors	Food Oils	Polyphenols	Vitamins	Enzymes	
Biopolymer							
Type	+	+	+	+	+	+	Dumoulin and Bimbenet (1988)
Emulsifying capability		+	+	n/a	n/a	n/a	Jafari *et al.* (2008)
Film-forming ability	+	+	+	+	+	+	Matsuno and Adachi (1992)
Infeed solids content	+	+	+	+	+	+	Sanguansri and Augustin (2010)
							Soottitantawat *et al.* (2005)
Core Material							
Molecular weight	–	+	+	+	+	+	Ananta *et al.* (2005)
Relative volatility	–	+	+	–	–	–	Desmond *et al.* (2001)
Polarity	n/a	+	+	n/a	n/a	n/a	Jafari *et al.* (2008)
Concentration	+	+	+	+	+	+	
Type of species and strain	+	–	–	–	–	–	
Growth phase	+	–	–	–	–	–	
Final Emulsification							
Droplet size	+	+	+	+	+	+	Castellar *et al.* (2003)
Viscosity	+	+	+	+	+	+	Dumoulin and Bimbenet (1988)
Stability	+	+	+	+	+	+	Jafari *et al.* (2008)
Method	+	+	+	+	+	+	Tonon *et al.* (2008)
pH	+	n/a	n/a	+	+	n/a	Sanguansri and Augustin (2010)
							Zbicinski *et al.* (2002)

(*Continued*)

Table 5.1 (Continued)

Type of factors	Type of Bioactive Substances						References
	Probiotics	Food Flavors	Food Oils	Polyphenols	Vitamins	Enzymes	
Spray-Drying Process							
Infeed temperature	+	+	+	+	+	+	Ananta *et al.* (2005)
Inlet and outlet air temperatures	+	+	+	+	+	+	Castellar *et al.* (2003)
							Dumoulin and Bimbenet (1988)
Feed flow rate	+	+	+	+	+	+	Ersus and Yurdagel (2007)
Humidity	+	+	+	+	+	+	Jafari *et al.* (2008)
Construction of spray-dryer	+	+	+	+	+	+	Jafari *et al.* (2013)
Stress adaptation	+	–	–	–	–	–	Tonon *et al.* (2008)
Nozzle pressure	+	+	+	+	+	+	Sun-Waterhouse *et al.* (2011)
Drying time	+	+	+	+	+	+	
Other Factors							
Water activity	+	+	+	+	+	+	Adamiec (2009)
Oxygen	+	+	+	+	n/a	n/a	Castellar *et al.* (2003)
Light	+	+	n/a	+	+	n/a	Desmond *et al.* (2001)
							Ersus and Yurdagel (2007)
							Hayashi (1989)
							Krishnan *et al.* (2005)
							Ruiz-Gutiérrez *et al.* (2014)
							Sanguansri and Augustin (2010)
							Wenrong and Griffiths (2000)

+, affects encapsulation efficiency; –, does not affect encapsulation efficiency; n/a, not applicable.

Primarily, wall material should provide protection for the core material. This choice should be mainly based on the physicochemical properties of a carrier material, such as solubility, molecular weight, good film-forming properties, glass and melting transitions, diffusibility, crystallinity, and emulsifying properties. This material should be also cheap, food grade, bland in taste, and biodegradable (Augustin and Hemar, 2009; Gharsallaoui *et al.*, 2007).

Many substances may be used to encapsulate bioactive materials. Materials most widely used for encapsulation for food applications are biomolecules. Encapsulation of food ingredients is usually accomplished with proteins, lipids, and polymers (Jafari *et al.*, 2013). Biopolymers commonly used are starch, cellulose, gum arabic, gum tragacanth, gum karaya, mesquite gum, locust bean gum, guar gum, tara gum, pectins, soluble soybean polysaccharide, carrageenans, alginian, xanthan, gellan, dextran, and chitosan (Wandrey *et al.*, 2010; Chen and Chen, 2007).

5.2.1 Preparation of feed solution

The first stage of spray-drying is the preparation of feed solution for dispersion, which contains bioactive substance and wall-forming material. The selection of wall material is one of the key steps in encapsulation by spray-drying (Bajsic and Kranjcevic, 2001). After wall material is selected, a carrier material must be dissolved or rehydrated (sometimes with heating) in water (Fang and Bhandari, 2012). The method of preparing feed solution depends on the nature of the active agent and coating materials. If a core material is water soluble, then it can be dissolved in the solution with a carrier material. If a core material is oil soluble or oil based, then an oil-in-water solution should be prepared. Particulates can be added into a solution containing wall material to form suspensions (Fang and Bhandari, 2012). However, if a core material is insoluble in water (e.g., oils), the feed solution should be emulsified before the spray-drying process begins (Bajsic and Kranjcevic, 2001).

The majority of flavors are in a liquid or gas state, but some materials in a solid state have a bad smell. Encapsulation of flavors is very desirable in the food industry. Emulsions with flavors are prepared before the spray-drying process (Zuidam and Shimoni, 2010). A major problem during encapsulation of flavors by spray-drying is that the majority of flavor compounds are volatile when in contact with water (Jafari, 2008). Interestingly, if the water evaporates from the drying droplets, volatile flavors undergo retention. This is known as the *selective diffusion* theory (Rulkens and Thijssen, 1972).

The retention of volatiles depends on their molecular size. If molecular size of the volatiles increases, then retention of the volatiles also increases (Bhandari and Howes, 1999). The feed solid concentration influences good flavor retention. If the feed solution is saturated, the level of volatile retention is high, because the time to form semi-permeable membrane around the flavor is shorter. However, if the solid concentration in feed is too high, viscosity of the feed increases and, as a result, atomization efficiency can decrease, film forming at the droplet surface slows down, and the flavors are lost. Generally, 20% to 25% of flavor concentration in total solids of the solution is used in microencapsulation of flavors by spray-drying (Ré and Liu, 1996). The retention rate of flavors during spray-drying also depends on the nature of flavor compounds (Jafari *et al.*, 2013). If the emulsion is stable, the retention level is high (Soottitantawat *et al.*, 2007). The retention level of hydrophilic flavors is high if before the spray-drying the flavors are entrapped within the inner water droplets of a water-in-oil-in-water double emulsion (Bruckner *et al.*, 2007).

5.2.2 Carriers

The main role of carriers is to reduce deactivation of bioactive compounds in the produced powders or reduce the stickiness (Chiou and Langrish, 2001). The main reason to use carriers is their ability to provide protection for the active compounds. Material coating bioactive substances causes reduction of the heat and oxidative stress during the spray-drying process (Yoshii *et al.*, 2008). Carriers can encapsulate bioactive compounds through their formation composition, morphology, or the specific material that is used in their formulation. After spray-drying, this wall material is a barrier against environmental factors that maintains the active substance until its desired release under specified conditions (Soottitantawat *et al.*, 2007). Generally, a mixture about 10% to 20% (w/w) carrier material concentration is used (Gharsallaoui *et al.*, 2007). If concentration of a carrier material is too high, particles size is larger and drying time takes longer. It leads to higher thermal inactivation of an active compound and less bacterial survival during the spray-drying process (Santivarangkna *et al.*, 2007).

There are two main reasons carriers can have an influence on the reduction of stickiness of the product. Firstly, carriers typically increase the glass-transition temperature of the mixture. Secondly, the sticky substance is encapsulated inside the nonsticky or less-sticky matrix of material (Chiou and Langrish, 2001). The molecular weight of the materials affects the increase of the glass-transition temperature. Compounds and molecules of greater molecular weight can absorb more energy before undergoing molecular change and interactions. For that reason, heavy-molecular-weight materials have a higher glass-transition temperature, and therefore a lot of compounds have the potential to be carriers that can reduce stickiness in products (Bhandari and Howes, 1999).

5.2.3 Atomization

Atomizers can generate microdroplets from liquids. Atomization leads to the formation of a very large surface area of liquid feed that is exposed in the drying chamber to the drying gas (Masters, 2002). Various devices achieve atomization: rotary wheel atomizers, pneumatic nozzles, and hydraulic (pressure) and ultrasonic nozzles (Figure 5.1) (Cal and Sollohub, 2010). The atomizers used for

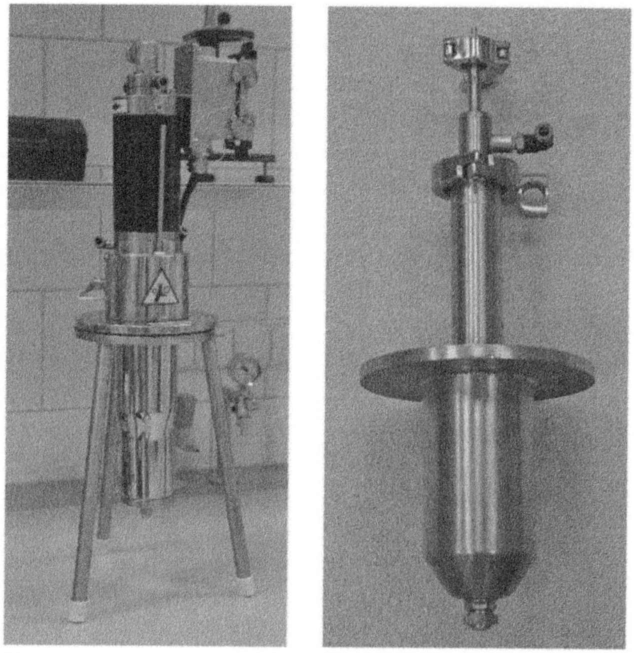

(a) (b)

Figure 5.1 Atomizers used in the spray-drying process. **a,** Rotary atomizer; **b,** two-fluid nozzle. (CC BY 3.0 by CBIMO).

spray-drying characterize the uniformity and homogeneity of the spray, which in turn have a significant effect on the particle size distribution of the final product (Masters, 2002).

Liquid feed is transported to the atomization device by different types of pumps (peristaltic pumps are the most commonly used). The feed flow rates are typically measured in milliliters per minute for small-scale dryers such as laboratory scale, whereas rates for industrial-sized dryers are typically measured liters per hour (Cal and Sollohub, 2010). The flow feed rate parameter is adjustable to ensure that each sprayed droplet reaches the desired drying level before it comes in contact with the drying hot medium (Zbicinski *et al.*, 2002). Large particle size of solid fill material or too-high viscosity can block the atomizers. The size of the atomized droplets depends on the viscosity and the surface tension of the liquid feed, pressure through the nozzle, and the velocity of the spray (Fang and Bhandari, 2012).

5.2.4 Drying medium, evaporation of solvent, and separation of product

The contact of the liquid with hot drying medium takes place during atomization in the drying chamber (Fang and Bhandari, 2012). Drying medium is used to evaporate the moisture from the feed solution and then carry the particles through the dryer into the receptacle system. Temperature of the drying medium is known as the drying temperature because this is the factor that encourages evaporation and results in the final dry product. Temperature of the drying medium can range from below room temperature to a temperature to which the heating system can heat up (Chiou and Langrish, 2001).

As a drying medium, air, nitrogen, or carbon dioxide can be used. The speed and volume of gas flow rate can also be controlled and changed. Spray dryers can work both in co-current and countercurrent gas flow paths, depending on the setup required of the system (Chiou and Langrish, 2001). In a co-current system, the droplets are sprayed in the same direction as the flow of hot drying medium through equipment. In a countercurrent system, the liquid is sprayed in the direction opposite to the flow of hot air. A countercurrent system is more often used than a co-current system for spray-drying of food ingredients and nutraceuticals (Fang and Bhandari, 2012) (Figure 5.2).

Achieving a large surface liquid area during atomization facilitates heat transfer from the heated drying gas to the atomized fluid particles. Thereby the solvent is evaporated in a few seconds and the mass is transferred back into the gas phase. For this reason, the drying material does not reach the inlet temperature of drying gas (Vehring, 2008). High heat, being transferred into the droplets, has contact with the wall material, and therefore the active compounds are exposed to a lesser degree to the hot drying medium (Jafari *et al.*, 2008). Most of the water is evaporated from the droplet surface, and as a result droplets are transformed into

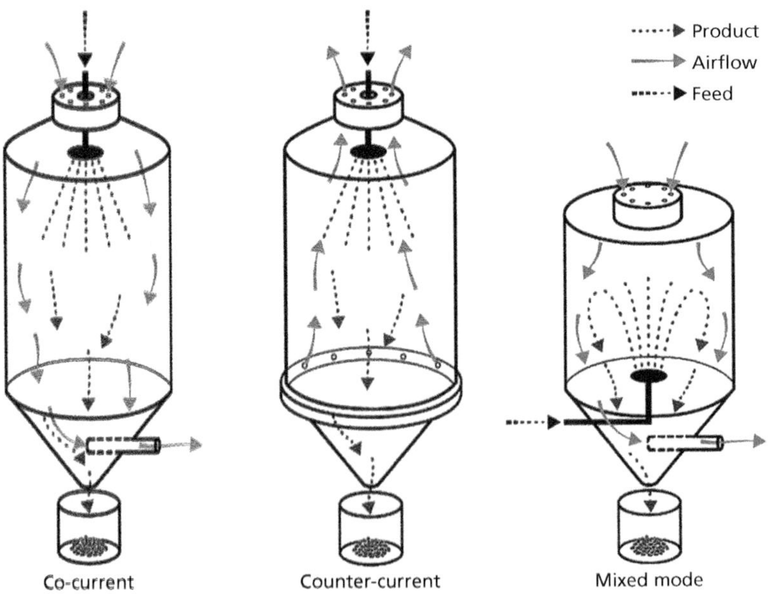

Figure 5.2 Spray contact with drying air: co-current, counter-current, and mixed mode. Reproduced with permission from Büchi Labortechnik AG, Switzerland.

dry powder. In these microcapsule particles, the core material is entrapped in a solid membrane of wall material (Gharsallaoui *et al.*, 2007). The drying medium carries the dried particles through the dryer into the cyclone, in which a powder is separated from the humid air. Spray dryers are commonly equipped with bag filters, which are used to remove the finest powder (Gharsallaoui *et al.*, 2007).

5.2.5 Properties of the product

Spray-drying involves many interactions that influence the quality of the final product. The physicochemical properties of this product mainly depend on inlet and outlet temperature, feed flow rate, viscosity, particle size, type of atomizer, and pressure (Tonon *et al.*, 2008). Diameters of product can range from 10 to 50 μm (very fine powder) to 2 to 3 mm (large particles). This size depends on the starting feed material and operating conditions (Gharsallaoui *et al.*, 2007). Concentration of the solid particles in the feed solution and the temperature affect viscosity and fluidity of the feed solution and its capacity to be homogenously sprayed. If the feed temperature is increased, then the droplet size is decreased. It influences degradation of the thermolabile compounds (Gharsallaoui *et al.*, 2007).

The difference between air inlet and air outlet temperature influences the microcapsule drying rate and the final water content of powders (Zbicinski *et al.*, 2002). If the air inlet temperature is too low, then the water evaporates slowly, leading to the formation of microcapsules with high-density membranes, poor fluidity, high water content, and easily forming agglomerates. However, air inlet temperature that is too high causes excessive evaporation, cracks of membrane, and, as a result, premature release and degradation or loss of encapsulated active agents.

The air inlet temperature can be set, whereas the air outlet temperature cannot (Gharsallaoui *et al.*, 2007). After setting the air inlet temperature, the air outlet temperature is controlled by the feed flow rate. During microencapsulation of bioactive compounds by spray-drying, the ideal air outlet temperature depends on the heat sensitivity of active agents and wall materials and on the property of the final product. The best conditions of spray-drying bioactive components is a combination of different factors (Bimbenet *et al.*, 2002).

5.3 Nutraceuticals in the food industry

Spray-drying can be applied to encapsulate different materials (e.g., food flavors, probiotics, polyphenols, lipids, vitamins, enzymes). Spray-drying is commonly used in the encapsulation of lipids. Numerous bioactive substances fall into the category of lipids. Lipids used in microencapsulation by spray-drying include fatty acids, phospholipids, acyloglycerols, phytosterols, and carotenoids

(McClements *et al.*, 2009). Lipid comprises a group of chemically diverse compounds that are insoluble (or soluble to only a small degree) in water but soluble in organic solvents. Moreover, lipids can be used themselves as solvents. They can be solvents of hydrophobic substances such as polyphenols, volatile aromatic compounds, and carotenoids. Lipids can also be used as a carrier for lipophilic compounds (Fang and Bhandari, 2012).

Microencapsulation of lipids by spray-drying can improve their stability, retard their auto- oxidation, help to control lipid-soluble flavor release, protect dissolved compounds against enzyme hydrolysis, and mask taste and smell of substances dissolved in lipids. The degree to which lipids are protective depends on different factors, including the nature of the wall materials, the lipids, and conditions of the encapsulation process (Table 5.1). Commonly used materials in microencapsulation of lipids by spray-drying are maltodextrins, modified starches, whey protein concentrate, gum arabic, and sodium caseinate (Jafari *et al.*, 2008; Matsuno and Adachi, 1992). During spray-drying of lipids, the surrounding membrane can crack, causing the droplets of lipids that are on the surface of particles to be released. Released lipids are more susceptible to oxidation because they are not already protected by microcapsules (Fang and Bhandari, 2012).

Microencapsulation by spray-drying is a valuable technique to encapsulate probiotic bacteria. For successful delivery in foods, probiotics must survive food processing and storage conditions during product maturation and shelf life and during passage through the gastrointestinal tract. The consumption of probiotics provides many benefits in the human body such as prevention and treatment of infectious diarrhea, alleviation of lactose intolerance, modulation of the immune response leading to prevention of the onset of allergic diseases, alleviation of constipation, reduction of serum cholesterol levels, and anticarcinogenic activity (Andersson *et al.*, 2001; Shanahan, 2000).

Powders that are obtained by spray-drying and that contain high levels of viable probiotic bacteria provide a convenient form of these cultures for storage purposes and applications in functional food products. However, the main problem during spray-drying of microorganisms is a loss of viable cells (Silva *et al.*, 2002). To produce the health benefits, probiotics must be alive and active in both the product and the host (Manojlović *et al.*, 2010). According to international standards (e.g., International Dairy Federation) the product may be referred to as a "probiotic product" if it contains a minimum of 10^7 viable probiotic bacteria per gram of product or 10^9 cells per serving size when sold, in order to provide 10^6 to 10^8 cells per gram of feces after consumption (Kailasapathy and Chin, 2000). In the food industry, probiotic products are mainly in the form of milk, cheese, drinking and frozen yogurt, ice cream, fermented soya products, and dairy spreads (Manojlović *et al.*, 2010).

The survival rate of probiotic bacteria during drying depends on numerous factors, including type of species, growth phase of the probiotics, type of carrier material and their concentration, protective agents, stress adaptation, nozzle pressure, inlet and outlet air temperature, and drying time (Table 5.1). The survival rate of probiotic bacteria is affected by temperature and time. Typically, if the drying temperature is lower and the drying time is shorter, then the survival rate of probiotics is better (Ananta *et al.*, 2005).

Polyphenols are another bioactive compound that can be spray-dried. These compounds have many health-benefit properties, including antioxidant, antiinflammatory, antibacterial, antiviral, and anticancer functions (Liang *et al.*, 2015). Polyphenols are sensitive to adverse environmental conditions including pH, light exposure, temperature, water activity, enzymes, and oxygen (Table 5.1). Spray-drying technology for microencapsulation of polyphenols is used to maintain their stability and antioxidant activity, as well as to mask their unpleasant taste (Fang and Bhandari, 2010; Sun-Waterhouse *et al.*, 2013). For microencapsulation of polyphenols by spray-drying, the most commonly used materials are modified starches, maltodextrin, chitosan, gum arabic, and sodium caseinate (Fang and Bhandari, 2010; Liang *et al.*, 2015).

Spray-drying technology is used also to produce solid enzyme preparations. Enzyme activity after this process is affected by the initial liquid to be evaporated, the process parameters (e.g., relatively low inlet and outlet air temperatures, suitable total solids content, small atomized droplets, and low shear during atomization), and the physicochemical character of the enzyme (Dumoulin and Bimbenet, 1988) (Table 5.1).

Spray-drying is also an attractive process for protecting vitamins. Vitamins are completely or partially denatured or damaged during the processing of foods. The spray-drying process can provide protection against light, pH, moisture, and temperature and also against their reaction with other ingredients (Sanguansri and Augustin, 2010) (Table 5.1).

5.4 Polymers and novel polymers used in the spray-drying process

Polymers play a very important role in everyday life. They are present everywhere: at home, at work, and in nature. Polymers are divided into natural, which are most the ones most commonly used in the food industry and paper industry, and synthetic, which have found application in the plastics industry.

The natural polymers (hydrocolloids) used in the spray-drying process can be extracted from plants and animals and can be obtained by biotechnological processes, such as xanthan or curdlan gum (Embuscado, 2011). Sometimes natural polymers are subjected to modifications (physicochemical and biochemical properties) that allow researchers to obtain novel polymers with improved properties enabling their use in the encapsulation process (Embuscado, 2011). These

Table 5.2 The most popular natural polymers used in spray-drying processes and their source.

Polymers	Source		
	Plant	Marine	Microbes, Animals
Carbohydrate	Starch and derivatives Cellulose and derivatives Gum arabic Pectin Chitosan	Alginate	Xanthan gum
Protein			Gelatin Casein Whey proteins
Lipid	Fatty acids and alcohols Glycerides		Fatty acids and alcohols Glycerides

procedures allow the best protection of nutraceutical compounds in food and beverage processing and production. The obtained material should be cheap, food grade, bland in taste, and biodegradable (Augustin and Hemar, 2009; Gharsallaoui *et al.*, 2007).

Many substances may be used to encapsulate bioactive materials. The encapsulation of food ingredients is usually accomplished with proteins, lipids, and polymers (Jafari *et al.*, 2013) (Table 5.2). Biopolymers commonly used include starch, cellulose, gum arabic, gum tragacanth, gum karaya, mesquite gum, locust bean gum, guar gum, tara gum, pectins, soluble soybean polysaccharide, carrageenan, alginian, xanthan, gellan, dextran, and chitosan (Chen and Chen, 2007; Wandrey *et al.*, 2010). However, regulations for food additives require that these substances be certified for food applications as "generally recognized as safe" (GRAS) materials. Actually, the whole food process should be designed to meet the safety requirements of government agencies such as the European Food Safety Authority (EFSA) or the U.S. Food and Drug Administration (FDA) (Wandrey *et al.*, 2010).

5.4.1 Well-known polymers

There are a number of carriers used in spray-drying of bioactive compounds. Commonly used wall materials for spray-drying include proteins (e.g., milk proteins, caseinates, skim milk powders), carbohydrates (e.g., starch, maltodextrins, cyclodextrins, and gums such as agar, acacia, xanthan, alginates), biopolymers (e.g., soluble soy polysaccharides, chitosan, modified celluloses). In the next subsection we focus on the most commonly used polymers, which are still used to create stable emulsions and shell-protected sensitive nutraceuticals during spray-drying.

5.4.1.1 Maltodextrins

Maltodextrin is a starch preparation obtained by enzymatic depolymerization of an aqueous suspension of potato starch that is then subjected to spray-drying. Maltodextrins are characterized by low sweetness and are readily digestible, highly soluble, and highly hygroscopic. With a wide range of starch depolymerization (DE) < 20, maltodextrins have a heterogeneous composition of the mixture of sugars; exhibit the properties of emulsifiers, fillers, stabilizers, gluing or raising agents; and they prolong freshness, reduce sweetness, enhance taste and smell, and delay the process of crystallization. Maltodextrins with DE <10 can be used as fat replacers in products such as ice cream; maltodextrin with DE >10 can be used as wall material. Maltodextrins, due to their composition and properties, have been widely used in various branches of the food industry:

- They are a universal carrier in the drying process of juices, colors, and flavors.
- Having a large surface area, they can serve as a carrier for flavors, colors, and fats.
- They can be used in the production of nutritional health drinks to deliver increased amounts of dry extract, decrease sweetness, and enhance the action of aromatic substances.
- They can be used in the production of medicinal preparations – tablets, syrups, expectorants, vitamin preparations – and mineral supplements.

Numerous studies have shown that maltodextrins as wall materials protect and stabilize nutritional compounds. The obtained powders are characterized by high stability during storage in different conditions, they do not agglomerate, and they do not lose color. Ersus and Yurdegel (2007) conducted a study in which they spray-dried anthocyanin extract from black carrot. The results showed that the use of maltodextrin with DE 20 to 21 as a wall material gave the highest anthocyanin content in powder. They also observed that the shelf life of spray-dried pigments stored at 4 °C increased three-fold in comparison with storage at 25 °C.

The positive effects of microencapsulation of pigments can also be observed in the case of colorant form *Opuntia stricta* fruits (Obon *et al.*, 2009), prickly-pear juice (Diaz *et al.*, 2006), betacyanin extract from red beetroot and *Amaranthus* (Azeredo *et al.*, 2007; Cai and Coke, 2000), bayberry fruit extracts (Fang and Bhandari, 2011), or *Garcinia cowa* fruit extract (Ezhilarasi *et al.*, 2014).

5.4.1.2 Gum arabic

Gum arabic is a mixture of polysaccharides obtained from the *Acacia senegal* tree. Primarily it is used as a thickener, stabilizer, and emulsifier. It also serves as a carrier and a substance for surface application. It facilitates the stabilization of food emulsions containing essential oils, oleoresin, vitamins, or lipid derivatives. It delays or prevents crystallization of sugar in confectionery, ice cream, and sorbet. A 30% solution of gum arabic is less viscous than a 1% solution of xanthan gum. The most interesting properties of gum arabic are its ability to create a good emulsion for spray-drying and its ability to act as an emulsifier (Vega and Roos, 2006). Gum arabic and other gums are used to encapsulate extracts, essential oils, antioxidants, colors, vitamins, and fatty acids.

Watanabe and colleagues (2004) showed that the use of gum arabic in encapsulation of arachidonic acid with ascorbic acid gave good oxidative resistance during storage. Another advantage of gum arabic is bixin encapsulation. Studies have shown that the dye is four times more stable than maltodextrin (Barbosa *et al.*, 2004). For encapsulation of cardamom oleoresin, gum arabic offered better encapsulation results than modified starch (Shaikh *et al.*, 2006). Brazilian scientists performed research on the suppression of lipid oxidation and resulting formation of unpleasant odor and taste for roasted coffee oil. Gum arabic inhibited lipid oxidation during spray-drying and did not show any increase in the peroxide value during storage of the product at 25 °C. The oxidation process was much lower, even at a temperature of 60 °C, as compared to nonencapsulated roasted coffee oil (Frascareli *et al.*, 2012).

5.4.1.3 Skim milk powder and whey proteins

Proteins can be good coating materials for microencapsulation by spray-drying. Two useful properties are high binding of flavor compounds (Gharsallaoui *et al.*, 2007) and the ability to form thermally irreversible gel above 70 °C (Wandrey *et al.*, 2010). The most commonly used proteins for encapsulating food ingredients by spray-drying are whey proteins and skim milk powder. Skim milk powder is obtained by removing water from pasteurized skim milk. It contains 5% or less moisture and 1.5% or less milk fat and a minimum milk protein content of 34%. Whey protein is a mixture of globular proteins isolated from whey. It is a byproduct of cheese production. It is commonly used during spray-drying as a carrier for probiotic bacteria *(Lactobacilli, Bifidobacteria)* and for protection against high temperatures (Corcoran *et al.*, 2004; Lian *et al.*, 2002). Proteins are also used in encapsulation of oregano essential oil and of aroma extracts of citronella and sweet marjoram. The efficiency of the encapsulation process for oregano oil, citronella aroma extract, and marjoram aroma extract with skim milk as coating material is, respectively, 80.2%, 69.4%, and 67.9%. When comparing these results with results for whey proteins (71.8%, 65.8%, and 54.3%), it is clear that skim milk leads to better properties of the product in terms of encapsulation efficiency and total oil content (Baranauskiene *et al.*, 2006).

5.4.1.4 Modified starch

The most common and best-known hydrocolloids are starches, the major carbohydrate constituents of corn, rice, wheat, potatoes, tapioca, and other agricultural crops. Starch is a relatively cheap and abundant hydrocolloid. For this reason, a number of ingredients used to protect flavors are derived from starch.

Native starches do not have emulsifying properties. In addition, the starch molecule is too large to form an enclosure around the very small oil particles in an emulsion, and after cooking it is too viscous for homogenization and spray-drying (Chavarri *et al.*, 2012). This is the reason starch molecules are modified. One popular reaction employed to prepare emulsifying starches is succinylation or esterification of starch using *n*-octenyl succinic anhydride (OSAn) (Embuscado, 2011). Studies show that when using OSAn starches as encapsulating agents for spray-drying, the levels of oil retention reached 94.75% (Murua-Pagola *et al.*, 2009).

Modified starch (OSAn) is used for encapsulating chlorophyll. In one study, the authors used 30% OSAn as a wall material. The obtained powder had the highest greenness value, total chlorophyll content, and antioxidant activity, as well as longer shelf life, compared with other powders (obtained with maltodextrin and gum arabic). The half-life for this powder was 462 days (Porrarud and Pranee, 2010). Rocha and colleagues (2012) used modified starch (Capsul) for encapsulating lycopene as a coloring agent. The results showed that encapsulation efficiency values varied between 21% and 29%, and lycopene was protected to a greater extent than in its free form. They also observed that the microcapsules were able to release pigment (Rocha *et al.*, 2012).

5.4.2 Novel polymers and mixtures of polymers

One limitation of the spray-drying process is the finite number of shell materials available. Scientists are therefore constantly searching for novel polymers, novel mixtures of well-known polymers, and novel applications that can be used to stabilize and protect nutraceuticals in storage conditions (Desai and Park, 2005). This subsection is devoted to polymers that are completely new or polymers that have been discovered for the spray-drying process.

5.4.2.1 Natural fibers: Inulin and β-glucan

Inulin is a fructo-oligosaccharide and is composed of fructose units with β(2–1) links with glucose units at the end of the chains. It belongs to the class of fructans and is prebiotic. Inulin is soluble in hot water. In plants, inulin is stored primarily in tubers, rhizomes, and the lower parts of the stems and in smaller amounts in the leaves. In vegetable raw materials, the average content of inulin (Kowalski and Wierciński, 2004) is

- *Silphium trifoliatum* roots: 38%
- Dandelion roots: 34%
- Chicory roots: 44%
- Roots of Oman: 34%
- Artichoke rhizomes: 52%

Usefulness of inulin for spray-drying applications is continuously confirmed. Inulin was used to encapsulate polyphenols such as quercetin and vanillin

(Sun-Waterhouse *et al.*, 2013). Studies have shown that inulin improved the efficiency of encapsulation and reduces water activity of the powder, thus preventing its stickiness. The final powder was characterized by high content of vanillin and quercetin, which were less susceptible to thermal degradation during spray-drying (Sun-Waterhouse *et al.*, 2013). Another example is the use of inulin to stabilize betalains and carotenoids in the form of dry pigments. Studies confirmed that inulin could also be used successfully as a carrier for dyes. Obtained powders showed high stability during storage under optimal conditions and at 60 °C, with only small differences between the freshly obtained and stored (44 days) product (Saenz *et al.*, 2009). Similar results were reported for blackcurrant polyphenols spray-dried with inulin. Antioxidant activity did not change after 12 months of storage at 25 °C and 8 °C (Bakowska-Barczak and Kołodziejczak, 2011). Inulin is also used for microencapsulation of bifidobacteria. According to the research of Corcoran and colleagues (2004), inulin should increase the survival rate of bacteria during spray-drying. Capsules produced with oligofructose-enriched inulin showed better protection for the bifidobacteria during storage (Fritzen-Freire *et al.*, 2012).

Another important natural fiber is β-glucan. This soluble fiber [(1–3) (1–4) β-D-glucan] is important for effects on blood glucose, reduction of serum cholesterol levels (Lazaridou and Biliaderis, 2009), and antimutagenic risk reduction of chronic diseases (Mantovani *et al.*, 2008). The use of soluble fibers for spray-drying of bioactive substances is an alternative method of exploiting the potential of fibers and increasing the value of food products. Ruiz-Gutierrez and colleagues (2014) used red pear cactus juice in their study. Results showed that a powder with higher bioactive compound content and good physical properties was obtained at 160 °C with addition of 22.5% of soluble fiber to red pear cactus juice. These conditions can be used to obtain powder for application as ingredients or colorants to develop food products high in antioxidant content (Ruiz-Gutierrez *et al.*, 2014). Chiou and Langrish (2007) for their study used milled citrus fiber and hibiscus extract, and they created a novel nutraceutical product suitable for a variety of applications in functional food manufacturing. The powder maintains a free-flowing form under appropriately controlled humidity conditions suitable for manufacturing purposes. The presence of the bioactive material in the fibers does not appear to significantly affect the product's size or shape (Chiou and Langrish, 2007).

5.4.2.2 Pectin and its mixtures

Pectin is a mixture of carbohydrates that occurs in the cell walls of many plants. Pectin is generally formed of polysaccharides and oligosaccharides of varying composition. There are two fractions of pectin, depending on the degree of esterification: high-methoxy (HM) pectin, with more than 50% of the carboxyl groups of the galacturonic acid residues esterified, and low-methoxy (LM) pectin, with the degree of esterification less than 50% (BeMiller 1986).

Pectin functionality depends on the form of the gel and the mechanism of gel formation, which result in many different applications. Pectin can be used in the spray-drying process because it produces stable emulsions at low concentrations. Another advantage of pectin is low cost, so it can be used as a substitute for expensive wall materials, such as proteins and gum arabic (Drusch, 2007). Sugar beet pectin produces a stable emulsion for spray-drying. A 2% concentration of the pectin solution, corresponding to a 15% concentration of gum arabic, decreased the oxidation of fish oil during drying (Leroux *et al.*, 2003). Pectin can be applied to spray-drying of oil, but it is very important to preserve the desired quantity of oil. Citrus and pumpkin pectin may be applied to spray-dried polyphenols (de Souza *et al.*, 2010).

Another option to increase the use of polymers in a new application is the formation of a mixture that contains pectin. Sansone and colleagues (2011) mixed two carbohydrates, apple pectin and maltodextrin, thus obtaining a multipurpose composition of carrier for the spray-drying process. This composition was applied for spray-drying of extracts from *Fadogia ancylantha, Melissa officinalis,* and *Tussilago farfara,* which are commonly used in the food and cosmetics industries. They obtained a nonsticky powder that was stable for 6 months under storage conditions and had improved solubility and no unpleasant smell. This solution may be suitable for successful production of functional components for foods or nutraceuticals (Sansone *et al.*, 2011). Another proposition is a modified method of encapsulation of iron molecules in composition based on low-methoxyl pectin and modified starch (Moslemi *et al.*, 2014). The product obtained in this way was characterized by encapsulation efficiency of 72.07%, low organoleptic changes, and better bioavailability. This method can be applied especially in dairy-based products for food fortification (Moslemi *et al.*, 2014).

Acknowledgements

We would like to thank Agnieszka Bednarczyk-Drąg for English-language editing of our chapter.

References

Adamiec, J. (2009). Drying of microorganisms for food applications. In: *Advances in Food Dehydration*, pp. 315–353. C. Ratti, ed. Boca Raton, FL: CRC.

Ananta, E., Volkert, M., and Knorr, D. (2005). Cellular injuries and storage stability of spray-dried *Lactobacillus rhamnosus* GG. *International Dairy Journal* 15: 399–409.

Andersson, H., Asp, N. G., Bruce, A., Roos, S., Wadstrom, T., and Wold, A. E. (2001). Health effects of probiotics and prebiotics: A literature review on human studies. *Scandanavian Journal of Nutrition* 45: 58–75.

Augustin, M. A., and Hemar, Y. (2009). Nano- and micro-structured assemblies for encapsulation of food ingredients. *Chemical Society Reviews* 38(4): 902–912.

Azeredo, H. M. C., Santos, A. N., Souza, A. C. R., Mendes, K. C. B, and Andrade, M. I. R. (2007). Batacyanin stability during processing and storage of a microencapsulated red beetroot extract. *American Journal of Food Technology* 2(4): 307–312.

Bajsic, I., and Kranjcevic, E. (2001). Automation of industrial spray dryer. *Instrumentation Science and Technology* 29: 201–213.

Bakowska-Baczak, A., and Kolodziejczyk, P. P. (2011). Black currant polyphenols: Their storage stability and microencapsulation. *Industrial Crops and Products* 34: 1301–1309.

Barbosa, M. I. M. J., Borsarelli, C. D., and Mercadante, A. Z. (2005). Light stability of spray-dried bixin encapsulated with different edible polysaccharide preparations. *Food Research International* 38: 989–994.

Baranauskiene, R., Venskutonis, P. R., Dewettinck, K., and Verhé, R. (2006). Properties of oregano (*Origanum vulgare* L.), citronella (*Cymbopogon nardus* G.) and marjoram (*Majorana hortensis* L.) flavors encapsulated into milk protein–based matrices. *Food Research International* 39: 413–425.

BeMiller, J. N. (1986). An Introduction to pectins – structure and properties. *ACS Symposium Series* 310: 2–12.

Bimbenet, J. J., Schuck, P., Roignant, M., Brulé, G., and Mejean, S. (2002). Heat balance of a multistage spray-dryer: Principles and example of application. *Le Lait* 82: 541–551.

Bhandari, B. R., and Howes T. (1999). Implication of glass transition for the drying and stability of dried foods. *Journal of Food Technology* 40: 71–79.

Bruckner, M., Bade, M., and Kunz, B. (2007). Investigations into the stabilization of a volatile aroma compound using a combined emulsification and spray drying process. *European Food Research and Technology* 226: 137–146.

Cal, K., and Sollohub, K. (2010). Spray drying technique. I: Hardware and process parameters. *Journal of Pharmaceutical Science* 99(2): 575–86.

Castellar, R., Obon, J., Alacid, M., and Fernández-López, J. (2003). Colour properties and stability of betacyanins from *Opuntia* fruits. *Journal of Agricultural and Food Chemistry* 51 L 2772–2776.

Cai, Y. Z., and Corke, H. (2000). Production and properties of spray dried *Amaranthus* betacyanin pigments. *Journal of Food Science* 65(7): 1248 –1252.

Chavarri, M., Maranon, I., and Villaran, M. C., (2012). Encapsulation Technology to Protect Probiotic Bacteria. In: *Probiotics*, pp. 501–540. E. C. Rigobelo, ed. Croatia: Intech.

Chen, M-J., and Chen, K.-N. 2007.Applications of Probiotic Encapsulation in Dairy Products. In: *Encapsulation and Controlled Release Technologies in Food Systems*, pp. 83–112. J. M. Lakkis, ed. Hoboken: Wiley.

Chiou, D., and Langrish, T. A. G. (2001). Application of Spray Drying Technology for Nutraceutical and Functional Food Product. In: *Handbook of Nutraceuticals Volume II: Scale- Up, Processing and Automation*, pp. 183–212. Y. Y. Pathak, ed. Boca Raton: CRC.

Concoran, B. M., Ross, R. P., Fitzgerald, G. F., and Stanton, C. (2004). Comparative survival of probiotics lactobacilli spray-dried in the presence of probiotic substances. *Journal of Applied Microbiology* 96: 1024–1039.

Desai, K. G. H., and Park, H. J. (2005). Recent developments in microencapsulation of food ingredients. *Drying Technology* 23: 1361–1394.

Desmond, C., Stanton, C., Fitzgerald, G. F., Collins, K., and Ross, R. P. (2001). Environmental adaptation of probiotic lactobacilli towards improvement of performance during spray drying. *International Dairy Journal* 11: 801–808.

de Souza, J. R. R., Feitosa, J. P. A., Ricardo, N. M. P. S., Trevisan, M. T. S., de Paula, H. C. B., *et al.* (2013). Spray-drying encapsulation of mangiferin using natural polymers. *Food Hydrocolloids* 33: 10–18.

Diaz, F., Santos, E. M., Filardo, S., Villagomez, R., and Scheinvar, L. (2006). Colorant extraction from a red prickly pear (*Opuntia lasiacantha*) for food application. *Electronic Journal of Environmental, Agricultural and Food Chemistry* 5: 1330–1337.

Drusch, S. (2007). Sugar beet pectin: A novel emulsifying wall component for microencapsulation of lipophilic food ingredients by spray-drying. *Food Hydrocolloids* 21: 1223–1228.

Dumoulin, E., and Bimbenet, J. J. (1988). Spray Drying and Quality Changes, In: *The Properties of Water in Foods: ISOPOW 6*, pp. 209–232. D. S. Reid, ed. New York: Blackie Academic and Professional.

Dziezak, J. D. (1988). Microencapsulation and encapsulated ingredients. *Food Technology* 42(4): 136–151.

Embuscado, M. E. 2011, Hydrocolloids in Flavor Stabilization; *Hydrocolloids in Food Processing*, Chapter 9, 215–242;

Ersus, S., Yurdagel, U. 2007. Microencapsulation of anthocyanin pigments of black carrot (Daucuscarota L.) by spray drier. *Journal of Food Engineering* 80, 805–812.

Ezhilarasi, P. N., Indrani, D., Jena, B. S., and Anandharamakrishnan, C. (2014). Microencapsulation of *Garcinia* fruit extract by spray drying and its effect on bread quality. *Journal of Agricultural and Food Chemistry* 94(6): 1116–1123.

Fang, Z., and Bhandari, B. (2010). Encapsulation of polyphenols – a review. *Trends in Food Science & Technology* 21: 510–523.

Fang, Z., and Bhandari, B. (2012). Spray drying, Freeze Drying and Related Process for Food Ingredient and Nutraceutical Encapsulation. In: *Encapsulation Technologies and Delivery Systems for Food Ingredients and Nutraceuticals*, pp. 72–109. N. Garti and D. J. McClements, eds. Philadelphia: Woodhead Publishing.

Frascareli, E. C., Silva, V. M., Tonon, R. V., and Hubinger, M. D. (2012). Effects of process conditions on the microencapsualtion of coffee oil by spray drying. *Food and Bioporoducts Processing* 90: 413–424.

Fritzen-Freire, C. B., Prudencio, E. S., Amboni, R. D. M. C., Pinto, S. S., Negrao-Murakami, A. N., and Murakami, F. S. (2012). Microencapsualtion of bifidobacteria by spray drying in the presence of probiotics. *Food Research International* 45: 306–312.

Gharsallaoui, A., Roudaut, G., Chambin, O., Voilley, A., and Saurel, R. (2007). Applications of spray-drying in microencapsulation of food ingredients: an overview. *Food Research International* 40: 1107–1121.

Hayashi, H. (1989). Drying technologies of foods- their history and future. *Drying Technology* 7(2): 315–369.

Jafari, S. M., Assadpoor, E., He, Y., and Bhandari, B. (2008). Encapsulation efficiency of food flavors and oils during spray drying. *Drying Technology* 26: 816–835.

Jafari, S. M., Beheshti, P., and Assadpour, E. (2013). Emulsification properties of a novel hydrocolloid (Angum gum) for D-limonene droplets compared with Arabic gum. *International Journal of Biological Macromolecules* 61: 182–188.

Kailasapathy, K., and Chin, J. C. (2000). Survival and therapeutic potential of probiotic organisms with reference to *Lactobacillus acidophilus* and *Bifidobacterium* spp. *Immunology & Cell Biology* 78: 80–88.

Kowalski, R., and Wierciński, J. (2004). Ocena niektórych gatunków *Silphium* jako surowców inulinowych [Evaluation of some *Silphium* species as alternative inulin raw materials]. *Polish Journal of Food and Nutrition Sciences* 13(4): 349–354.

Lazaridou, A., and Biliaderis, C. G. (2009). Concurrent phase separation and gelation in mixed oat β-glucans/sodium caseinate and oat β-glucans/pullulan aqueous dispersion. *Food Hydrocolloid* 23: 886–895.

Leroux, J., Langendorff, V., Schick, G., Vaishnav, V., and Mazoyer, J. (2003). Emulsion stabilizing properties of pectin. *Food Hydrocolloids* 17: 455–462.

Lian, W.-C., Hsiao, H.-C., Chou, C.-C. (2002). Survival of bifidobacteria after spray drying. *International Journal of Food Microbiology* 74: 79–86.

Liang, H., Zhou, B., He, L., An, Y., Lin, L., *et al.* (2015). Fabrication of zein quaternized chitosan nanoparticles for the encapsulation and protection of curcumin. *RSC Advances* 5: 13891–13900.

Manojlović, V., Nedović, V. A., Kailasapathy, K., Zuidam, N. J. (2010). Encapsulation of Probiotics for use in Food Products. In: *Encapsulation Technologies for Active Food Ingredients and Food Processing*, pp. 269–302. N. J. Zuidam and V. A. Nedović, eds. New York: Springer.

Mantovani, M. S., Bellini, M. F., Angeli, J. P. F., Oliviera, R. J., Silva, A. F., and Ribeiro, L. R. (2008). β-Glucans in promoting health: Prevention against mutation and cancer. Mini-review. *Mutation Research* 658: 154–161.

Masters, K. (2002). *Spray Drying in Practice*. Charlottenlund: Spray Dry Consult International ApS.

Matsuno, R., and Adachi S. (1992). Lipid encapsulation technology – techniques and applications to foods. *Trends Food Science & Technology* 4: 256–261.

McClements, D. J., Decker, E. A., Park, Y., and Weiss, J. (2009). Structural design principles for delivery of bioactive components in nutraceuticals and functional foods. *Critical Reviews in Food Science and Nutrition* 49(6): 577–606.

Moslemi, M., Hosseini, H., Erfan, M., Mortazavian, A. M., Fard, R. M. N., *et al.* (2014). Characterisation of spray-dried microparticles containing iron coated by pectin/resistance starch. *Food Science and Technology* 49: 1736–1742.

Mujumdar, A. S. (2000). Dryers for particulate solids, slurries and sheet-form materials. In: *Mujumdar's Practical Guide to Industrial Drying*, pp. 37–71. S. Devahastion, ed. Montreal: Exergex.

Murúa-Pagola, B., Beristain-Guevara, C.I., and Martínez-Bustos, F. (2009). Preparation of starch derivatives using reactive extrusion and evaluation of modified starches as shell materials for encapsulation of flavouring agents by spray drying. *Journal of Food Engineering* 91(3): 380–386.

Porrarud, S., and Pranee, A. (2010). Microencapsulation of Zn–chlorophyll pigment from Pandan leaf by spray drying and its characteristic. *International Food Research Journal* 17: 1031–1042.

Ré, M. I., and Liu, Y. J. (1996). Microencapsulation by spray drying: Influence of wall systems on the retention of the volatiles compounds. *Drying '96 – Proceedings of the 10th International Drying Symposium*, 541–549.

Rocha, G. A., Fávaro-Trindade, C. S., and Grosso, C. R. F. (2012). Microencapsulation of lycopene by spray drying: Characterization, stability and application of microcapsules. *Food and Bioproducts Processing* 90: 37–42

Ruiz-Gutiérrez, M. G., Amaya-Guerra, C. A., Quintero-Ramos, A., de Jesús Ruiz-Anchondo, T., Gutiérrez-Uribe, J. A., *et al.* (2014). Effect of soluble fiber on the physicochemical properties of cactus pear *(Opuntia ficus indica)* encapsulated using spray drying. *Food Science Biotechnology* 23: 755–763

Rulkens, W. H., and Thijssen, H. A. C. (1972).The retention of organic volatiles in spray-drying aqueous carbohydrate solutions. *International Journal of Food Science & Technology* 7: 95–105.

Saenz, C., Tapia, S., Chavez, J., and Robert, P. (2009). Microencapsulation by spray drying of bioactive compounds from cactus pear *(Opuntia ficus-indica)*. *Food Chemistry* 114: 616–622.

Sanguansri, L., and Augustin, M. A. (2010). Microencapsulation in Functional Food Product Development. In: *Functional Food Product Development*, pp. 3–23. J. Smith and E. Charter, eds. Hoboken: Wiley.

Sansone, F., Mencherini, T., Picerno, P., d'Amore, M., Aquino, R. P., and Lauro, M. R. (2011). Maltodextrin/pectin microparticles by spray drying as carrier for nutraceutical extracts. *Journal Food Engineering* 105: 468–476.

Santivarangkna, C., Kulozik, U., and Foerst, P. (2007). Alternative drying processes for the industrial preservation of lactic acid starter cultures. *Biotechnology Progress* 23(2): 302–315.

Shahidi F., Han X. Q. (1993). Encapsulation of food ingredients. *Critical Review in Food Science and Nutrition* 33: 501–547.

Shaikh, J., Bhosale, R., and Singhal, R. (2006). Microencapsulation of black pepper oleoresin. *Food Chemistry* 94: 105–110.

Shanahan, F. (2000). Probiotics and inflammatory bowel disease: Is there a scientific rationale? *Inflammatory Bowel Disease* 6: 107–112.

Silva, J., Carvahlo, A. S., Teixeira, P., and Gibbs, P. A. (2002). Bacteriocin production by spray dried lactic acid bacteria. *Letters in Applied Microbiology* 34(2): 77–81.

Soottitantawat, A., Peigney, J., Uekaji, Y., Yoshii, H., Furuta, T., *et al.* (2007). Structural analysis of spray-dried powders by confocal laser scanning microscopy. *Asia-Pacific Journal of Chemical Engineering* 2: 41–46.

Soottitantawat, A., Takayama, K., Okamura, K., Muranaka. D., Yoshii, H., *et al.* (2005). Microencapsulation of L-menthol by spray drying and its release characteristics. *Innovative Food Science & Emerging Technologies* 6: 163–170.

Sun-Waterhouse, D., Sivam, A. S., Cooney, J., Zhou, J., Perera, C. O., and Waterhouse, G. I. N. (2011). Effects of added fruit polyphenols and pectin on the properties of finished breads revealed by HPLC/LC–MS and size-exclusion HPLC. *Food Research International* 44(9): 3047–3056.

Sun-Waterhouse, D., Wadhwa, S. S., and Waterhouse, G. I. N. (2013). Spray-drying microencapsulation of polyphenol bioactives: A comparative study using different naturalfibre polymers as encapsulants. *Food Bioprocess Technology* 6: 2376–2388.

Tonon, R. V., Brabet, C., and Hubinger, M. D. (2008). Influence of process conditions on the physochemical properties of acai (*Euterpe oleraceae* Mart.) powder produced by spray drying. *Journal of Food Engineering* 88(3): 411–418.

Vega, C., and Roos, Y. H. (2006). Invited review: Spray-dried dairy and dairy-like emulsion – composition considerations. *Journal of Dairy Science* 89: 383–401.

Vehring, R. 2008. Pharmaceutical particle engineering via spray drying. *Pharmaceutical Research* 25: 999–1022.

Wandrey, C., Bartkowiak, A., and Harding, S. E. (2010). Materials for Encapsulation. In: *Encapsulation Technologies for Active Food Ingredients and Food Processing*, pp. 31–100. N. J. Zuidam and V. A. Nedović, eds. New York: Springer.

Watanabe, Y., Fang, X., Adachi, S., Fukami, H., and Matsuno, R. (2004). Oxidation of 6-*O*-arachidonoyl-ascorbate microencapsulated with a polysaccharide by spray-drying. *Lebensmittel- Wissenschaft und-Technologie* 37: 395–400.

Yoshii, H., Buche, F., Takeuchi, N., Terrol, C., Ohgawara, M., and Furuta, T. (2008). Effects of protein on retention of ADH enzyme activity encapsulated in trehalose matrices by spray drying. *Journal of Food Engineering* 87(1): 34–39.

Zbicinski, I., Dela, A., Strumillo, C., and Adamiec, J. (2002). Advanced experimental analysis of drying kinetics in spray drying. *Chemical Engineering Journal* 86: 207–216.

Zuidam, N. J., and Shimoni, E. (2010). Overview of Microencapsulates for Use in Food Products or Processes and Methods to Make Them. In: *Encapsulation Technologies for Active Food Ingredients and Food Processing*, pp. 3–30. N. J. Zuidam and V. A. Nedović, eds. New York: Springer.

CHAPTER 6

The use of encapsulation to guarantee the stability of phenolic compounds

Maria Inês Dias[1,2], Cristina Caleja[1,2], Isabel C. F. R. Ferreira[1], and Maria Filomena Barreiro[2]

[1] *Mountain Research Centre (CIMO), ESA, Polytechnic Institute of Bragança, Campus Santa Apolónia Ap. 1172, 5301-855, Bragança, Portugal*

[2] *Laboratory of Separation and Reaction Engineering (LSRE), Associate Laboratory LSRE/LCM, Polytechnic Institute of Bragança, Campus Santa Apolónia Ap. 1134, 5301-857, Bragança, Portugal*

6.1 Introduction

Society is increasingly concerned with well-being and health issues. Knowing the long-term effects of a poor diet, tobacco and alcohol consumption, sedentary life, and high levels of stress, consumers are becoming more attracted to food products with recognized beneficial health effects. Phenolic compounds, including anthocyanins, have been described as powerful antioxidants, and are said to have other bioactive attributes such as antimicrobial or even antitumoral properties, usually correlated with the presence of these compounds in food products (Carocho and Ferreira, 2013a; Carocho and Ferreira, 2013b; Martins *et al.*, 2015). There are numerous food matrices naturally enriched with phenolic compounds, but nowadays, with the increasing market demand, these extracts or their isolated individual compounds are being incorporated into many other products. However, some of these molecules are naturally instable and/or susceptible to degradation during food processing or storage. In general, phenolic compounds with high molecular weight have very poor solubility and stability in water (Li *et al.*, 2015).

To overcome the problems related with the direct use of bioactives in their free form in food matrices, the microencapsulation technique, through the development of micro-sized particle systems, will ensure protection of the bioactive compounds and, additionally, functional properties to the final product. The organoleptic characteristics of phenolic extracts and isolated compounds are other important factors that drive researchers to study encapsulation of phenolic compounds, because many of them have bitter or astringent tastes, due to the

New Polymers for Encapsulation of Nutraceutical Compounds, First Edition.
Edited by Jorge Carlos Ruiz Ruiz and Maira Rubi Segura Campos.

presence of terpenes and glycosylates (Drewnowski and Gomez-Carneros, 2000). This factor is a decisive point for the food industry that must be considered when developing novel products, because acceptance by consumers is ultimately the most important reason for these studies. Controlled and targeted delivery-release studies are also crucial to understanding how the microspheres will interact and behave as they transit the gastrointestinal tract, because it is important to know if the bioactive form of the encapsulated phenolic compounds is maintained (Dias *et al.*, 2015).

In this chapter the fragility of phenolic compounds is discussed, starting from their intrinsic chemical characteristics, continuing to stability during processing and storage steps, and concluding with their behavior after ingestion. Microencapsulation technique is presented as a reliable tool to overcome the problems of using phenolic compounds in their free form, supported by studies dealing with the microencapsulation of these compounds. The understanding of the controlled release or targeted delivery behavior of the microparticles (microspheres or microcapsules) is crucial to understanding how they will act in the gastrointestinal tract, specifically if the bioactive properties of the phenolic compounds are maintained.

6.2 Phenolic compounds

6.2.1 Stability and bioavailability of free phenolic compounds

Phenolic compounds are a well-known group of secondary metabolites naturally produced by plants, having as their main function defense and protection against biotic and abiotic stress (Boudet, 2007; Quideau *et al.*, 2011). Structurally, these compounds are formed by a benzene ring with a hydroxyl substitute containing a functional group derivative (Cohen and Kennedy, 2010); they can have various biological functions often associated to the well-being of human consumers (Carocho and Ferreira, 2013). Therefore, the bioavailability and stability of phenolic compounds after consumption has become one of the most-discussed topics in research and review articles in order to understand the mechanisms behind phenolic action in the organism (Crozier *et al.*, 2010).

The bioavailability of any compound is measured by the fraction that reaches the circulatory system, which depends on its degree of absorption (Carbonell-Capella *et al.*, 2014). The absorption of the majority of phenolic compounds into the circulatory system occurs in the small intestine and is associated with the hydrolysis of the molecules, releasing the aglycone from the sugar component by the action of lactase-phlorizin hydrolase (LPH), reaching the blood stream by diffusion passage, due to the high lipophilicity and proximity with the cell membrane (Crozier *et al.*, 2010; Del Rio *et al.*, 2013). A different approach was also proposed in which the hydrolysis step occurs in the epithelial cells reaching the blood stream that conducts them into the liver, initiating phase II of metabolism, where the metabolites undergo conversions and some enterohepatic recirculation (excreted by bile) (Crozier *et al.*, 2010; Del Rio *et al.*, 2013). The metabolite that reaches the liver for conversion is estimated to be between 90% and 95% of the phenolics in the blood stream; the remainder is metabolized in the intestinal mucosa (Lutz *et al.*, 2014).

The majority of dietary phenolic compounds are aglycones bound to the matrix wall and also linked to sugar moieties; however, they can also be found as free compounds (flavan-3-ols and proanthocyanidins), as monomers, or in a polymeric form (Crozier *et al.*, 2010; Santos-Buelga *et al.*, 2012). There are thousands of phenolic compounds, divided into flavonoids and nonflavonoids, that present an immense diversity of chemical structures that not only influence their behavior in the organism when consumed but also influence their stability, functionality, and, consequently, bioavailability, which can be a limiting factor for their applicability as a functional compound and/or additive in food products (Holst and Williamson, 2008; Leong and Oey, 2012).

Figure 6.1 describes the main points that characterize the stability and bioavailability of phenolic compounds. Their distribution in plant tissues is not equal, and this affects their stability and limits the protocols for their extraction (Santos-Buelga *et al.*, 2012). The low- and medium-molecular-weight phenolics are considered extractable polyphenols because their extraction can be achieved by several solvents, whereas nonextractable phenolics are the ones with high molecular weight and are normally bound to dietary fiber and proteins, lowering their solubility (Bravo, 1998).

Despite the extensive literature on the beneficial effects of consuming foods rich in phenolic compounds, the phenolics bound to the matrix wall have very low bioavailability (Germanò *et al.*, 2006). Therefore, many researchers conduct their studies to increase the bioavailability of bound-phenolic compounds by breaking down the linkage between phenolic and

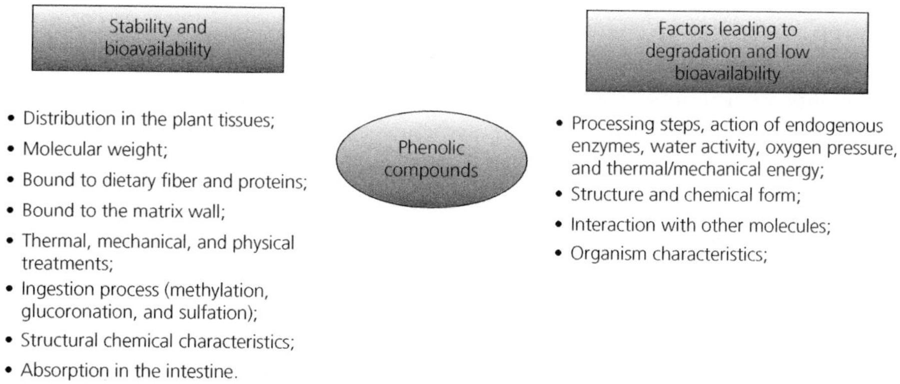

Figure 6.1 Main characteristics for stability and bioavailability of phenolic compounds and main factors conducting to their degradation and low bioavailability.

cell, such as the study by Martínez-Huélamo *et al.* (2015) in tomato using mechanical and thermal treatments or by Wang *et al.* (2014) in cereal grains by using thermal and extrusion treatments. Both groups reached the same conclusion: that these aggressive treatments, although liberating the phenolic compounds, increasing their bioavailability, compromise their stability by changing their chemical structure.

The influence of postharvest processing and storage of foodstuffs on the bioavailability of flavonoids and phenolic acids has been thoroughly discussed by Cermak *et al.* (2009). However, and despite the use of thermal, mechanical, and physical treatments to enhance the bioavailability of phenolic compounds during ingestion and after the passage to the blood stream, the sulfotransferase (SULT), uridine-5′-diphospho-glucuronosyltransferase (UGT), and catechol-*O*-methyltransferase (COMT) enzymes act on the free metabolites, forming methylated, glucoronated, and sulfated compounds that can lead to the loss of the bioactive characteristics of the phenolics (Crozier *et al.*, 2010; Heleno *et al.*, 2015). Glucoronidation is one of the most important factors for the loss of bioavailability in phenolic compounds. Research studies have developed protocols to inhibit the enzymes responsible for the chemical transformation (UGTs), increasing the bioavailability of the compounds after ingestion (Wu *et al.*, 2011).

The structural chemical characteristics of the phenolic compounds are also very important to consider when discussing their bioavailability. Karakaya (2004) extensively revised the bioavailability of some phenolic compound classes, such as phenolic acids, flavonoids (flavones, flavonols, flavanols), anthocyanins, and chalcones, listing a series of factors that could affect their bioavailability and absorption. The sugar molecules linked to the phenolic compound is one of the factors that most influences the absorption in the intestine, regarding their nature and number. For instance, phenolics containing a rhamnose moiety in their structure are not absorbed in the intestine due to the action of rhamnoside enzymes, whereas acylated flavonoids (epicatechin and epigallocatechin) are well absorbed in the intestine without deconjugation and hydrolysis (Karakaya, 2004). Karakaya also reached to the conclusion that the partition coefficients of phenolic compounds greatly influence their solubility in the microflora of the gastrointestinal gut and consequently their absorption in the lumen; minor variations in the structure of the compounds can cause a major difference in their behavior inside the human organism (Karakaya, 2004). The absorption of phenolic compounds in the intestine not only is influenced by the intrinsic characteristics of the compounds, but also may be related to external factors. For example, the human organism lacks many specific receptors in the small intestinal epithelial cell surface for various phenolic compounds, which limits their absorption, so that they are excreted in the urine and feces (Li *et al.*, 2015). pH changes in the medium could also affect anthocyanin compounds (Fernandes *et al.*, 2014).

Several methods are used to assess the bioavailability of bioactive compounds – in this case, phenolic compounds – and can be categorized as *in vitro* (e.g., simulated gastrointestinal digestion, artificial membranes), *ex vivo* (e.g., laboratory-scale gastrointestinal organs), *in situ* (e.g., intestinal perfusion in live animals), and *in vivo* (e.g., animal and human trials) models (Carbonell-Capella *et al.*, 2014). However, many of these studies have an incomplete conclusion, requiring further studies to understand the mechanisms leading to the loss or gain of the phenolic compounds' bioavailability (García-Villalba *et al.*, 2014; Hole *et al.*, 2012; Pérez-Jiménez *et al.*, 2009; Rubió *et al.*, 2014; Stalmach *et al.*, 2012; Zhang *et al.*, 2012).

6.2.2 Factors leading to degradation of phenolic compounds

The loss of bioactivity of phenolic compounds can come from a set of adverse conditions regarding processing steps, action of endogenous enzymes, water activity, oxygen pressure, and thermal/mechanical action. Moreover, the structure and chemical form of the phenolic compounds, as well as their interaction with other molecules present in the food product and the organism's characteristics, influence their stability and, consequently, their bioavailability (Figure 6.1) (Holst and Williamson, 2008; Leong and Oey, 2012; Dias *et al.*, 2015).

The processing steps after harvesting, which include thermal and mechanical treatments, can be responsible for the loss of bioavailability of phenolic compounds. As described in the previous section, thermal and mechanical treatments can be used to break the linkages between phenolics and cells; however, most of those treatments could lead to the degradation of the compounds, modifying their chemical structure (Cermak *et al.*, 2009). For instance, the degradation of anthocyanins is very complex, and using thermal treatments above 50 °C can affect the levels of these compounds in fruits and vegetables or can modify their chemical structure (Patras *et al.*, 2010).

Anthocyanins are among the phenolic compounds prone to conversion during the processing steps of food products, leading to the loss of stability and color (Cheynier, 2005). As previously mentioned, the chemical structure of phenolic compounds greatly influences their bioavailability, especially those linked to some types of sugar moieties (Karakaya, 2004). Also, some phenolic compounds are susceptible to degradation and transformation during the digestive process by the action of several enzymes carrying out a series of chemical reactions – glucuronidation, methylation, and sulfation – leading to the loss of some bioactive properties (Crozier *et al.*, 2010; Heleno *et al.*, 2015). The interactions between phenolic compounds and other molecules in the food products is also a very important factor for the degradation of phenolic compounds, in the way that some biochemical and chemical processes are involved in those steps. The enzymatic oxidation is one of the main factors leading to loss of structural integrity of the phenolic compounds, to the detriment of the quality of the food product (Cheynier, 2005).

6.3 Microencapsulation process

6.3.1 Techniques and materials used to encapsulate phenolic compounds

Microencapsulation is a technique in which an active principle is encapsulated using an encapsulating material, preferably a natural polymer. The main objective is to protect it from the action of oxygen, light, hydrolysis, and other external conditions (Gharsallaoui *et al.*, 2007). It also allows a higher stability, solubility, and dispersability of the encapsulated compounds (Wang *et al.*, 2014). Microencapsulation has been mostly applied in the pharmaceuticals field (68%), and the food industry accounts for only a share of 13% (Dias *et al.*, 2015). Nowadays, this tendency is changing: Microencapsulation is increasingly applied in the development of novel functional food products (Colla and Morales, 2006). Besides the advantage of maintained the biological and bioactive characteristics of extracts and compounds, microencapsulation also masks some organoleptic characteristics that are less appreciated by consumers (Martins *et al.*, 2014). However, rigid parameters for the production of microencapsulated food products must be followed to ensure its safety for human consumption (Nedovic *et al.*, 2011). The microencapsulation techniques and encapsulation materials should be chosen depending on the final product to be developed. The specific characteristics of the bioactive extracts and compounds should also be taken into account (Lachman *et al.*, 2001).

As previously explained, phenolic compounds are prone to degradation, and to prevent that, many studies propose microencapsulation to protect and stabilize the extracts and compounds as well as offering a controlled release and targeted delivery (Dias *et al.*, 2015). Studies regarding the microencapsulation of phenolic extracts or pure compounds are listed in Tables 6.1, 6.2, 6.3, and 6.4.

To better understand the potential of this technology, it is essential to know the main characteristics of the different microencapsulation processes, the properties of the encapsulation materials, and the release mechanisms of the encapsulated bioactives (Lachman *et al.*, 2001).

The compounds are protected in small capsules with sizes ranging from 1 to 1000 μm, allowing various applications, only being released under specific conditions (Fang and Bhandari, 2010). Microencapsulation protects the core material and also influences the delivery behavior after ingestion (Nedovic *et al.*, 2011). The choice of the encapsulation material is a very important step because its nature could affect the stability of the encapsulated compound. The choice must take into account the physical and chemical characteristics of the bioactive compounds and extracts, the microencapsulation method, and the intended application (Suave *et al.*, 2006). The material can be natural, semi-natural, or synthetic (Gharsallaoui *et al.*, 2007), but mainly it must be biocompatible and nontoxic. The most used are water-soluble polymers followed by water-soluble nonpolymers (Dias *et al.*, 2015). Examples are polysaccharides (maltodextrin,

Table 6.1 Examples of microencapsulated phenolic compounds using spray-based processes.

Phenolic compounds	Source	Encapsulation Material	Reference
(–)-Hydroxycitric acid	*Garcinia cowa* Roxb fruit rinds	Whey protein and maltodextrin	Ezhilarasi *et al.* (2013b)
(–)-Hydroxycitric acid	*Garcinia cowa* Roxb fruit rinds	Whey protein and maltodextrin	Ezhilarasi *et al.* (2013a)
(–)-Hydroxycitric acid	*Garcinia cowa* Roxb. fruit	Whey protein	Pillai *et al.* (2012)
Anthocyanin	*Daucus carota* L. roots	Maltodextrin and glucodry	Ersus and Yurdagel (2007)
Anthocyanin	*Garcinia indica* Choisy fruit pulp	Maltodextrin	Nayak and Rastogi (2010)
Anthocyanin	*Bactris guineensis* L. fruits	Maltodextrin	Osorio *et al.* (2012)
Anthocyanins	*Myrciaria cauliflora* (Mart.) fruit peel	Ca-alginate	Santos *et al.* (2013)
Anthocyanins	*Vaccinium* genus fruits	Maltodextrin, citric acid, pectins and caffeine	Berg *et al.* (2012)
Anthocyanins	*Euterpe oleracea* Mart. Fruit pulp	Maltodextrin, gum arabic and tapioca starch.	Tonon *et al.* (2010)
Anthocyanins	*Myrciaria jaboticaba* (Mart.) fruit peel	Maltodextrin, arabic gum and Capsul™	Silva *et al.* (2013)
Bioactive compounds	Quercus resinosa leaves	Lactose–sodium caseinate	Rocha-Guzmán *et al.* (2010)
Bioactive compounds	Paeonia rokii roots	Chitosan	Sansone *et al.* (2014)
Catechins	*Camellia sinensis L.*tea	Maltodextrin	Jung *et al.* (2013)
Ellagitanins	*Rubus chamaemorus* L. fruits	Maltodextrin	Laine *et al.* (2008)
Gallic acid	Commercial	Chitosan, β-cyclodextrin and xanthan	Rosa *et al.* (2013)
Gallic acid	Commercial	Mucilage extract of *Opuntia ficus indica*	Medina-Torres *et al.* (2013)
Gallic acid	Commercial	Native and acetylated starch and inulin	Robert *et al.* (2012)
Mangiferin	*Mangifera indica* L.	Pectin and chitosan	Souza *et al.* (2013)
Naringenin and quercetin	Commercial	Cellulose acetate phthalate	Sansone *et al.* (2011a)
Phenolic compounds	*Punica granatum* L. fruit	Maltodextrin or soybean protein	Robert *et al.* (2010)
Phenolic compounds	*Vitis labrusca* L. skeen and seeds	Maltodextrin	Souza *et al.* (2014)
Phenolic extracts	*Rubus ulmifolius* Schott flowers	Alginate	Martins *et al.* (2014)
Polyphenols	*Ilex paraguariensis* A. St. Hil. aerial parts	Ca-alginate and Ca-alginate-chitosan	Deladino *et al.* (2008)

(Continued)

Table 6.1 (Continued)

Phenolic compounds	Source	Encapsulation Material	Reference
Polyphenols	Cabernet Sauvignon fruits	Maltodextrin	Sanchez *et al.* (2011)
Polyphenols	*Camellia sinensis* L. tea	Chitosan	Liang *et al.* (2011)
Polyphenols	*Hypericum perforatum* L. Leaves and flowers	β-cyclodextrin	Kalogeropoulos *et al.* (2010)
Polyphenols	*Ribes nigrum* L. pomace	Maltodextrin and inulin	Bakowska-Barczaka and Kolodziejczykb (2011)
Polyphenols	*Punica granatum* L. peels	Maltodextrin	Çam *et al.* (2014)
Polyphenols	*Quercus resinosa* Liebm. leaves	k-Carrageenan and maltodextrin	Gallegos-Infante *et al.* (2013)
Polyphenols	*Orthosiphon stamineus* Benth leaves	Whey protein and maltodextrin	Pang *et al.* (2014)
Polyphenols and betalains	*Opuntia ficus-indica* fruit	Maltodextrin or inulin	Saénz *et al.* (2009)
Quercetin and vanillin	Commercial	Sodium alginate, methyl-β-cyclodextrin, hydroxypropylmethycellulose and inulin	Sun-Waterhouse *et al.* (2013)

Table based on Dias *et al.* (2015).

Table 6.2 Examples of microencapsulated phenolic compounds using emulsion-based process.

Phenolic Compounds	Source	Encapsulation Material	Reference
Anthocyanins	*Vaccinium myrtillus* L. fruits	Whey proteins	Betz & Kulozika, 2011
Antochianins	*Vaccinium myrtillus* L. fruits	Pectin and PGPR	Frank et al., 2012
Curcumin	Commercial	Surfactants (SDS STAB, Tween 20 and poloxamer) and solvents (cotton seed oil)	Malik et al., 2014
Curcumin and retinol	Commercial	Casein protein	Pan et al., 2014
Isoflavone	Commercial	Polyglycerol monostearate	Seok et al., 2003
Phenolic extract	*Vaccinium myrtillus* L. fruits	Whey protein	Betz et al., 2012
Polyphenols	*Aristotelia chilensis* [Molina] Stuntz leaves	Gum arabic and liquid Vaseline	Vidal et al., 2012

Table based on Dias *et al.* (2015).

Table 6.3 Examples of microencapsulated phenolic compounds using liposom process.

Phenolic Compounds	Source	Encapsulation Material	Reference
Curcumin	Commercial	Lecithin	Hasan *et al.* (2014)
Ellagic acid	Commercial	Lecithin/chitosan–dextran sulfate	Madrigal-Carballo *et al.* (2010)
Fatty acid	Commercial	Soybean phospholipids	Rasti *et al.* (2012)
Polyphenols	Commercial	Labrafac, Phospholipon 90G, Solutol H515	Barras *et al.* (2009)
Polyphenols	*Vitis vinifera* L. seed	Soy lecithin	Gibis *et al.* (2014)
Polyphenols	Commercial	Tween 60	Tavano *et al.* (2014)
Polyphenols and oils	Commercial	DPPC and PEG_{2000}-DSPE	Coimbra *et al.* (2011)

Table based on Dias *et al.* (2015).

dextrose, alginate), gums (gum arabic), and proteins (gelatin and milk proteins) (Gharsallaoui *et al.*, 2007).

The main encapsulating agent used in the food industry is maltodextrin (Saénz *et al.*, 2009). Maltodextrin is obtained from the acid or enzymatic hydrolysis of various starches, being structurally characterized by glucose units linked together by glycosidic bonds of α $(1 \rightarrow 4)$ type (Madene *et al.*, 2006). Maltodextrin is highly soluble in water, has a pleasant flavor, is colorless, and has low viscosity and cost, justifying its broad use in the food industry (Ersu and Yurdagel, 2007; Robert *et al.*, 2010). Several studies report the use

Table 6.4 Examples of microencapsulated phenolic compounds using other microencapsulation technologies.

Phenolic Compounds	Method	Source	Encapsulation Material	Reference
Anthocyanins	Rapid Extraction of Supercritical Solution	*Myrciaria cauliflora* (Mart.) fruit peel	Polyethyleneglycol/ethanol	Santos *et al.* (2013)
Caffeine	Nanoparticules/Spray-drying	Commercial	Whey proteins/alginate	Bagheri *et al.* (2014)
Chlorogenic acid	Inclusion	*Nicotiana tabacum* L. leaves	Cyclodextrin	Zhao *et al.* (2010)
Citric acid	Microwave	Commercial	Casein and inulin	Abbasi *et al.* (2009)
Polyphenols	Electrostatic extrusion	*Urtica dioica* L. leaves	Alginate–chitosan	Belščak-Cvitanović *et al.* (2011)
Polyphenols	Electrostatic extrusion	*Crategus laevigata* (Poir.) Dc. aerial parts	Alginate–chitosan	Belščak-Cvitanović *et al.* (2011)
Polyphenols	Electrostatic extrusion	*Rubus idaeus* L. leaves	Alginate–chitosan	Belščak-Cvitanović *et al.* (2011)
Polyphenols	Electrostatic extrusion	*Olea europea* L. leaves	Alginate–chitosan	Belščak-Cvitanović *et al.* (2011)
Polyphenols	Electrostatic extrusion	*Achillea millefolium* L. aerial parts	Alginate–chitosan	Belščak-Cvitanović *et al.* (2011)
Polyphenols	Electrostatic extrusion	*Glechoma hederacea* L. aerial parts	Alginate–chitosan	Belščak-Cvitanović *et al.* (2011)
Polyphenols	Extrusion		Ethylene vinyl acetate and low-density polyethylene	Barbosa-Pereira *et al.* (2014)
Polyphenols	Phase separation method	*Myrica* genus fruit	Ethyl cellulose	Zheng *et al.* (2011)
Polyphenols	Supercritical antisolvent process	*Rosmarinus officinalis* L. leaves	Poloxamers	Visentin *et al.* (2012)
Polyphenols	Ultrasonication	*Prunus cerasus* L. pomace	Maltodextrin and gum arabic	Cilek *et al.* (2012)
Quercetin	Nanoprecipitation	Commercial	Eudragit E and polyvinyl alcohol	Wu *et al.* (2008)
Quercitrin	Solvent evaporation	*Albizia chinensis* L. flowers	Poly-D,L-lactide (PLA)	Kumari *et al.* (2010)
Resveratrol	Response surface methodology	*Arachis hypogaea* L. sprout	Medium-chain triacylglycerol/ whey protein, maltodextrin, and gum arabic	Lee *et al.* (2013)
Resveratrol	Ultrasound	*Polygonum cuspidatum* Siebold & Zucc roots	Cyclodextrins	Mantegna *et al.* (2012)
Rutin and anthocyanins	Spinning disc reactor	*Hibiscus sabdariffa* L. dried calyx	High and low HLP lypophilic polimeric emulsifiers	Akhtar *et al.* (2014)

Table based on Dias *et al.* (2015).

of maltodextrins for microencapsulation purposes, mainly for those highly unstable in the presence of oxygen (Saénz *et al.*, 2009). Maltodextrin is also used in the pharmaceutical and nutritional fields as a supplement for improving athletic and mental performance. Its binder properties and moisture-retaining capacity make it very appealing also for pharmaceutical uses (Ferrari *et al.*, 2013; Sousdaleff *et al.*, 2013).

Alginates are another example of polymers used for microencapsulation purposes. Alginates are derived from bacteria and algae, but brown algae is the most common source of these compounds. Their physical and chemical properties allow their commercial application in several fields. In the food industry, for instance, alginates are used as a stabilizer and thickener agent for jams and beverages (Goh *et al.*, 2012). These properties are due to the ability of alginates to form a gel when in an aqueous solution in the presence of a bivalent cation such as Ca^{2+}. The use of alginate in the food industry is allowed by the U.S. Food and Drug Administration (FDA), which classifies it as nontoxic for oral administration (George and Abraham, 2006).

Alginates are very appealing to use as microencapsulating materials, allowing the controlled release of the protected compounds under the moderate alkaline pH conditions normally occurring in the intestinal tract. The release of the bioactive molecules from the alginate microparticles is avoided at the acidic pH found in the gastric environment. However, when transiting into the higher-pH environment of the intestinal tract, the polymer network is disrupted, converting the alginate into a soluble polymer, thus releasing the compounds (George and Abraham, 2006).

It is worth noting that the morphological characteristics of the encapsulating agent, such as texture and shape, as well as the trigger mechanism for the release of the phenolic compounds, are parameters that significantly influence the choice of microencapsulation technique (Bansode *et al.*, 2010).

There are numerous methodologies for encapsulating bioactive compounds (Dias *et al.*, 2015). These can be classified by the microcapsules' formation mechanism, by their consolidation method, or even by the specific equipment used for microencapsulation. There is not a clear categorization into physical, chemical, or physical–chemical methods. However, a novel approach by Dias and colleagues (2015) proposed coacervation, extrusion-based processes, spray-based processes, emulsion-based processes, liposomes, supercritical fluid–based processes, ultrasound-based processes, and others, as general categories to encompass the vast array of microencapsulation techniques. Each one presents a set of parameters and characteristics that determine their use according to the intended objective (Suave *et al.*, 2006).

The most widely used techniques for microencapsulation of phenolic compounds are, as expected, spray-based processes (Table 6.1), emulsion-based processes, and liposomes (Dias *et al.*, 2015; Munin and Edwards-Lévy, 2011). Some other techniques are also referred to in the literature but are used to a more modest extent (e.g., extrusion, ultrasound, supercritical fluids, and microwave-based processes) (Dias et al., 2015).

Spray drying is the most commonly used microencapsulation technique, being a fast and easily available technique (Fang and Bhandari, 2011). It allows continuous production of microencapsulated compounds, which makes it economically feasible for industry due to the low associated costs. It also produces microspheres with high quality, low water activity, and low weight, resulting in an easier storage and transportation (Murugesan and Orsat, 2012). However, this method has some limitations, such as constraints related to the encapsulating material, which must be sufficiently soluble in water, and the high cost of the equipment (Estevinho *et al.*, 2013; Martins *et al.*, 2014). It is most commonly used in the food and pharmaceuticals industry (Fang and Bhandari, 2010; Ré, 1998). Microspheres are formed by the atomization of the solution containing the active principle and the encapsulating material through a nozzle. The microspheres' consolidation occurs by contacting with heated gas (air or nitrogen), which promotes evaporation of the solvent. After deposition, the microparticles are collected in a cyclone or in a filter (Fang and Bhandari, 2010; Murugesan and Orsat, 2012).

Emulsion technology is also commonly used for food, pharmaceutical, and nutraceutical applications (Table 6.2). It has been successfully used to encapsulate bioactive molecules such as phenolic compounds (Dias *et al.*, 2015; Fang and Bhandari, 2010). An emulsion involves the use of two or more immiscible liquids (usually designated by oil and water phases) that, due to mutual incompatibility, generate a biphasic system composed of small droplets incorporating the bioactive dispersed within a continuous external phase. These small droplets constitute the embryonic microcapsules that could be further coated by a material and then consolidated (Friberg *et al.*, 2004; McClements, 2005). Emulsion often constitutes the first step of an encapsulation process.

Liposomes are by definition spherical structures consisting of one or more phospholipid bilayers enclosing an aqueous core (Table 6.3) (Zeisig and Cämmerer, 2001). Because the process is easy and encapsulation is highly efficient, giving rise to stable entities, the potential applications for liposomes are vast, and several examples can be found in the literature (Gouin, 2004). The pharmaceuticals and cosmetics industries regularly use liposome technology for targeted delivery of therapeutic agents and for inclusion of stabilizers in creams and lotions, respectively. The food industry is another area that foresees the potential of this technique, which can find applications such as encapsulating poorly soluble compounds, protecting sensitive ingredients, and increasing the bioavailability of bioactive molecules (Barras *et al.*, 2009; Hasan *et al.*, 2014; Madrigal-Carballo *et al.*, 2010). However, due to chemical and physical instability during storage and the high cost, its applicability in the food industry is still very limited (Zuidam *et al.*, 2003). Other methodologies, not so common, in the microencapsulation of phenolic compounds, such as electrostatic extrusion, ultrasound-based processes, supercritical fluid–based processes, and even microwaves, have been also used (Table 6.4).

6.3.2 Controlled release and targeted delivery

One of the main goals of microencapsulation is the delivery of the encapsulated compound in its original form to a target tissue, to ensure the maintenance of the bioactive properties. In the case of ingestion, the delivery should be targeted (e.g., stomach or intestine) and triggered (e.g., temperature or pH stimulus). Thus the release of bioactive compounds depends on several factors, such as the physical and chemical properties of the wall material, the molecular bonding between core and wall material, and the external trigger stimulus (e.g., temperature, moisture, pH, and shear) (Ko and Gunasekaran, 2014). For that manner, it is necessary to monitor the behavior of the enriched microcapsules after ingestion, because their release through the gastrointestinal tract could be affected by several circumstances. Several methodologies are used for that purpose, one being a pH-based method that measures the fraction of free fatty acids released from triacylglycerols over time. This method is usually applied to characterize the *in vitro* digestibility of lipids under simulated small intestine conditions (Frank *et al.*, 2012; Li and McClements, 2010).

Dialysis is a purification process adapted from the protein purification process. Through this technique it is possible by selective and passive diffusion to remove small, low-molecular-weight solutes by passing them through a semipermeable membrane. Dialysis is characterized by a simple and cheap technique used to separate the colloid particles from the nonencapsulated particles. There are, however, some limitations to applying this purification technique: It is only effective for small molecules, the dialysate solution must be changed many times (which causes problems when some compounds need special disposal), and a long time is required to complete the purification. Temperature, the molecules' concentration in the solution, and the molecular weight are some of the several factors that influence the time for purification (Nguyen *et al.*, 2014; Rosenberg, 2005).

In the study of the controlled release of a bioactive compound, it is important to understand the mechanism behind the procedure. According to the literature there are three main controlled-release mechanisms: diffusion, mechanical, rupture and dissolution (Figure 6.2) (Uhrich *et al.*, 1999). The most important mechanism of controlled release for food ingredients is diffusion, in which the dissolution fluid penetrates the shell or matrix material, fomenting the liberation of the active principle through the interstitial channels. This mechanism controls the release speed of the core material into the matrix. The release is influenced by different factors, including the solubility and the permeability of the active component with the food matrix (Korsmeye *et al.*, 1983; Madene *et al.*, 2006).

Mechanical rupture is the mechanism by which the microcapsule suffers an external physical stress (e.g., pressure, shearing force, ultrasound radiation) or

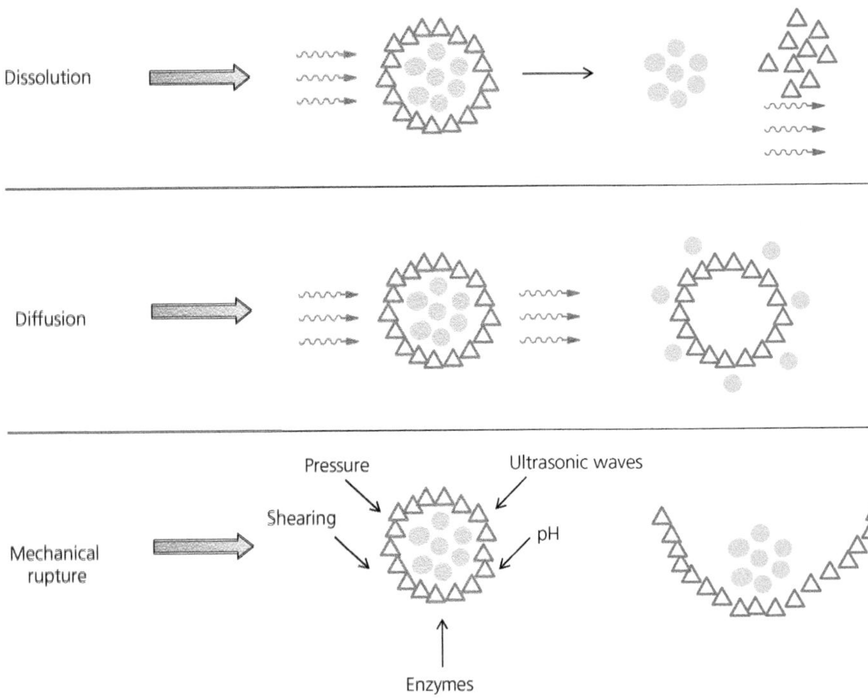

Figure 6.2 Main controlled release mechanisms of microencapsulated compounds.

an internal stimulus (e.g., pH, enzymes), breaking the structure, which enables the encapsulated core material to be released to the surrounding media or to a targeted area (Allen and Cullis, 2013).

Another type of controlled release mechanism is dissolution. The literature defines dissolution as the easiest system in comparison to other controlled-release mechanisms (Risch and Reineccius, 1995). In this case, the release rate of the active ingredient from the microcapsule depends on the dissolution rate of the wall material in the surrounding fluid (Nuppor and Rathore, 2012). The solubility and the thickness of coat are factors influencing the release rate (Costa and Lobo, 2001). The literature describes two types of dissolution. In the capsule dissolution controlled system, the active principle is coated by a shell of a slowly dissolving material (e.g., carbohydrates, lipids, and proteins). In this case, the dissolution rate depends on the physicochemical properties of the capsule and the solubility of the active principle. In the matrix dissolution controlled system, the active materials are homogeneously dispersed throughout a matrix. (Siepmann and Siegel, 2012; Wise, 2000).

It is important to note that controlled release of a bioactive compound with impact in the food industry must be studied in aqueous media and under different pHs mimicking those of the gastrointestinal tract. The release of the bioactive compounds from the microspheres is very complex and gradual, which may require more than one trigger signal to unlock the core material. For instance, depending on the encapsulation material used, as in the case of alginates, the stomach pH (low pH) helps to stabilize the microsphere; in the small intestine, where the pH is higher, the bioactive material is released from the medium. This complexity of the controlled-release mechanism allows a variety of applications for bioactive compounds in the pharmaceuticals and food industries (Ko and Gunasekaran, 2014).

Regarding the controlled released of encapsulated phenolic compounds, there is an enormous lack of information on the subject. Most of the microencapsulation studies performed refer to the optimization of the encapsulation method or the evaluation of the bioactive properties of the compounds after encapsulation. Some controlled-release studies were already performed for other types of encapsulated compounds such as vitamins, riboflavin (Chen and Subirade, 2006; Wichchukit *et al.*, 2013), folic acid (Prasertmanakit *et al.*, 2009), fish oil, resveratrol and tributyrin (Augustin *et al.*, 2011), and even probiotics (Anal and Singh, 2007). These *in vitro* assays have the main advantage of enabling the study of absorption of bioactive compounds and, therefore, allowing researchers to comprehend the potential beneficial health effects that these compounds could present after ingestion (Carbonell-Capella *et al.*, 2014).

As previously mentioned, there is a lack of *in vitro* release studies of microencapsulated phenolic compounds, but some studies have been made, such as the ones presented by Tavano and coworkers (2014), in which they demonstrated an improved solubility of microencapsulated curcumin and quercetin in niosomes. The anthocyanin extract of *Vaccinium myrtillus* L. was also tested using an *in vitro* gastrointestinal model, having improved the stability in adverse pH conditions during digestion, being only released in the intestinal mucosa (Frank *et al.*, 2012; Park *et al.*, 2014). A similar result was obtained for a commercial isoflavone incorporated into an emulsion of polyglycerol monostearate in which a higher stability of the bioactive molecule was observed, and even after incorporation into a food matrix (milk) the organoleptic characteristics were not affected and the release in the intestinal mucosa was also enhanced (Seok *et al.*, 2003). Controlled-release studies have been also applied in the cosmetics industry, in which flavanols and phenolic acids were tested for their bioavailability in human trials using cocoanut creams with microencapsulated extracts (Vitaglione *et al.*, 2013).

6.4 Concluding remarks and future perspectives

Phenolic compounds are a large group of biomolecules with recognized beneficial health effects. These compounds have been extensively used for their antioxidant, antimicrobial, antitumoral, and cytotoxic effects. Being naturally present in food products or artificially added to them, phenolic compounds have been used as food ingredients to stabilize or preserve the food matrix, adding benefits beyond their nutritional and health effects. Nevertheless, the stability, bioavailability, and related bioactivity of these compounds can be seriously compromised by several factors, and therefore many efforts have been made to enhance or maintain the stability and bioavailability of these compounds, sometimes leading to their degradation. For that reason, the microencapsulation process emerges a reliable response to overcome the problems related to the use of free bioactive compounds. Although the food industry only represents 13% of the applied studies for microencapsulation technologies, it is its potential is increasing. Water-soluble polymers (maltodextrins and alginates already approved by the FDA) are the most-used wall materials, followed by water-soluble nonpolymers. The most widely used techniques for the encapsulation of phenolic compounds are spray-based processes, followed by emulsions and liposomes.

The main goal of a microencapsulation protocol is the delivery of the bioactive compounds into the target sites of absorption, usually stomach and intestines. The absorption of the bioactive occurs mainly in the stomach cells and intestinal mucosa, usually triggered by temperature or pH, releasing the molecules into the medium for metabolism. Several methodologies have been used to track the gastrointestinal effects of food products, bioactive extracts, isolated compounds, and microencapsulated bioactives. Among those methods, dialysis is one of the most used for its simplicity and fast results. The release mechanism of the microencapsulated bioactive can be performed through diffusion, mechanical rupture, and dissolution into the medium, being dependent on the wall material used and dissolution rate in the medium. However, there is a huge lack of information regarding controlled targeted delivery of microencapsulated bioactives, and further studies are needed to understand if microencapsulated phenolic compounds maintain their stability and bioavailabity after ingestion.

References

Abbasi, S., Rahimi, S., and Azizi, M. (2009). Influence of microwave-microencapsulated citric acid on some sensory properties of chewing gum. *Journal of Microencapsulation* 26: 90–96.

Akhtar, M., Murray, B. S., Afeisume, E. I., Khew, S. H. (2014). Encapsulation of flavonoid in multiple emulsion using spinning disc reactor technology. *Food Hydrocolloids* 34: 62–67.

Allen, T. M., and Cullis, P. R. (2013). Liposomal drug delivery systems: From concept to clinical applications. *Advanced Drug Delivery Reviews* 65: 36–48.

Anal, A. K., and Singh, H. (2007). Recent advances in microencapsulation of probiotics for industrial applications and targeted delivery. *Trends in Food Science & Technology*, 18: 240–251.

Augustin, M. A., Abeywardena, M. Y., Patten, G., Head, R., Lockett, T., *et al.* (2011). Effects of microencapsulation on the gastrointestinal transit and tissue distribution of a bioactive mixture of fish oil, tributyrin and resveratrol. *Journal of Functional Foods* 3: 25–37.

Bagheri, L., Madadlou, A., Yarmand, M., and Mousavi, M. E. (2014). Spray-dried alginate microparticles carrying caffeine-loaded and potentially bioactive nanoparticles. *Food Research International* 62: 1113–1119.

Bakowska-Barczak, A. M., and Kolodziejczyk, P. P. (2011). Black currant polyphenols: Their storage stability and microencapsulation. *Industrial Crops and Products* 34: 1301–1309.

Bansode, S. S., Banarjee, S. K., Gaikwad, D. D., Jadhav, S. L., and Thorat, R. M. (2010). Microencapsulation: A review. *International Journal of Pharmaceutical Sciences Review and Research* 1: 38–43.

Barbosa-Pereira, L., Angulo, I., Lagarón, J. M., Paseiro-Losada, P., and Cruz, J. M. (2014). Development of new active packaging films containing bioactive nanocomposites. *Innovative Food Science & Emerging Technologies* doi: 10.1016/j.ifset.2014.06.002.

Barras, A., Mezzetti, A., Richard, A., Lazzaroni, S., Roux, S., *et al.* (2009). Formulation and characterization of polyphenol-loaded lipid nanocapsules. *International Journal of Pharmaceutics* 379: 270–277.

Belščak-Cvitanović, A., Stojanović, R., Manojlović, V., Komes, D., Cindrić, I. J., *et al.* (2011). *Food Research International* 44: 1094–1101.

Berg, S., Bretz, M., Hubbermann, E. A., and Schwarz, K. (2012) Influence of different pectins on powder characteristics of microencapsulated anthocyanins and their impact on drug retention of shellac coated granulate. *Journal of Food Engineering* 108: 158–165.

Betz, M., and Kulozik, U. (2011). Microencapsulation of bioactive bilberry anthocyanins by means of whey protein gels. *Procedia Food Science* 1: 2047–2056.

Betz, M., Steiner, B., Schantz, M., Oidtmann, J., Mäder, K., *et al.* (2012). Antioxidant capacity of bilberry extract microencapsulated in whey protein hydrogels. *Food Research International* 47: 51–57.

Bravo, L. (1998). Polyphenols: Chemistry, dietary sources, metabolism, and nutritional significance. *Nutrition Reviews* 56: 317–333.

Çam, M., İçyer, N. C., and Erdoğan, F. (2014). Pomegranate peel phenolics: Microencapsulation, storage stability and potential ingredient for functional food development. *LWT – Food Science and Technology* 55: 117–123.

Carbonell-Capella, J. M., Buniowska, M., Barba, F. J., Esteve, M. J., and Frígola, A. (2014). Analytical methods for determining bioavailability and bioaccessibility of bioactive compounds from fruits and vegetables: A review. *Comprehensive Reviews in Food Science and Food Safety* 13: 155–171.

Carocho, M., and Ferreira, I. C. F. R. (2013a). A review on antioxidants, prooxidants and related controversy: natural and synthetic compounds, screening and analysis methodologies and future perspectives. *Food and Chemical Toxicology* 51: 15–25.

Carocho, M., and Ferreira, I. C. F. R. (2013b). The role of phenolic compounds in the fight against cancer – a review. *Anti-Cancer Agents in Medicinal Chemistry* 13: 1236–1258.

Cermak, R., Durazzo, A., Maiani, G., Böhm, V., Kammerer, D. R., *et al.* (2009). The influence of postharvest processing and storage of foodstuffs on the bioavailability of flavonoids and phenolic acids. *Molecular Nutrition & Food Research* 53: 184–193.

Chen, L., and Subirade, M. (2006). Alginate–whey protein granular microspheres as oral delivery vehicles for bioactive compounds. *Biomaterials* 27: 4646–4654.

Cheynier, V. (2005). Polyphenols in foods are more complex than often thought. *American Journal of Clinical Nutrition* 81: 223–229.

Cilek, B., Luca, A., Hasirci, V., Sahin, S., and Sumnu, G. (2012). Microencapsulation of phenolic compounds extracted from sour cherry pomace: Effect of formulation, ultrasonication time and core to coating ratio. *European Food Research and Technology* 235: 587–596.

Coimbra, M., Isacchi, B., Bloois, L. V., Torano, J. S., Keta, A., *et al.* (2011). Improving solubility and chemical stability of natural compounds for medicinal use by incorporation into liposomes. *International Journal of Pharmaceutics* 416: 433–442.

Costa, P., and Lobo, J. M. S. (2001). Modeling and comparison of dissolution profiles. *European Journal of Pharmaceutical Sciences* 13: 123–133.

Crozier, A., Del Rio, D., and Clifford, M. N. (2010). Bioavailability of dietary flavonoids and phenolic compounds. *Molecular Aspects of Medicine* 31: 446–467.

Del Rio, D., Rodriguez-Mateos, A., Spencer, J. P. E., Tognolini, M., Borges, G., and Crozier, A. (2013). Dietary (poly)phenolics in human health: Structures, bioavailability, and evidence of protective effects against chronic diseases. *Antioxidants & Redox Signaling* 18: 1818–1892.

Deladino. L., Anbinder, P. S., Navarro, A. S., and Martino, M. N. (2008). Encapsulation of natural antioxidants extracted from *Ilex paraguariensis*. *Carbohydrate Polymers* 71: 126–134.

Dias, M. I., Ferreira I. C. F. R., and Barreiro M. F. (2015). Microencapsulation of bioactives for food applications. *Food &Function* doi: 10.1039/c4fo01175a.

Drewnowski, A., and Gomez-Carneros, C. (2000). Bitter taste, phytonutrients, and the consumer: A review. *American Journal of Clinical Nutrition* 72: 1424–1435.

Ersus, S., and Yurdagel, U. (2007). Microencapsulation of anthocyanin pigments of black carrot (*Daucus carota* L.) by spray drier. *Journal of Food Engineering* 80: 805–812.

Estevinho, B. N., Rocha, F., Santos, L., and Alves, A. (2013). Microencapsulation with chitosan by spray drying for industry applications – A review. *Food Science & Technology* 31: 138–155.

Ezhilarasi, P. N., Indrani, D., Jena, B. S., and Anandharamakrishnana, C. (2013a). Microencapsulation of *Garcinia* fruit extract by spray drying and its effect on bread quality. *Journal of the Science of Food and Agriculture*, 94: 1116–1123.

Ezhilarasi, P. N., Indrani, D., Jena, B. S., and Anandharamakrishnana, C. (2013b). Freeze drying technique for microencapsulation of *Garcinia* fruit extract and its effect on bread quality. *Journal of Food Engineering* 117: 513–520.

Fang, Z., and Bhandari, B. (2010). Encapsulation of polyphenols – a review. *Food Science and Technology* 21: 510–523.

Fang, Z. X., and Bhandari, B. (2011). Effect of spray drying and storage on the stability of bayberry polyphenols. *Food Chemistry* 129: 1139–1147.

Fernandes, I., Faria, A., Calhau, C., Freitas, V., and Mateus, N. (2014). Bioavailability of anthocyanins and derivatives. *Journal of Functional Foods* 7: 54–66.

Ferrari, C., Germer, S., Alvim, I., and Aguirre, J. (2013). Storage stability of spray-dried blackberry powder produced with maltodextrin or gum arabic. *Drying Technology: An international Journal* 31: 470–478.

Frank, K., Walz, E., Gräf, V., Greiner, R., Köhler, R., and Schuchmann, H. P. (2012). Stability of anthocyanin-rich W/O/W-emulsions designed for intestinal release in gastrointestinal environment. *Journal of Food Science* 77: 50–57.

Friberg, S., Larsson, K., and Sjoblom, J. (2004). *Food Emulsions*, 4th ed. New York: Marcel Dekker.

Gallegos-Infante, J. A., Rocha-Guzmán, N. E., González-Laredo, R. B., Medina-Torres, L., Gomez-Aldap, C. A., *et al.* (2013). Physicochemical properties and antioxidant capacity of oak *(Quercus resinosa)* leaf infusions encapsulated by spray-drying. *Food Bioscience* 2: 31–38.

García-Villalba, L., Larrosa, M., Possemiers, S., Tomás-Barberán, F. A., and Espín, J. C. (2014). Bioavailability of phenolics from an oleuropein-rich olive *(Olea europaea)* leaf extract and its acute effect on plasma antioxidant status: Comparison between pre- and postmenopausal women. *European Journal of Nutrition* 53: 1015–1027.

George, M., and Abraham, T. E. (2006). Polyionic hydrocolloids for the intestinal delivery of protein drugs: Alginate and chitosan — a review. *Journal of Controlled Release* 114: 1–14.

Germanò, M. P., D'Angelo, V., Biasini, T., Sanogo, R., De Pasquale, R., and Catania, S. (2006). Evaluation of the antioxidant properties and bioavailability of free and bound phenolic acids from *Trichilia emetica* Vahl. *Journal of Ethnopharmacology* 105: 368–373.

Gharsallaoui, A., Roudaut, G., Chambin, O., Voilley, A., and Saurel, R. (2007). Applications of spray-drying in microencapsulation of food ingredients: An overview. *Food Research International* 10: 1107–1121.

Gibis, M., Thellmann, K., Thongkaew, C., and Weiss, J. (2014). Interaction of polyphenols and multilayered liposomal-encapsulated grape seed extract with native and heat-treated proteins. *Food Hydrocolloids* 41: 119–131.

Goh, C. H., Heng, P. W. S., and Chan, L. W. (2012). Alginates as a useful natural polymer for microencapsulation and therapeutic applications. *Carbohydrate Polymers* 88: 1–12.

Gouin, S. (2004). Microencapsulation: Industrial appraisal of existing technologies and trends. *Trends in Food Science & Technology* 15: 330–347.

Gunasekaran, S., and Ko, S. (2014). Rationales of Nano- and Microencapsulation for Food Ingredients. In: *Nano- and Microencapsulation for Foods*, 1st ed., pp. 3, 43–64. H.-S. Kwak, ed. Chicester, UK: Wiley–Blackwell.

Hasan, M., Belhaj, N., Benachour, H., Barberi-Heyob, M., Kahn, C. J. F., *et al.* (2014) Liposome encapsulation of curcumin: Physico-chemical characterizations and effects on MCF7 cancer cell proliferation. *International Journal of Pharmaceutics* 461: 519–528.

Heleno, S. A., Martins, A., Queiroz, M. J. R. P., and Ferreira, I. C. F. R. (2015). Bioactivity of phenolic acids: Metabolites vs. parent compounds. *Food Chemistry* 173: 501–513.

Hole, A. S., Rud, I., Grimmer, S., Sigl, S., Narvhus, J., and Sahlstrøm, S. (2012). Improved bioavailability of dietary phenolic acids in whole grain barley and oat groat following fermentation with probiotic *Lactobacillus acidophilus, Lactobacillus johnsonii,* and *Lactobacillus reuteri. Journal of Agriculture and Food Chemistry* 60: 6369–6375.

Holst, B., and Williamson, G. (2008). Nutrients and phytochemicals: From bioavailability to bioefficacy beyond antioxidants. *Current Opinion in Biotechnology* 19: 73–82.

Jung, M. H., Seong, P. N., Kim, M. H., Myong, N., and Chang, M. (2013). Effect of green tea extract microencapsulation on hypertriglyceridemia and cardiovascular tissues in high fructose-fed rats. *Nutrition Research and Practice* 7: 366–372.

Kalogeropoulos, N., Yannakopoulou, K., Gioxari, A., Chiou, A., and Makris, D.P. (2010). Polyphenol characterization and encapsulation in β-cyclodextrin of a flavonoid-rich *Hypericum perforatum* (St John's wort) extract. *LWT – Food Science and Technology* 43: 882–889.

Ko, S., and Gunasekaran, S. (2014). Controlled Release of Food Ingredients. In: *Nano- and Microencapsulation for Foods,* 1st ed., pp. 13, 347–348. H.-S. Kwak, ed. Chicester, UK: Wiley–Blackwell.

Korsmeye, R. W., Gurny, R., Doelker, E. M., Buri, P., and Peppas, N. A. (1983). Mechanism of solute release from porous hydrophilic polymers. *International Journal of Pharmaceutics* 15: 25–35.

Kumari, A., Yadav, S. K., Pakade, Y. B., Kumar, V., Singh, B., *et al.* (2010). Nanoencapsulation and characterization of *Albizia chinensis* isolated antioxidant quercitrin on PLA nanoparticles. *Colloids and Surfaces B: Biointerfaces* 82: 224–232.

Lachman, L., Lieberman, H. A., and Kaning, J. L. (2001). *Teórica e Prática na Indústria Farmacêutica,* vols. I e II. Lisboa: Fundação Calouste Gulbenkian, pp. 707–711.

Laine, P., Kylli, P., Heinonen, M., and Jouppila, K. (2008). Storage stability of microencapsulated cloudberry *(Rubus chamaemorus)* phenolics. *Journal of Agricultural and Food Chemistry* 56: 11251–11261.

Lee, Y., Ahn, S., and Kwak, H. (2013). Optimizing microencapsulation of peanut sprout extract by response surface methodology. *Food Hydrocolloids* 30: 307–314.

Leong, S. Y., and Oey, I. (2012). Effects of processing on anthocyanins, carotenoids and vitamin C in summer fruits and vegetables. *Food Chemistry* 133: 1577–1578.

Li, Y., and McClements, D. J. (2010). New mathematical model for interpreting pH-Stat digestion profiles: Impact of lipid droplet characteristics on *in vitro* digestibility. *Journal of Agricultural and Food Chemistry* 58(13): 8085–8092.

Li, Z., Jiang, H., Xu, C., and Gu, L. (2015). A review: Using nanoparticles to enhance absorption and bioavailability of phenolic phytochemicals. *Food Hydrocolloids* 43: 153–164.

Liang, J., Li, F., Fang, Y., Yang, W., An, X., *et al.* (2011). Synthesis, characterization and cytotoxicity studies of chitosan-coated tea polyphenols nanoparticles. *Colloids and Surfaces B: Biointerfaces* 82: 297–301.

Lutz, M., Castro, E., García, L., and Henríquez, C. (2014). Bioavailability of phenolic compounds in grape juice cv. Autumn Royal. *CyTA – Journal of Food* 12: 48–54.

Madene, A., Jacquot, M., Scher, J., and Desobry, S. (2006). Flavour encapsulation and controlled release – a review. *International Journal of Food Science and Technology* 41: 1–21.

Madrigal-Carballo, S., Lim, S., Rodriguez, G., Vila, A. O., Krueger, C. G., *et al.* (2010). Biopolymer coating of soybean lecithin liposomes via layer-by-layer self-assembly as novel delivery system for ellagic acid. *Journal of Functional Foods* 2: 99–106.

Malik, P., Ameta, R. K., and Singh, M. (2014). Preparation and characterization of bionanoemulsions for improving and modulating the antioxidant efficacy of natural phenolic antioxidant curcumin. *Chemico-Biological Interactions* 222: 77–86.

Mantegna, S., Binello, A., Boffa, L., Giorgis, M., Cena, C., and Cravotto, G. (2012). A one-pot ultrasound-assisted water extraction/cyclodextrin encapsulation of resveratrol from *Polygonum cuspidatum*. *Food Chemistry* 130: 746–750.

Martínez-Huélamo, M., Tulipani, S., Estruch, R., Escribano, E., Illán, M., *et al.* (2015). The tomato sauce making process affects the bioaccessibility and bioavailability of tomato phenolics: A pharmacokinetic study. *Food Chemistry* 173: 864–872.

Martins, A., Barros, L., Carvalho, A. M., Santos-Buelga, C., Fernandes, I. P., *et al.* (2014). Phenolic extracts of *Rubus ulmifolius* Schott flowers: Characterization, microencapsulation and incorporation into yogurts as nutraceutical sources. *Food & Function* 5: 1091–1100.

Martins, N., Barros, L., Henriques, M., Silva, S., and Ferreira, I. C. F. R. (2015). Activity of phenolic compounds from plant origin against *Candida* species. *Industrial Crops and Products* 74: 648–670.

McClements, D. J. (2005). *Food Emulsions: Principles, Practice, and Techniques*, 2nd ed. Boca Raton: CRC Press.

Medina-Torres, L., García-Cruz, E.E., Calderas, F., Laredo, R. F. G., Sánchez-Olivares, G., *et al.* (2013). Microencapsulation by spray drying of gallic acid with nopal mucilage *(Opuntia ficus indica)*. *LWT – Food Science and Technology* 50: 642–650.

Munin, A., and Edwards-Lévy, F. (2011). Encapsulation of natural polyphenolic compounds: A review. *Pharmaceutics* 3: 793–829.

Murugesan, R., and Orsat, V. (2012). Spray drying for the production of nutraceutical ingredients – A review. *Food Bioprocess Technology* 5: 3–14.

Nayak, C. A., and Rastogi, N. K. (2010). Effect of selected additives on microencapsulation of anthocyanin by spray drying. *Drying Technology* 28: 1396–1404.

Nedovic, V., Kalusevic, A., Manojlovic, V. Levic, S., and Bugarski, B. (2011). An overview of encapsulation technologies for food applications. *Procedia Food Science* 1: 1806–1815.

Nguyen M.-H., Aripin, N. F. K., Chen, X. G., and Park H.-J. (2014). Methodologies Used for the Characterization of Nano- and Microcapsules. In: *Nano- and Microencapsulation for Foods*, 1st ed., pp. 4, 65–88. H.-S. Kwak, ed. Chicester, UK: Wiley–Blackwell.

Nuppor, S., and Rathore, K. S. (2012). A review on microencapsulation: A new multiutility advanced technology. *International Journal of Advanced Research in Pharmaceutical & Bio Science* 1: 477–489.

Osorio, C., Acevedo, B., Hillebrand, S., Carriazo, J., Winterhalter, P., and Morales, A. L. (2012). Microencapsulation by spray-drying of anthocyanin pigments from corozo *(Bactris guineensis)* fruit. *Journal of Agriculture and Food Chemistry* 58: 6977–6985.

Pan, Y., Tikekar, R. V., Wang, M. S., Avena-Bustillos, R. J., and Nitin, N. (2015). Effect of barrier properties of zein colloidal particles and oil-in-water emulsions on oxidative stability of encapsulated bioactive compounds. *Food Hydrocolloids* 43: 82–90.

Pang, S. F., Yusoff, M. M., and Gimbun, J. (2014). Assessment of phenolic compounds stability and retention during spray drying of *Orthosiphon stamineus* extracts. *Food Hydrocolloids* 37: 159–165.

Park, K. M., Sung, H., Choi, S. J., Choi, Y. J., and Chang, P. (2014). Double-layered microparticles with enzyme-triggered release for the targeted delivery of water-soluble bioactive compounds to small intestine. *Food Chemistry* 161: 53–59.

Patras, A., Brunton, N. P., O'Donnell, C., and Tiwari, B. K. (2010). Effect of thermal processing on anthocyanin stability in foods; mechanisms and kinetics of degradation. *Trends in Food Science & Technology* 21: 3–11.

Pérez-Jiménez, J., Serrano, J., Tabernero, M., Arranz, S., Díaz-Rubio, M.E., *et al.* (2009). Bioavailability of phenolic antioxidants associated with dietary fiber: Plasma antioxidant capacity after acute and long-term intake in humans. *Plant Foods for Human Nutrition* 64: 102–107.

Pillai, D. S., Prabhasankar, B., and Jena, B. S., Anandharamakrishnan, C. (2012). Microencapsulation of garcinia cowa fruit extract and effect of its use on pasta process and quality. *International Journal of Food Properties* 15: 590–604.

Prasertmanakit, S., Praphairaksit, N., Chiangthong, W., and Muangsin, N. (2009). Ethyl cellulose microcapsules for protecting and controlled release of folic acid. *AAPS PharmSciTech* 10: 1104–1112.

Rasti, B., Jinap, S., Mozafari, M. R., and Yazid, A. M. (2012). Comparative study of the oxidative and physical stability of liposomal and nanoliposomal polyunsaturated fatty acids prepared with conventional and Mozafari methods. *Food Chemistry* 135: 2761–2770.

Ré, M. I. (1998). Microencapsulation by spray drying. *Drying Technology: An International Journal* 16(6): 1195–1236.

Risch, S. J., and Reineccius, G. A. (1995). Controlled release techniques in the food industry. In: *Encapsulation and Controlled Release of Food Ingredients*. G.A. Reineccius, ed. Washington, DC: American Chemical Society.

Robert, P., García, P., Reyes, N., Chávez, J., and Santos, J. (2012). Acetylated starch and inulin as encapsulating agents of gallic acid and their release behaviour in a hydrophilic system. *Food Chemistry* 134: 1–8.

Robert, P., Gorena, T., Romero, N., Sepulveda, E., Chavez, J., and Saenz C. (2010). Encapsulation of polyphenols and anthocyanins from pomegranate *(Punica granatum)* by spray drying. *International Journal of Food Science and Technology* 45: 1386–1394.

Rocha-Guzmán, N. E., Gallegos-Infante, J. A., González-Laredo, R. A., Harte, F., Medina-Torres, L., *et al.* (2010). Effect of high-pressure homogenization on the physical and antioxidant properties of *Quercus resinosa* infusions encapsulated by spray-drying. *Journal of Food Science* 75: 57–61.

Rosa, C. G., Borges, C. D., Zambiazi, R. C., Nunes, M. R., Benvenutti, E. V., *et al.* (2013). Microencapsulation of gallic acid in chitosan, β-cyclodextrin and xanthan. *Industrial Crops and Products* 46: 138–146.

Rosenberg, I. M. (2005). Getting Started with Protein Purification. In: *Protein Analysis and Purification: Benchtop Techniques*, 2nd edn, pp. 118–152. Boston: Birkhauser.

Rubió, L., Macià, A., Castell-Auví, A., Pinent, M., Blay, M. T., *et al.* (2014). Effect of the co-occurring olive oil and thyme extracts on the phenolic bioaccesibility and bioavailability assessed by *in vitro* digestion and cell models. *Food Chemistry* 149: 277–284.

Saénz, C., Tapia, S., Chávez, J., and Robert, P. (2009). Microencapsulation by spray drying of bioactive compounds from cactus pear *(Opuntia ficus-indica)*. *Food Chemistry* 144: 616–622.

Sanchez, V., Baeza, R., Galmarini, M. V., Zamora, M. C., and Chirife, J. (2011). Freeze-drying encapsulation of red wine polyphenols in an amorphous matrix of maltodextrin. *Food Bioprocess Technology* doi:10.1007/s11947-011-0654-z

Sansone, F., Picerno, P., Mencherini, T., Porta, A., Lauro, M. R., *et al.* (2014). Technological properties and enhancement of antifungal activity of a *Paeonia rockii* extract encapsulated in a chitosan-based matrix. *Journal of Food Engineering* 120: 260–267.

Sansone, F., Picerno, P., Mencherini, T., Villecco, F., D'Ursi, A. M., *et al.* (2011a). Flavonoid microparticles by spray-drying: Influence of enhancers of the dissolution rate on properties and stability. *Journal of Food Engineering* 103: 188–196.

Santos, D. T., Albarelli, J. Q., Beppu, M. M., and Angela, M. (2013). Stabilization of anthocyanin extract from jabuticaba skins by encapsulation using supercritical CO_2 as solvent. *Food Research International* 50: 617–624.

Santos-Buelga, C., Gonzalez-Manzano, S., Dueñas, M., and Gonzalez-Paramas, A. M. (2012). Extraction and Isolation of Phenolic Compounds. In: *Natural Products Isolation* (Methods in Molecular Biology). S. D. Sarkar and L. Nahar, eds. Totowa, NJ: Humana Press.

Seok, J. S., Kim, J. S., and Kwak, H. S. (2003). Microencapsulation of water-soluble isoflavone and physico-chemical property in milk. *Archives of Pharmacal Research* 26: 426–431.

Siepmann, J., and Siegel, R. A. (2012). Overview of controlled release mechanism. In: *Fundamentals and Applications of Controlled Release Drug Delivery*. M. J. Rothbone, ed. New York: Springer.

Silva, P. I., Stringheta, P. C., Teófilo, R. F., and Oliveira, I. R. N. (2013). Parameter optimization for spray-drying microencapsulation of jaboticaba *(Myrciaria jaboticaba)* peel extracts using simultaneous analysis of responses. *Journal of Food Engineering* 117: 538–544.

Sousdaleff, M., Baesso, M., Neto, A., Nogueira, A., Marcolino, V., and Matioli, G. (2013). Microencapsulation by freeze-drying of potassium norbixinate and curcumin with maltodextrin: stability, solubility, and food apllication. *Journal of Agricultural and Food Chemistry* 61: 955–965.

Souza, J. R. R., Feitosa, J. P. A., Ricardo, N. P. S., Trevisan, M. T. S., Paula, H. C. B., *et al.* (2013). Spray-drying encapsulation of mangiferin using natural polymers. *Food Hydrocolloids* 33: 10–18.

Stalmach, A., Edwards, C. A., Wightman, J. D., and Crozier, A. (2012). Gastrointestinal stability and bioavailability of (poly)phenolic compounds following ingestion of Concord grape juice by humans. *Molecular Nutrition & Food Research* 56: 497–509.

Suave, J., Dall'agnol, E. C., Pezzin, A. P. T., Silva, D. A. K., Meier, M. M., and Soldi, V. (2006). Microencapsulação: Inovação em diferentes areas. *Health and Environment Journal* 7: 12–20.

Sun-Waterhouse, D., Wadhwa, S. S., and Waterhouse, G. I. N. (2013). Spray-drying microencapsulation of polyphenol bioactives: A comparative study using different natural fibre polymers as encapsulants. *Food and Bioprocess Technology* 6: 2376–2388.

Tavano, L., Muzzalupo, R., Picci, N., and Cindio, B. (2014). Co-encapsulation of antioxidants into niosomal carriers: Gastrointestinal release studies for nutraceutical applications. *Colloids and Surfaces B: Biointerfaces* 114: 82–88.

Tonon, R. V., Brabet, C., and Hubinger, M. D. (2010). Anthocyanin stability and antioxidant activity of spray-dried açai (*Euterpe oleracea* Mart.) juice produced with different carrier agents. *Food Research International* 43: 907–914.

Uhrich, K. E., Cannizzaro, S. M., Langer, R. S., and Shakesheff, K. M. (1999). Polymeric systems for controlled drug release. *Chemical Reviews* 99: 3181–3198.

Vidal, J. L., Avello, L. M., Loyola C. C., Campos P. J., Aqueveque M. P., *et al.* (2012). Microencapsulation of maqui (*Aristotelia chilensis* [Molina] Stuntz) leaf extracts to preserve and control antioxidant properties. *Chilean Journal of Agricultural Research* 73: 17–23.

Visentin, A., Rodríguez-Rojo, S., Navarrete, A., Maestri, D., and Cocero, M.J. (2012). Precipitation and encapsulation of rosemary antioxidants by supercritical antisolvent process. *Journal of Food Engineering* 109: 9–15.

Vitaglione, P., Lumaga, R. B., Ferracane, R., Sellitto, S., Morelló, J. R., *et al.* (2013). Human bioavailability of flavanols and phenolic acids from cocoa-nut creams enriched with free or microencapsulated cocoa polyphenols. *British Journal of Nutrition* 109: 1832–1843

Wang, T., He, F., and Chen, G. (2014). Improving bioaccessibility and bioavailability of phenolic compounds in cereal grains through processing technologies: A concise review. *Journal of Functional Foods* 7: 101–111.

Wichchukit, S., Oztop, M. H., McCarthy, M. J., and McCarthy, K. L. (2013). Whey protein/alginate beads as carriers of a bioactive component. *Food Hydrocolloids* 33: 66–73.

Wise, D. L. (2000). Drug Release from the Swelling-Controlled System. In: *Handbook of Pharmaceutical Controlled Release Technology*, vol. 1. Boca Raton, FL: CRC Press.

Wu, B., Kulkarni, K., Basu, S., Zhang, S., and Hu, M. (2011). First-pass metabolism via UDP-glucuronosyltransferase: A barrier to oral bioavailability of phenolics. *Journal of Pharmaceutical Sciences* 100: 3655–3681

Wu, T., Yen, F., Lin, L., Tsai, T., Lin, C., and Cham, T. (2008) Preparation, physicochemical characterization, and antioxidant effects of quercetin nanoparticles. *International Journal of Pharmaceutics* 346: 160–168.

Zeisig, R., and Cämmerer, B. (2001). Liposomes in the food industry. In *Microencapsulation of Food Ingredients*, pp. 101–119. P. Vilstrup, ed. London: Leatherhead Publishing.

Zhang, H., Zheng, J., Liu, X., Ding, Q., Jiang, L., *et al.* (2012). Milk protein and fat play different roles in affecting the bioavailability and the antioxidant activity of jujube juice phenolics in rats. *Molecular Nutrition & Food Research* 56: 1511–1519.

Zhao, M., Wang, H., Yang, B., and Tao, H. (2010). Identification of cyclodextrin inclusion complex of chlorogenic acid and its antimicrobial activity. *Food Chemistry* 120: 1138–1142

Zheng, L., Ding, Z., Zhang, M., and Sun, J. (2011). Microencapsulation of bayberry polyphenols by ethyl cellulose: Preparation and characterization. *Journal of Food Engineering* 104: 89–95.

Zuidam, N. J., VanWinden, E., De Vrueh, R., and Crommelin, D. J. A. (2003). Stability, Storage and Sterilization of Liposomes. In: *Liposomes*, pp. 149–165. V. P. Torchilin and V. Weissig, eds. Oxford: Oxford University Press.

CHAPTER 7

Fortification of dairy products by microcapsules of polyphenols extracted from pomegranate peels

Wissam Zam

Department of Analytical and Food Chemistry, Faculty of Pharmacy, Al-Andalus University for Medical Sciences, Tartus, Al Qadmus P.O. Box 101, Syrian Arab Republic

7.1 Extraction procedure

The extraction of compounds from plant materials is the first step in using phytochemicals to prepare dietary supplements or nutraceuticals, food ingredients, pharmaceuticals, and cosmetic products (Dai and Mumper, 2010). Solvent extractions are the most commonly used procedures to extract phenolic compounds from their plant sources and to liberate theme from the vacuolar structures where they are found due to their ease of use, efficiency, and wide applicability (Escribano-Bailon and Santos-Buelga, 2003). It is generally known that the yield of chemical extraction depends on the type of solvents with varying polarities, extraction time, and temperature, as well as on the chemical composition and physical characteristics of the samples.

An efficient method for extracting polyphenols from pomegranate peel was performed: 20 g of dried and ground peel were placed in a thermostatic water bath shaker with 1000 ml of deionized (DI) water at 50 °C for 20 minutes. The liquid extract was separated from solids by centrifugation at 2000 rpm for 10 minutes. The supernatant was transferred to a 1000-mL flask, and DI water was added to make the final volume 1000 mL. The stability of polyphenols in the extract can be maintained for more than 2 weeks by storing the extract in freezer.

7.1.1 Determining total polyphenol content

The total polyphenol content in the extract was determined by the Folin–Ciocalteu method according to the method described by the International Organization for Standardization (2005). In this determination, 250 μL of the extract was diluted with distilled water to 10 mL. Aliquots of 1 mL of samples

New Polymers for Encapsulation of Nutraceutical Compounds, First Edition.
Edited by Jorge Carlos Ruiz Ruiz and Maira Rubi Segura Campos.

were mixed with 5 mL of 10-fold-diluted Folin–Ciocalteu reagent. After 3 minutes, 4 mL of 7.5% sodium carbonate was added (Zahin *et al.*, 2009). The mixtures were allowed to stand for 30 minutes at 40° C temperature (water bath) before the absorbance was measured at 734 nm. The total polyphenol content in the extract was calculated and expressed as gallic acid equivalents (GAE; g/100 g dry mass) using a gallic acid (0–120 mg/L) standard curve.

The total polyphenol yield after five successive extraction was 21.79 ± 1.28% of dry matter.

7.1.2 DPPH radical-scavenging activity

The antioxidant activity of different extracts was measured in term of hydrogen-donating or radical-scavenging ability using the stable DPPH method according to the method proposed by Brand-Williams and colleagues (1995). For this measurement, 250 μL of the extract was diluted with distilled water to 10 mL. Aliquots of 200 μL of samples were mixed with 2 mL of 100 μM DPPH methanolic solution. The mixture was placed in the dark at room temperature for 60 minutes. The absorbance of the resulting solution was then read at 520 nm. The antiradical activity was expressed in terms of the percentage reduction of the DPPH. The ability to scavenge the DPPH radical was calculated using the following equation:

$$\text{DPPH scavenging effect}(\%) = \left[\left(A_0 - A_1\right) / A_0\right] * 100 \tag{7.1}$$

Where A_0 is the absorbance of the control at 60 minutes and A_1 is the absorbance of the sample at 60 minutes (Kim *et al.*, 2010).

The extract was able to scavenge 82.53 ± 3.57% of the DPPH solution.

7.2 Formulation of pomegranate peels' polyphenol microbeads and their *in vitro* release

Many factors affect the stability of polyphenols during processing and storage. These compounds are very sensitive to oxygen, light, acid, and alkali, but they are relatively less sensitive to heat. Microencapsulation is an economical method for preserving natural antioxidants by entrapping the ingredients in a coating material. Sodium alginate and pectin are of the most important carrier and coating agents used for encapsulating water-soluble drugs, so it is important to evaluate the encapsulation of polyphenols in these materials. The ionic gelation process, one of the physicochemical methods used in microencapsulation, consists of extruding an aqueous solution of polymer through a syringe needle or a nozzle, in which the active material is dissolved or dispersed. Droplets are received in a dispersant phase and are transformed, after reaction, into spherical gel particles (Vandamme *et al.*, 2007).

Alginate is a linear unbranched polysaccharide composed of varying proportion of 1,4- linked β-D mannuronic acid (M) and α-L glucuronic acid (G) residues. Alginate has a unique gel-forming property in the presence of multivalent cations, such as calcium ions in an aqueous medium, which takes place mainly at junctions in the G-G sequence–rich chain region known as *egg box junctions* (Khazaeli *et al.*, 2008). Varying proportions of pectin were used in the formulations with alginate.

Pectin is a heterogeneous anionic polysaccharide present in the cell wall of most plants. It is nontoxic, almost totally degraded by colonic bacteria, and not digested by gastric enzymes. Pectin forms water-insoluble complexes with several drugs and may be a useful additive for sustained-release preparations (Aydin and Akbuga, 1996). The low-methoxy polysaccharide, pectin with the degree of esterification less than 50%, can form rigid gels by the action of calcium ions that cross-link the galacturonic acid chains of pectin to yield hydrogels that are stable at low pH (Mishra and Pathak, 2008).

The main objective is to formulate polyphenols in sodium alginate or/and pectin beads to protect them from degradation. The effect of some formulation parameters on polyphenol loading efficiency and the use of pectin and sodium alginate combination was investigated. The *in vitro* release studies of alginate gel beads was evaluated in both simulated gastric fluid (SGF) and simulated intestinal fluid (SIF).

7.2.1 Capsule formulation

Beads were obtained by mixing 10 mL of the active component with 10 mL of the sodium alginate solution at the best concentration. Once the mixture was homogenized, 10 mL of calcium chloride solution at the best concentration was added to the alginate solution and was cured for different durations to optimize curing time at 25 °C. The beads formed in this process were maintained in the gelling bath to harden. Then they were centrifuged at 4000 rpm and 4 °C for 15 minutes (Anbinder *et al.*, 2011).

7.2.2 Loading efficiency

The amount of lyophilized extract loaded in beads was estimated ,as described by Deladino and colleagues (2007) by dissolving the capsules obtained from 10 mL extract in sodium citrate (10% w/v) during 20 minutes for alginate capsules in a shaker at 37 °C and 125 rpm. The concentrations of lyophilized extract loaded in the beads were determined by Folin–Ciocalteu and butanol assay method. A blank of sodium citrate was also performed. The percentage of loading efficiency was calculated with the following equation:

$$\text{Loading efficiency}(\%) = (L / L_0) * 100 \tag{7.2}$$

where L is the amount of extract determined on the solution of sodium citrate and L_0 is the initial amount of extract dissolved in the alginate solution (Deladino *et al.*, 2007).

7.2.3 Optimization of loading efficiency

7.2.3.1 Sodium alginate concentration

The formulation of the calcium alginate beads is based on both the concentration of sodium alginate and on the ability of calcium ions to cross-link with sodium alginate. The degree of cross-linking is dependent on both the concentration of the calcium chloride solution and the time of contact of the beads with this solution. To optimize the parameters affecting the formulation of beads, various factors were evaluated: sodium alginate concentration (1–4.5%), calcium chloride concentration (0.01–0.1 M), calcium chloride exposure time (5–60 min), and gelling bath time maintaining (5–60 min).

Results obtained showed that increasing sodium alginate concentration from 1% to 3% elevated loading efficiency from approximately 8% to 33% (Figure 7.1). As reported by El-Kamel and colleagues (2003), this may be attributed to the greater availability of active calcium-binding sites in the polymeric chains and, consequently, the greater degree of cross–linking as the quantity of sodium alginate increased.

Higher concentration of sodium alginate is accompanied by increase in viscosity and decrease in loading efficiency.

7.2.3.2 Calcium chloride concentration

Alginate solution droplets in this experiment are gelled by contact with calcium chloride solution droplets. The concentration of calcium chloride has an important influence on the characteristics of the resulting alginate beads.

Results obtained showed that increasing calcium chloride concentration from 0.01 M to 0.05 M elevated loading efficiency from approximately 20% to 34% (Figure 7.2). This may be explained by the increase in the gel strength as the calcium ions increased. These results are in agreement with Takka and colleagues (1999) and Mirghani and colleagues (2000).

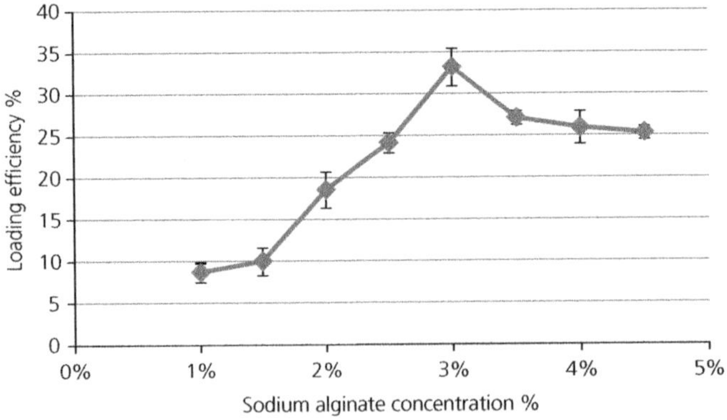

Figure 7.1 Effect of sodium alginate concentration on total extractable polyphenol loading efficiency. Values are mean ± SDs, ($n=3$).

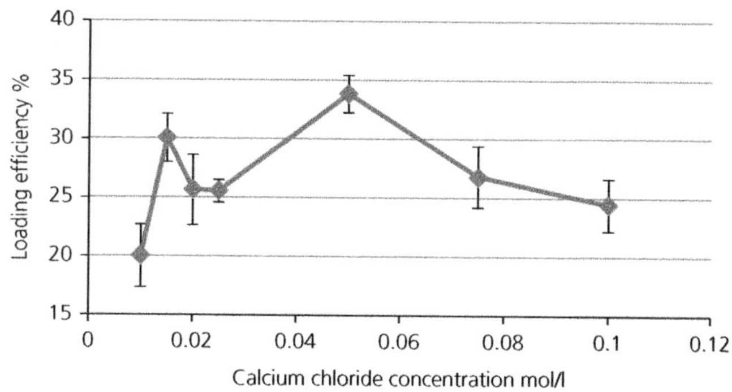

Figure 7.2 Effect of calcium chloride concentration on total extractable polyphenol loading efficiency. Values are mean ± SD, (n=3).

The loading efficiency was found to decrease at concentrations of more than 0.05 M, which may indicate damage of microcapsules due to possible saturation of calcium-binding sites in the glucuronic acid chain, preventing further calcium ion entrapment as reported by Ostberg's group (1994) or osmotic stress as reported by Takayuki and colleagues (2009). Based on these results, we adopted a concentration of 0.05 M in subsequent experiments.

7.2.3.3 Calcium chloride exposure time

When calcium and alginate solutions come in contact, a gel is formed immediately at the interface; thus matrix homogeneity depends on the calcium diffusion through the gel network. Continuous exposure of the alginate to the calcium solution will increase the firmness of the gel, as more calcium diffuses into the gel and binds to the G blocks within the alginate structure (Lamkey, 2009). Diffusion of calcium chloride toward the bead core, at 5, 10, 15, 20, 25, 30, 45, and 60 minutes, was examined, and loading efficiency values were demonstrated as shown in Figure 7.3.

Thus, 20 minutes in air was enough to get the best loading efficiency for the total extractable polyphenols. Patel and colleagues (2006) showed that the loading efficiency of calcium alginate beads containing metronidazole decreased with increase in curing time. The explanation for this could be that longer times could cause the shift of the bounded calcium ions by alginate as reported by Deladino and colleagues (2007), or it may be due to the increased release of polyphenols from the matrix as reported by El-Kamel and coworkers (2003).

7.2.3.4 Gelling bath time

The beads formed were maintained in the gelling bath to harden for different times (5–60 min).

Results obtained showed that increasing maintaining time from 5 minutes to 15 minutes elevated loading efficiency from approximately 28% to 37% (Figure 7.4). This may be explained by the increase in the gel strength as the time increased.

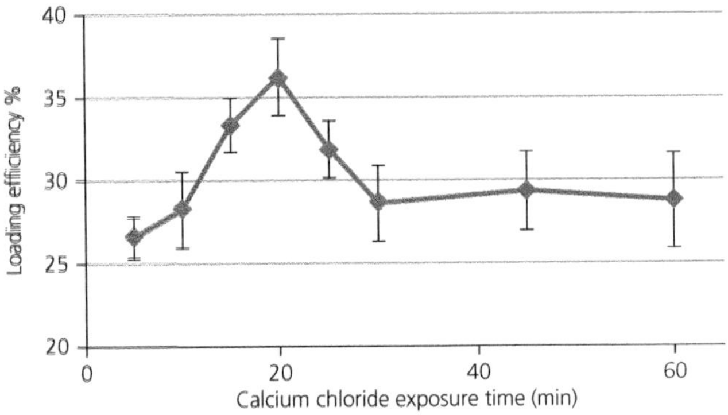

Figure 7.3 Effect of calcium chloride exposure time on total extractable polyphenol loading efficiency. Values are mean ± SD, (n=3).

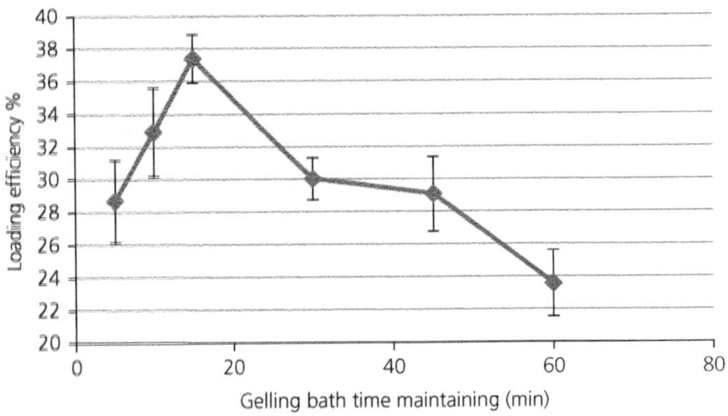

Figure 7.4 Effect of gelling bath time on total extractable polyphenol loading efficiency. Values are mean ± SD, (n=3).

Results also showed that the loading efficiency of calcium alginate beads decreased with an increase in maintaining time in the gelling bath. The explanation for this could be that longer times could increase the release of polyphenols from the matrix. These results are in agreement with those of Anbinder's group (2011).

7.2.4 Preparation of beads with sodium alginate and pectin blend

Beads were obtained by mixing 10 mL of the active component with 10 mL solution containing a combinations of sodium alginate and pectin sodium alginate (1:2, 1:1, 2:1). Once the mixture was homogenized, 10 mL of calcium chloride solution 0.05 M was added to the solution and was cured for 20 minutes at 25 °C.

Table 7.1 Effect of copolymer combination on the loading efficiency of extracted polyphenols.

Ratio of Sodium Alginate to Pectin	Loading Efficiency of Polyphenols (%)*
0:3	34.97 ± 0.011
1:2	35.23 ± 0.007
1:1	37.78 ± 0.012
2:1	50.20 ± 0.010
3:0	43.92 ± 0.006

*Values are mean ± standard deviation ($n = 3$).

The beads formed in this process were maintained in the gelling bath to harden for 15 minutes. Then they were centrifuged at 4,000 rpm and 4 °C for 15 minutes.

Gelation occurred due to intermolecular cross-linking between the divalent calcium ions and the negatively charged carboxyl groups of pectin and sodium alginate molecules.

Our results, presented in Table 7.1, indicate that the loading efficiency was less when the beads were prepared with a single type of polymer, in comparison with the beads prepared with two types of polymers (sodium alginate and pectin). These results are in agreement with those of Dahiya and Tyagi (2008). This might be due to the presence of two types of protective layers in beads, one of calcium pectinate, which prevented the diffusion of polyphenols more effectively than a single type of layer only.

Another factor that affected the loading efficiency is the alginate pectin ratio. As the proportion of alginate was reduced, the polyphenol content started to reduce. These results were in agreement with those of Jaiswal and colleagues (2009) and Danish and colleagues (2011). It can be explained that in combination of two layers, the calcium alginate layer was more effective in preventing diffusion of polyphenols than the calcium pectinate layer, but there was an optimum ratio of these two polymers (sodium alginate to pectin: 2:1), which was responsible for the maximum loading efficiency.

7.2.5 *In vitro* dissolution studies

The ability of the prepared microcapsules to release the polyphenols in the physiological environment of the stomach and the small intestine was assessed by conducting release studies in simulated stomach and small intestinal pH, respectively. Dissolution test was conducted in duplicate using USP dissolution apparatus (paddle method) at 75 rpm and 37 ± 0.5 °C.

The beads prepared from 100 mL pomegranate peel extract were placed in the basket. Initial release studies were conducted in 150 mL of 0.1 N HCl (pH 1.2)

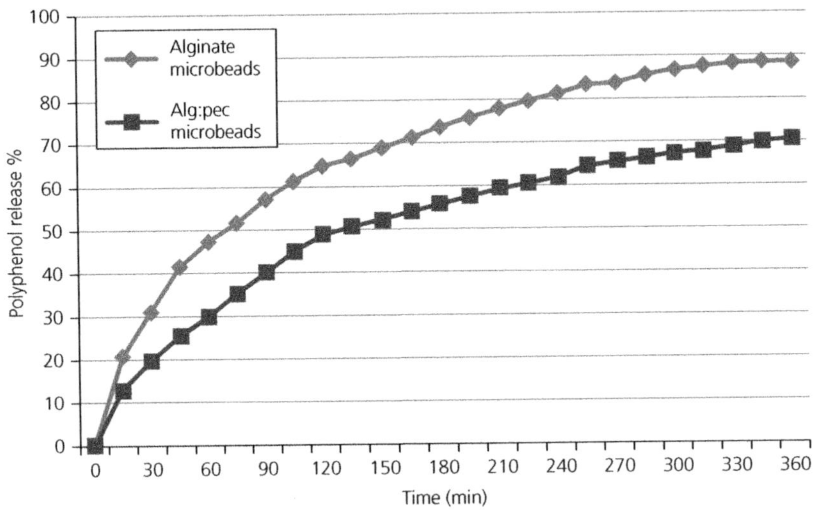

Figure 7.5 Dissolution profile of polyphenols from sodium alginate and pectin–sodium alginate microbeads.

as simulated gastric fluid (SGF) for 2 hours. After this, 50 mL of 0.2 M trisodium phosphate was added to the dissolution media as simulated intestinal fluid (SIF) and the pH was adjusted to 6.8; the study at a pH of 6.8 was continued for 4 hours. Samples were withdrawn at specified time intervals, and volume was replaced immediately with an equal amount of fresh medium. Samples were suitably diluted, and polyphenol release was analyzed using the Folin–Ciocalteu method.

The polyphenol release pattern was affected by the nature of the polymer as shown in (Figure 7.5. In both cases there was an initial burst release. This may be due to the water-soluble nature of polyphenols. It may also be possible that polyphenol particles were dragged on the surface of the beads during curing in aqueous surrounding medium, which resulted in initial burst release.

The release pattern of polyphenol from microbeads prepared with a combination of polymers (sodium alginate and pectin) was entirely different from that prepared with a single polymer (sodium alginate). The release of polyphenol from calcium alginate microbeads was found to be 64.87% ± 0.05% in pH 1.2 within 2 hours. After 2 hours, the calcium alginate microbeads disintegrated and lost remaining polyphenol within 3 hours in the SIF dissolution medium (pH 6.8). With the addition of pectin with sodium alginate, the release of entrapped polyphenol during first 2 hours in SGF was significantly reduced. Only 48.81% ± 0.06% of polyphenol was released in pH 1.2 within 2 hours. This was expected, because interaction between two polymers had occurred, forming a closer network, which decreased the diffusion of polyphenols outward from the interiors of the microbeads.

7.3 Fortification of dairy products with polyphenol microcapsules

Functional foods provide health benefits in addition to normal nutrition (Mollet and Lacroix, 2007). They must generally be made available to consumers in forms that are consumed within the usual daily dietary pattern of the target population group. Consumers expect functional foods to have good organoleptic qualities and to be of similar qualities to the traditional foods in the market (Klahorst, 2006).

Functional dairy products account for 42.9% of the functional food market (Watson *et al.*, 2003). Dairy products have been the most popular delivery vehicles for a number of functional and healthy ingredients, from vitamin and mineral fortification to addition of bioactives to promote health benefits. Because milk and dairy products are a normal part of our daily diet, in all life stages, any new product launched can be expected to gain some market share.

Although some reports on milk enriched with polyphenols can be found in the literature (Axten *et al.*, 2008; Servili *et al.*, 2011), there is to our knowledge none developed using polyphenols extracted from pomegranate peels. These peels are usually discarded as waste even though a significant portion of polyphenols are often present in high concentrations in the outer parts of fruits. In addition, it has been considered that no less than 1 to 2 g of polyphenols should be consumed daily to produce their health benefits such as the prevention of cardiovascular disease, cancer, osteoporosis, diabetes mellitus, arthritis, and neurodegenerative diseases, which are associated with oxidative stress and chronic inflammation (Cicerale *et al.*, 2012; Williamson and Manach, (2005). An average diet cannot provide this quantity of polyphenols (Cieslik *et al.*, 2006).

In light of this, the aim of our research was the development of a new milk product fortified with natural polyphenols extracted from pomegranate peels and microencapsulated by ionic gelation using sodium alginate or a combination of sodium alginate and pectin (2:1).

Three different milk beverages fortified with 150 mg of polyphenols per serving (250 mL) were prepared. The first beverage was prepared by adding 200 mL of aqueous extract to 800 mL of milk (sample 1). The second was prepared by suspending microbeads of polyphenols prepared with sodium alginate (sample 2), and the last one was prepared by suspending microbeads prepared with a combination of sodium alginate and pectin (sample 3).

All beverages were kept in the refrigerator, and the shelf-life of milk beverages in terms of polyphenol content and radical scavenging activity quality was studied.

7.3.1 Shelf life of milk beverages

There has been evidence that polyphenols possess a high binding affinity for proteins (Papadopoulou and Frazier, 2004; Siebert *et al.*, 1996), particularly proline-rich proteins such as caseins (Luck *et al.*, 1994). This affinity is strongly influenced by the structural differences of dietary polyphenols (Xiao *et al.*, 2011).

Results demonstrated in Figure 7.6 were in agreement with this evidence, as polyphenol content rapidly decreased in milk fortified with the direct addition of pomegranate peel aqueous extract. After 2 days of storage, 49.37% of polyphenols remained stable in fortified milk, and only 5.47% of polyphenol remained after 11 days of storage.

As shown in Figure 7.7 and Figure 7.8, the addition of polyphenol microbeads was more effective for the fortification of milk beverages compared with the addition of pomegranate peels aqueous extract.

Results also indicated that the stability of microbeads was less when prepared with a single type of polymer, in comparison of the beads prepared with two types of polymers (sodium alginate and pectin). Only 38.13% of polyphenols remained stable in sample 2, whereas 62.23% of polyphenols remained stable in sample 3, after 11 days of cold storage. This is due to the presence of two types of protective layers in beads, one of calcium pectinate and other one of calcium alginate, which prevented the diffusion of polyphenols more effectively than a single type of layer only.

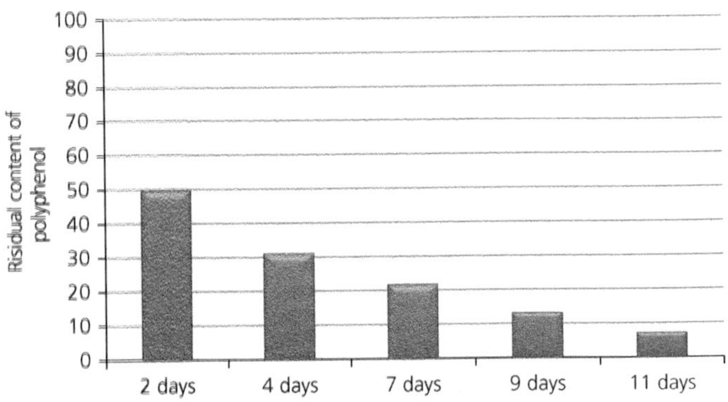

Figure 7.6 Residual content of polyphenols in milk beverage (sample 1).

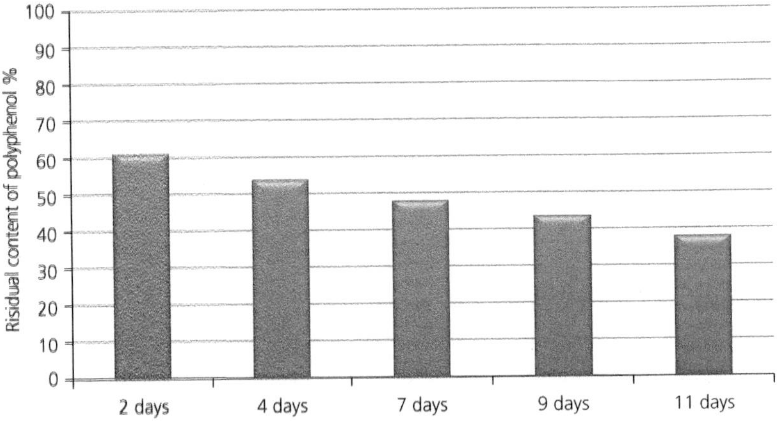

Figure 7.7 Residual content of polyphenols in milk beverage (sample 2).

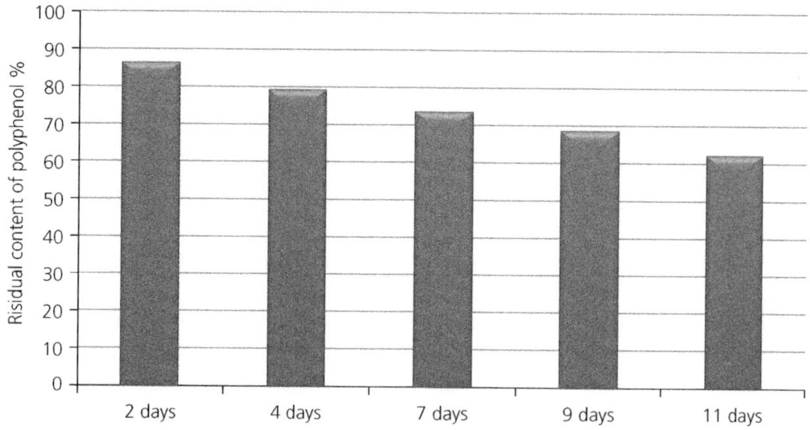

Figure 7.8 Residual content of polyphenols in milk beverage (sample 3).

Table 7.2 Antioxidant activity of the extract and the fortified milk (sample 3) before and after digestion.

Sample	Antioxidant activity (%)
Extract	58.48
Milk + extract	27.67
Milk + extract after digestion	40.56

7.3.2 *In vitro* digestibility assay

The method consists of a pepsin/HCl digestion with shaking to simulate gastric conditions. In this assay, 315 units per mL of pepsin was added to the fortified milk (sample 3), and then the pH was adjusted to 1.7 with HCl (Mollet and Lacroix, 2007). The digestion was carried out for 2 hours at 37 °C with shaking. After the 2 hours, the antioxidant activity of the mixture was quantified.

As shown in Table 7.2, the antioxidant activity of polyphenols decreased directly from 58.48% to 27.67% after being mixed with the milk sample. After digestion, the antioxidant activity raised again to 40.56%, which could be attributed to the partial degradation of complex and the release of polyphenols.

From Table 7.2 it is possible to observe that after digestion the antioxidant activity of polyphenols is less than its activity initially present in the extract. This means that some complexes formed are more resistant to the digestion conditions performed in this study. Soares and colleagues (2015) have already demonstrated that complexes formed with the lowest polymerized tannins (monomers, dimers and trimers) could be disrupted by gastric digestion, leading to the release of tannins, whereas the complexes formed by tannin tetramers and pentamers were significantly more resistant to stomach conditions (Soares *et al.*, 2015). These results could explain the findings of our study.

References

Anbinder, P. S., Deladino, L., Navarro, A. S., Amalvy, J. I., and Martino, M. N. (2011). Yerba mate extract encapsulation with alginate and chitosan systems: Interactions between active compound encapsulation polymers. *Journal of Encapsulation and Adsorption Sciences* 1: 80–87.

Axten, L. G., Wohlers, M. W., and Wegrzyn, T. (2008). Using phytochemicals to enhance health benefits of milk: Impact of polyphenols on flavor profile. *Journal of Food Science* 73(6): H122–H126.

Aydin, Z., and Akbuga, J. (1996). Preparation and evaluation of pectin beads. *International Journal of Pharmaceutics* 137: 133–136.

Brand-Williams, W., Cuvelier, M. E., and Berset, C. (1995). Use of a free radical method to evaluate antioxidant activity. *LWT – Food Science and Technology* 28(1): 25–30.

Cicerale, S., Lucas, L. J., and Keast, R. S. J. (2012). Antimicrobial, antioxidant and anti-inflammatory phenolic activities in extra virgin olive oil. *Current Opinion in Biotechnology* 23: 129–135.

Cieslik, E., Greda, A., and Adamus, W. (2006). Contents of polyphenols in fruit and vegetables. *Food Chemistry* 94: 135–142.

Dahiya, S., and Tyagi, L. (2008). Preparation and evaluation of oxytetracycline of hydrochloride microbeads for delayed release. *Pakistan Journal of Pharmaceutical Science* 21(2): 103–108.

Dai, J., and Mumper, R. J. (2010). Plant phenolics: extraction, analysis and their antioxidant and anticancer properties. *Molecules* 15: 7313–7352.

Danish Khan, A., and Bajpai, M. (2011). Formulation and evaluation of floating beads of verapamil hydrochloride. *International Journal of PharmTech Research* 3(3): 1537–1546.

Deladino, L., Anbinder, P. S., Navarro, A. S., and Martino, M. N. (2007). Encapsulation of natural antioxidants extracted from *Ilex paraguariensis*. Carbohydrate Polymers 71(1): 126–134.

El-Kamel, A. H., Al-Gohary, O. M. N., and Hosny, E. A. (2003). Alginate–diltiazem hydrochloride beads: Optimization of formulation factors, *in vitro* and *in vivo* availability. *Journal of Microencapsulation* 20(2): 211–225.

Escribano-Bailon, M. T., and Santos-Buelga, C. (2003). Polyphenols Extraction from Foods. In: *Methods in Polyphenol Analysis*, pp. 1–16. C. Santos-Buelga and G. Williamson, eds. Cambridge: UK: Royal Society of Chemistry.

International Organization for Standardization (ISO). (2005). ISO 14502-1:2005. Determination of substances characteristic of green and black tea. Part 1: Content of total polyphenols in tea. Colorimetric method using Folin–Ciocalteu reagent. http://www.iso.org/iso/home/store/catalogue_tc/catalogue_detail.htm?csnumber=31356

Jaiswal, D., Bhattacharya, A., Yadav, I.K., Singh, H.P., Chandra, D., and Jain, D. A. (2009). Formulation and evaluation of oil entrapped floating alginate beads of ranitidine hydrochloride. *International Journal of Pharmacy and Pharmaceutical Sciences* 1(1): 128–140.

Khazaeli, P., Paradakhty, A., and Hassanzadeh, F. (2008). Formulation of Ibuprofen beads by ionotropic gelation. *Iranian Journal of Pharmaceutical Research* 7(3): 163–170.

Kim, N. Y., Jang, M. K., Lee, D. G., Yu, K. H., Jang, H. J., and Kim, M. (2010). Comparison of methods for proanthocyanidin extraction from pine *(Pinus densiflora)* needles and biological activities of the extracts. *Nutrition Research and Practice* 4(1): 16–22.

Klahorst, S. J. (2006). Flavour and innovation meet. *World of Food Ingredients* 26–30.

Lamkey, J. W. (2009). Nonstarch Hydrocolloids. In: *Ingredients in Meat Products: Properties, Functionality and Applications*, pp. 57–82. T. Rodrigo, ed. New York: Springer.

Luck, G., Liao, H., Murray, N. J., Grimmer, H. R., Warminski, E. E., and Williamson, M. P. (1994). Polyphenols, astringency and proline-rich proteins. *Phytochemistry* 37: 357–371.

Mirghani A., Idkaidek, N. M., Salem, M. S., and Najib, N. M. (2000). Formulation and release behavior of diclofenac sodium in compritol matrix beads encapsulated in alginate. *Drug Development and Industrial Pharmacy* 26: 791–795.

Mishra, S. K., and Pathak, K. (2008). Formulation and evaluation of oil entrapped gastroretentive floating gel beads of Loratadine. *Acta Pharmaceutica* 58: 187– 197.

Mollet, B., and Lacroix, C. (2007). Where biology and technology meet for better nutrition and health. *Current Opinion in Biotechnology* 18: 154–155.

Ostberg, T., Lund, E. M., and Graffner, C. (1994). Calcium alginate matrices for oral multiple unit administration IV. Release characteristics in different media. *International Journal of Pharmaceutics* 112(3) 241–248.

Papadopoulou, A., and Frazier, R. A. (2004). Characterization of protein–polyphenol interactions. *Trends in Food Science and Technology* 15: 186–190.

Patel, Y. L., Sher, P., and Pawar, A. P. (2006). The effect of drug concentration and curing time on processing and properties of calcium alginate beads containing metronidazole by response surface methodology. *AAPS Pharmscitech* 7(4): 86.

Servili, M., Rizzello, C. G., Taticchi, A., Esposto, S., Urbani, S., *et al.* (2011). Functional milk beverage fortified with phenolic compounds extracted from olive vegetation water, and fermented with functional lactic acid bacteria. *International Journal of Food Microbiology* 147(1): 45–52.

Siebert, K. J., Troukhanova, N. V., and Lynn, P. Y. (1996). Nature of polyphenol–protein interactions. *Journal of Agricultural and Food Chemistry* 44: 80–85.

Soares, S., Brandao, E., Mateus, N., and de Freitas, V. (2015). Interaction between red wine procyanidins and salivary proteins: Effect of stomach digestion on the resulting complexes. *RSC Advances* 5: 12664.

Takka, S., Ocak, O. H., Acarturk, F. (1998). Formulation and investigation of nicardipine HCl–alginate gel beads with factorial design-based studies. *European Journal of Pharmaceutical Sciences* 6: 241–246.

Vandamme, T. F., Poncelet, D., and Subra-Paternault, P. (2007). *Microencapsulation: Des Sciences aux Technologies*. Paris: Lavoisier Tec & Doc.

Watson, E., Carvalho, A., Green, R., Britton, S., and Scott, S. (2006). Functional ingredients. *Food Manufacture*. 81(11): 4–19.

Williamson, G., and Manach, C. (2005). Bioavailability and bioefficacy of polyphenols in humans. II. Review of 93 intervention studies. *American Journal of Clinical Nutrition* 81: 243S–255S.

Xiao, J., Mao, F., Yang, F., Zhao, Y., Zhang, C., and Yamamoto, K. (2011). Interaction of dietary polyphenols with bovine milk proteins: Molecular structure-affinity relationship and influencing bioactivity aspects. Molecular Nutrition and Food Research 55(11): 1637–1645.

Zahin, M., Aqil, F., and Ahmad, I. (2009). The *in vitro* antioxidant activity and total phenolic content of four Indian medicinal plants. *International Journal of Pharmacy and Pharmaceutical Sciences* 1(1): 88–95.

TOPIC 3

Application of encapsulated compounds with modified polymers in functional food systems

CHAPTER 8

Encapsulation technologies for resveratrol in functional food

María Chávarri and María Carmen Villarán
Bioprocesses & Preservation Area, Health Division, TECNALIA, Parque Tecnológico de Álava, c/Leonardo Da Vinci N° 11, 01510, Miñano (Álava), Spain

8.1 Introduction

The food industry has generally been regarded as a low-tech industry (Bigliardi and Galati, 2003). However, this is changing, and the industry possesses high potential for future economic growth (Menrad, 2004). Following the trends observed in consumer demand, the food industry has introduced a new category of products called *functional foods* – foods that bring science and high-technology into everyday life by promising certain health benefits Niva, 2007). This interest has been fueled by increased media attention and an increasing number of consumers determined to take greater responsibility for their own health.

Food industry marketers perceive that consumers want foods that are convenient, fresh (less processed and less packaged), all natural and with no preservatives (a so-called clean label), without a perceived negative component (i.e., foods without high fat, high salt, and high sugar, and foods low in calories), and healthy. Moreover, today consumers demand food products not only to satisfy the appetite and to provide the necessary nutrients, but also to prevent nutrition-related diseases (Bigliardi and Galati, 2003). Newer foods with bioactive compounds needed by the body to stave off the progression of diseases associated with aging or to enhance physical performance attract the consumers' attention and sell well in today's marketplace Zink, (1997).

The food industry is starting to innovate specifically with respect to new scientific and technical approaches in food processing and to the development of functional food (Bigliardi and Galati, 2003). Functional foods, being one of the major food categories of the global health and wellness market, are becoming a major focus of new product development in the food industry (Khan *et al.*, 2013).

Today, manufacturers and others in the food industry are looking for newer and better ways to enhance the value of their products as well as differentiate

New Polymers for Encapsulation of Nutraceutical Compounds, First Edition.
Edited by Jorge Carlos Ruiz Ruiz and Maira Rubi Segura Campos.

themselves in the marketplace. Encapsulation is being seen by many as an effective technology for achieving these goals (Veršič, 2014).

The encapsulation process, although complex and efficient, cannot be described as good or bad, only as appropriate or inappropriate to meet the specific requirements of each application. Further, the suitability of encapsulation cannot be determined without taking a close, careful look at the viability of the economics of using this cutting-edge process (Veršič, 2014).

By analyzing and considering all of the economic factors involved with encapsulation, today's food makers can put themselves in a position to clearly determine if this technology will work for them. If the economics are viable, this could dramatically improve their ability to add new ingredients, develop more novel foodstuffs with advanced properties, provide more protection for processed food products, penetrate new market segments, and achieve other important goals.

8.2 Functional foods

Recent studies have also established that diet has a strong influence on the etiology of several diseases. These dietary guidelines normally emphasize dietary modifications and use of certain types of food and food groups, which, because of their unusual content of nutrients or non-nutrient components, may have a protective influence on diseases. Functional foods can include specific foods and food with ingredients that exert a beneficial effect on human health and/or reduce the risk of chronic disease beyond basic nutritional functions (Ali Khan *et al.*, 2014).

The functional foods concept started in Japan in the early 1980s with the launch of three large-scale government-funded research programs on systematic analyses and development of functional foods, analyses of physiological regulation of functional food, and analyses of functional foods and molecular design (Pravst, 2012).

In 1991 in Japan, in an effort to reduce the escalating cost of health care, a category of foods with potential health benefits was called FOSHU (foods for specified health use) (Ashwell, 2002; Burdock *et al.*, 2006; Menrad, 2003), and this class of product could be seen on the food label with a FOSHU symbol (Siró *et al.*, 2008). There is no doubt that the Japanese interest in functional foods has also brought awareness for the need of such products in Europe and the United States. However, in these places, the question is more about a concept: Functional food means adding functionality to an existing traditional food product (often a mainstream product), and such food products do not create a separate group (Fern, 2007; Hilliam, 1998; Kotilainen *et al.*, 2006). In the United States, evidence-based health or disease-prevention claims have been allowed since 1990, when the Nutrition Labelling and Education Act was adopted; claims have

Table 8.1 Practical examples of functional foods.

Definition	Examples
A natural food, fruit or grain, which may or may not be modified	Vitamin E–enriched vegetable oils Vitamin A–enriched, genetically engineered, "golden" rice
A food to which a component has been added	A spread with added phytosterols
A food from which a component has been removed or reduced	Yogurt with reduced fat
A food in which one component (or several components) has been modified, replaced, or enhanced to improve its health properties	Juice drink with enhanced antioxidant content Yogurt with added prebiotic or probiotic

to be approved by the U.S. Food and Drug Administration (FDA) (Arvanitoyannis and Van Houwelingen-Koukaliaroglou, 2005). In the European Union, harmonization was achieved in 2006 with Regulation (EC) No. 1924/2006 on nutrition and health claims made on foods, which requires authorization of all health claims before entering the market (Pravst, 2012).

A functional food is defined as food that is a part of the human diet and is demonstrated to provide health benefits and to decrease the risk of chronic diseases beyond those provided by adequate nutrition (Al-Sheraji *et al.*, 2013). A functional food must remain in a normal food form rather than pills or capsules, and it must demonstrate its effects in amounts that can be consumed in the diet. A functional food can be a natural food, or it can be a food that one or more components have been added to or removed from (International Life Sciences Institute, 1999; Roberfroid, 2002). The functional foods include usual foods with naturally occurring bioactive substances (e.g., polyphenols), foods supplemented with bioactive substances (e.g., probiotics, antioxidants), and conventional foods with food-derived ingredients (e.g., prebiotics). Functional food should have a novel prospective, rather than merely being a food product. Functional foods are not medicines such as pills or capsules but are consumed as part of a normal daily diet Grajek *et al.*, 2005). Some examples of functional food are shown in Table 8.1 (Assmann *et al.* (2014); Kotilainen *et al.*, 2006); Spence, 2006).

8.3 Resveratrol

Resveratrol is a natural polyphenolic compound (*trans*-3,5,4′-trihydroxystilbene) from the stilbens family of aromatic phytochemicals Amri *et al.*, 2012). Resveratrol exists in two geometric isomers, *cis*- and *trans*- (Montsko *et al.*, 2008). The *trans*- form is present in many plants, including blueberries, peanuts, cocoa, pistachios, nuts, red grapes, and the roots of *Polygonum cuspidatum* (Aluyen *et al.*, 2012; Burns *et al.*, 2002; Kristl *et al.*, 2009; Ndiaye *et al.*, 2011; Neves *et al.*, 2012; Walle *et al.*, 2004).

The *trans-* isomer is the natural form and the more stable and more active form (Augustin *et al.*, 2013; Rius *et al.*, 2010). Chemical degradation often involves the isomerization of resveratrol: *trans*-resveratrol to the *cis*-isomer when exposed to sunlight, high-intensity white light, or ultraviolet (UV) light, at 360 and 254 nm (López-Hernández *et al.*, 2007; Montsko *et al.*, 2008). In the absence of light, *trans*-resveratrol was shown to be stable for at least 28 days in the pH range of 1 to 7 (Trela and Waterhouse, 1996).

Resveratrol is highly soluble in alcohols, but it is soluble in only trace amounts in aqueous or lipid phase. The molecular structure of *trans*-resveratrol is highly hydrophobic, with a partition coefficient (log $Po_{/w}$) of 3.1 and an aqueous solubility of 0.021 to 0.030 g/L (SciFinder, 2013). Despite its poor aqueous solubility, the compound is expected to demonstrate high membrane permeability due to its lipophilicity. On the other hand, resveratrol shows markedly high solubility in organic solvents such as ethanol (50 g/L) and dimethyl sulfoxide (DMSO) (16 g/L) (Davidov-Pardo and McClements, 2014), and it is moderately soluble in triacylglycerol oils (0.18 mg/mL) (Hung *et al.*, 2006). Consequently, it is difficult to incorporate relatively high levels of resveratrol into aqueous-based food products. In addition, resveratrol is sensitive to chemical degradation within food products. Resveratrol may be chemically degraded when exposed to elevated temperatures (Lyons *et al.*, 2003; Schmidt *et al.*, 2005) pH changes (Allan *et al.*, 2009), ultraviolet light (Rodriguez *et al.*, 2012); Trela and Waterhouse, 1996), or certain types of enzymes (Pinto *et al.*, 2003).

Resveratrol is of interest to the food and pharmaceuticals fields due to its potential beneficial effects on human health. Resveratrol is a well-known bioactive compound that has various biological effects, including cardioprotective (Hung *et al.*, 2000), neuroprotective (Bhavnani, 2003; Valenzano *et al.*, 2006; Wang *et al.*, 2006), antioxidant (Frankel *et al.*, 1993; Frémont *et al.*, 1999), antiinflammatory (Pace-Asciak *et al.*, 1995), antibiotic (Neves *et al.*, 2013), anticarcinogenic and antiobesity effects (Lai *et al.*, 2015), lifespan extension (Howitz *et al.*, 2003), and inhibition of platelet aggregation (Bertelli *et al.*, 1995; Chung *et al.*, 1992).

Resveratrol has emerged as an extremely promising natural molecule due to its therapeutic prospects. However, the potential of resveratrol is immensely hindered by its poor pharmacokinetic properties. The oral absorption of resveratrol in humans is about 75% and occurs primarily through transepithelial diffusion (Walle *et al.*, 2004; Walle, 2011).

The actual bioavailability of resveratrol is less than 1% due to extensive metabolism in the intestine and liver involving glucuronic acid conjugation and sulfation to generate the key metabolites, *trans*-resveratrol-3-O-glucuronide and *trans*-resveratrol-3-sulfate, respectively (Cottart *et al.*, 2010; Rotches-Ribalta *et al.*, 2012; Walle, 2011; Yu *et al.*, 2002). Following resveratrol's absorption, rapid metabolism in the liver, with an initial short plasma half-life of 8 to 14 minutes, accounts for its insufficient bioavailability (Walle, 2011).

It has been estimated that the current daily intake of resveratrol is around 4 mg/day (Vang *et al.*, 2011). Increasing this level could lead to improvements in human health due to the mechanisms mentioned above. Toxicology studies suggest that resveratrol is safe when consumed at doses up to 5 g per day in healthy humans, but that doses of 2.5 to 5 g can cause mild to moderate gastrointestinal symptoms (Brown *et al.*, 2010).

Despite the potential health benefits of resveratrol, its use within the food industry as a nutraceutical ingredient is currently limited due to its poor water solubility, photosensitivity, low oral bioavailability, and rapid metabolism. Therefore, exploitation of resveratrol as a functional food may be overcome when it is encapsulated in a delivery system that is capable of stabilizing it, protecting it from degradation, and solubilizing it in water, while preserving its biological activities and enhancing its bioavailability. However, until now, only a few studies have addressed the suitability of delivering encapsulated resveratrol to the site of action, and the main research focus has been its biological activity, especially in synergy with the consumption of other diet and beverage components.

8.4 Encapsulation technology

Many encapsulation procedures have been proposed but none of them can be considered as a universally applicable procedure for bioactive food components. This is because individual bioactive food components have their own characteristic molecular structure (Augustin and Hemar, 2009). However, compatibility with the bioactives is not the only requirement an encapsulation procedure has to meet. It also should have specific characteristics to withstand influences from the environment (Augustin and Hemar, 2009). An important requirement is that the encapsulation system has to protect the bioactive component from chemical and physical degradation (e.g., oxidation or hydrolysis) to keep the bioactive component fully functional. A major obstacle in the efficacious delivery of bioactive food components is not only the hazardous events that occur during passage through the gastrointestinal tract but also the deleterious circumstances during storage in the product that serves as vehicle for the bioactive components (de Vos *et al.*, 2010). Many food components can interfere with the bioactivity of the added bioactive food component. It is therefore mandatory that the encapsulation procedure protects the bioactive component during the whole period of foodstuff processing, storage, and transport (Gibbs *et al.*, 1999).

The effectiveness of polyphenols depends on preserving their stability, bioactivity, and bioavailability. The use of encapsulated polyphenols, instead of free compounds, can effectively alleviate some deficiencies (Leonard, 2000). Another limit on the application of most of phenolic compounds is their unpleasant taste when they are used at higher concentrations. Another problem is that only a small proportion of the molecules remain available following oral administration, due to insufficient gastric residence time and low permeability and solubility within the gut. In addition, their instability under conditions encountered in food processing and storage (temperature, oxygen, light) or in the gastrointestinal tract (pH, enzymes, presence of other nutrients), are limiting for activity and potential health benefits of components like polyphenols (Leonard, 2000). Therefore, manufacturers have to provide protective mechanisms that can maintain the active ingredients until the time of consumption, enabling delivery to the physiological target in an organism (Chen *et al.*, 2006).

From the literature, it is clear that use of encapsulated polyphenols instead of free compounds can lead to improvements in both the stability and bioavailability of the compounds *in vivo* and *in vitro*. A number of techniques are available for encapsulation of food compounds. Because encapsulating compounds are very often in a liquid form, many technologies are based on drying. Different techniques like spray-drying, spray-bed-drying, fluid-bed coating, spray-chilling, spray-cooling, or melt injection are available to encapsulate active agents (Gibbs *et al.*, 1999; Zuidam and Heinrich, (2010).Although most of the encapsulation technologies employed for various compounds have been adopted, there are still some technologies that have not been yet applied for polyphenols, including spray-cooling/chilling, spinning-disk extrusion, and centrifugal coextrusion. However, this does not necessarily mean that these technologies are not suitable for polyphenol encapsulation (Fang and Bhandari, 2010). Future research of polyphenol encapsulation is likely to focus on aspects of delivery and the potential use of coencapsulation methodologies, where two or more bioactive ingredients can be immobilized together simultaneously in order to provide synergistic activity of those bioactives. It can be foreseen that with a deep understanding of the health benefits of polyphenols and new strategies for stabilizing fragile nutraceuticals, encapsulated polyphenols will play an important role in increasing the efficacy of functional foods.

Research is being undertaken to overcome the challenges of using resveratrol as a bioactive agent. However, much of this research has been carried out from a pharmaceutical perspective (Amri *et al.*, 2012; Santos *et al.*, 2011). In food applications, a number of additional factors need to be considered when designing effective encapsulation systems (McClements *et al.*, 2009). First, all the components used to assemble a delivery system should be food-grade generally recognized as safe (GRAS) ingredients. Actually, the whole food process should be designed to meet the safety requirements of government agencies such as the European Food Safety Authority (EFSA) or the FDA (Nedovic *et al.*, 2011). Second, the fabrication method should be economically viable and robust so that it can be used commercially for large-scale production in the food industry. Third, the delivery system should not adversely affect the organoleptic properties of the food product, such as appearance, texture, or flavor. Fourth, the delivery system should remain physically stable during food processing, transport, and storage and should prevent undesirable interactions with the food matrix. Finally, the resveratrol should remain in a metabolically active form within the food or beverage product (Sessa *et al.*, 2011) and should prevent degradation until the product is delivered to specific sites within the consumer's body, such as the mouth, stomach, small intestine, or colon Lesmes and McClements, 2009). Thus, resveratrol would be kept fully functional. Also, this technology may provide barriers between sensitive bioactive materials and the environment, and thus, to allow taste and aroma differentiation, mask bad taste or smell, stabilize food ingredients, or increase bioavailability.

Most microcapsules are small spheres with diameters ranging between a few micrometers and a few millimeters. However, many of these microcapsules bear little resemblance to these simple spheres. In fact, both the size and shape of formed microparticles depend on the materials and methods used to prepare them. The different types of microcapsules and microspheres are produced from a wide range of wall materials like monomers and/or polymers (Poshadri and Kuna, 2010). Depending on the physicochemical properties of the core, the wall composition, and the microencapsulation technique used, different types of particles can be obtained: A simple sphere surrounded by a coating of uniform thickness; a particle containing an irregularly shaped core; several core particles embedded in a continuous matrix of wall material; several distinct cores within the same capsule and multiwalled microcapsules.

The choice of the wall material is very important for encapsulation efficiency and microcapsule stability. The criteria for selecting a suitable wall material are mainly based on its physicochemical properties such as solubility, molecular weight, glass/melting transition, crystallinity, diffusibility, film-forming and emulsifying properties, and cost. The most-used wall materials are biopolymers of various sources, such as natural gums (gum arabic, alginates, carrageenans), proteins (milk or whey proteins, soy proteins, gelatin), starches, maltodextrins with different dextrose equivalents, corn syrup, and waxes and their derivatives (Gharsallaoui *et al.*, 2007).

The functionality and bioavailability of resveratrol as nutraceutical and preventive or therapeutic agent is strongly affected by its chemical properties, and they can be reduced or compromised during processing due to the instability from oxygen, temperature, and light, as well as to the environmental conditions during its passage through the gastrointestinal tract (Landete, 2011; Manach *et al.*, 2004; Munin and Edwards-Lévy, 2011). Encapsulation of resveratrol can effectively mitigate these limitations (Amri *et al.*, 2012; Gürbüz *et al.*, 2007; Kolouchová-Hanzlíková *et al.*, 2010; Peng *et al.*, 2010; Saiko *et al.*, 2008) and it can represent a promising option and could be a way to develop functional foods with resveratrol (Fang and Bhandari, 2010).

Resveratrol is currently marketed as a nutritional supplement available in traditional dosing forms including tablets, capsules, and powders, although data regarding their efficacy is scarce (Rossi *et al.*, 2012). Novel drug-delivery systems, such as polymeric nanoparticles, cyclodextrins, micelles, and liposomes, provide

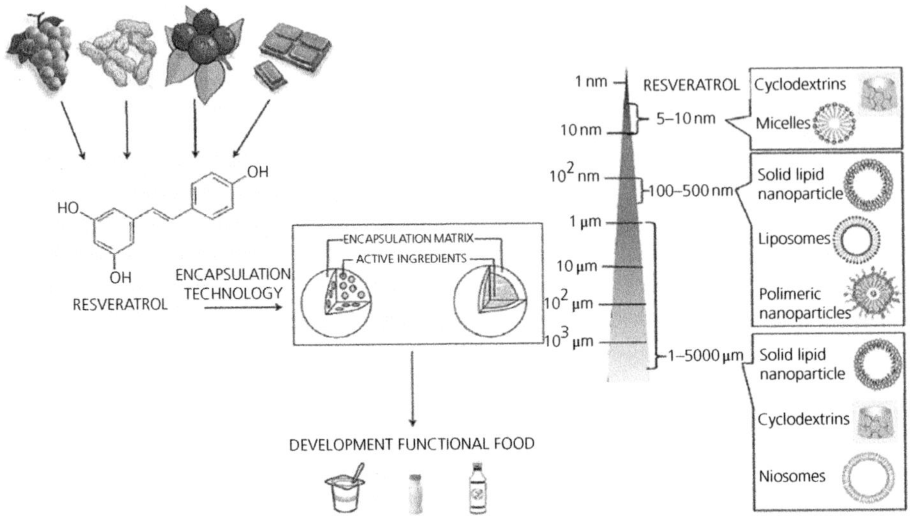

Figure 8.1 Schematic representation of various resveratrol encapsulated formulations to develop functional food.

several advantages over traditional forms, including the ability to enhance resveratrol's aqueous solubility and bioavailability, improve physicochemical stability, and enable targeted and controlled drug release (da Rocha Lindner *et al.*, 2013; Sanna *et al.*, 2015; Venuti*et al.*, 2014). Figure 8.1 shows the molecular structure of *trans*-resveratrol that is found in several plant species. To achieve development of functional foods with resveratrol, it is necessary to employ encapsulation technologies, either micro- or nanoencapsulation.

8.5 Microencapsulation

Microencapsulation is defined as a technology for packaging solids, liquids, or gases in miniature, sealed capsules that can release their contents at controlled rates under specific conditions (Desai and Park, 2005). Microencapsulation is based on the embedding effect of a polymeric matrix, which creates a microenvironment in the capsule able to control the interactions between the internal part and the external one (Borgogna *et al.*, 2010). Microencapsulation allows the protection of a wide range of materials of biological interest, from small molecules and protein (enzymes, hormones) to cells of bacterial, yeast, and animal origin (Thies, 2005). The same characteristics make microencapsulation suitable for food industry applications, in particular for the production of high-value food and nutraceuticals.

Studies have addressed a broad array of questions and challenges related to microencapsulation in four main research directions: microencapsulating materials, wall (matrix) materials for microencapsulation, processes for microencapsulation, and properties and functionality of encapsulated systems.

Microencapsulated delivery systems, such as emulsion-based systems, inclusion complexes, niosomes, and biopolymeric gelled microspheres, have the potential to protect bioactives, mask taste of undesirable components, and release the bioactives upon ingestion (Augustin and Hemar, 2009; Drusch, and Mannino, 2009; McClements *et al.*, 2009; Sagalowicz and Leser, 2010). Moreover, the stability, bioavailability, and bioefficacy of active substances strongly depend on the food matrix and the chosen (micro)encapsulation or delivery system (Acosta, 2009; Folmer *et al.*, 2009; Palzer, 2009; Tamayo-Esquivel *et al.*, 2006).

Several studies have focused on the development of microparticles to stabilize and protect resveratrol, to increase its water solubility, to achieve a controlled release, and to improve its effectiveness as antioxidant, anticarcinogenic, and so on (Li *et al.*, 2011; Lu *et al.*, 2012; Sanna *et al.*, 2013a). For example (Table 8.2), single-emulsion droplets containing resveratrol demonstrated an improved systemic bioavailability in the blood and liver (Augustin *et al.*, 2011), double-emulsion droplets increased its stability (Matos *et al.*, 2014; Sanna *et al.*, 2015), use of cyclodextrins to protect resveratrol and to increase its solubility, stability, and bioactivity was applied in several studies (Kumpugdee-Vollrath, 2012; Li *et al.*, 2010; Lu *et al.*, 2009; Lucas-Abellán *et al.*, 2007), resveratrol niosomes increased entrapment efficiencies (Pando *et al.*, 2013), and chitosan microspheres containing resveratrol were able to control the release and stabilization of resveratrol (Peng *et al.*, 2010).

8.5.1 Single-emulsion droplet

An emulsion is the dispersion of two immiscible liquids in the presence of a stabilizing compound or emulsifier. When the core phase is aqueous, this is termed a water-in-oil emulsion (w/o), and a hydrophobic core phase is termed an oil-in-water emulsion (o/w). Emulsions are simply produced by the addition of the core phase to a vigorously stirred excess of the second phase that contains, if necessary, the emulsifier (Chávarri *et al.*, 2012). Specifically, in the study of Augustin and colleagues (2011), resveratrol is encapsulated in an oil in-water emulsion system stabilized by a heated mixture of a milk protein, glucose, and a modified resistant starch was used as the single delivery vehicle for fish oil, tributryin, and resveratrol (Table 8.2.). In concrete, for resveratrol, a single emulsion formulation is advantageous due to increased bioavailability in the blood and liver (Augustin *et al.*, 2011).

8.5.2 Double-emulsion droplets

The simplest multiple emulsions are called double emulsions, and they are ternary systems, having either a water-in-oil-in-water (w1/o/w2) or an oil-in-water-in-oil (O1/W/O2) structure, whereby the dispersed droplets contain smaller droplets of a different phase (Aserin, 2008). One problem of resveratrol is maintaining stability for long periods of time. In this sense, Sanna's group (2015) demonstrated that PLGA (poly-lactic-co-glycolic acid) microcapsules

Table 8.2 Properties of resveratrol microencapsulation.

Microencapsulation Detail	Materials	Size (μm)	Encapsulation Efficiencies	Improved Characteristic	References
Emulsion Based					
Oil-in-water emulsion	fish oil	7 to 9		Solubility, bioavailability	Augustin *et al.* (2011)
Water-in-oil emulsion chemical cross-linking method	Chitosan cross-linked with vanillin	53 to 311	94%	Stability, Protected from light and heat	Sanna *et al.* (2015)
Water-in-oil-in-water double emulsion	chitosan (CS) and poly(D,L-lactic-co-glycolic acid) (PLGA)	11 to 20	40–52%	Stability (6 months), long-term protection	Matos *et al.* (2014)
Water-in-oil-in-water double emulsion. Mechanical agitation	polyglycerol polyrici-noleate (inner emulsifier)	1	33%	Stability (2 weeks)	Matos *et al.* (2014)
Inclusion Complexes					
Complexation	α-Cyclodextrin			Thermal stability, solubility	Li *et al.* (2010)
	β-Cyclodextrin			Antioxidant, solubility	Li *et al.* (2011)
	Hydroxypropyl-β-cyclodextrin			Antioxidant, solubility	Lu *et al.* (2009)
	Hydroxypropyl-β-cyclodextrin			Anticarcinogenic	Lu *et al.* (2012)
	α-, β-, γ-, 2-hydroxy propyl-β-, dimethyl-β-cyclodextrin			Solubility, stability	Kumpugdee-Vollrath (2012)
Niosomes					
Two-stage technique: mechanical agitation and sonication	Surfactant concentration in the range 1%–4% (w/v) (Span 80 niosomes)	8.5	13%	Stability	Pando *et al.* (2013)
	Surfactant concentration in the range 0.5%–2% (w/v) (Span 60-cholesterol niosomes)	4.5	44%	Stability	

with a 4% w/w of chitosan were able to ensure a good retention and stability of encapsulated resveratrol up to 6 months (Table 8.2) (Sanna *et al.*, 2015). Matos and colleagues (2014) developed w1/o/w2 double emulsions of food-grade formulation to encapsulate resveratrol, which could be used for the development of functional foods, but more tests would have to be conducted to improve the encapsulation ability of these emulsions (Table 8.2) (Matos *et al.*, 2014).

8.5.3 Cyclodextrins

Cyclodextrins are cyclic oligosaccharides arising from the degradation of starch, which can be a viable option as encapsulation technique. Cyclodextrins are inexpensive, friendly to humans (Davis and Brewster, 2004; Matsuda and Arima, 1999; Shulman *et al.*, 2011), and capable of improving the biological, chemical, and physical properties of bioactive molecules (Pinho *et al.*, 2014). In several studies cyclodextrins were employed to protect resveratrol and to increase its solubility, stability, and bioactivity (Kumpugdee-Vollrath, 2012; Li *et al.*, 2011; Li *et al.*, 2010; Lu *et al.*, 2012; Lu *et al.*, 2009; Lucas-Abellán *et al.*, 2007; Sapino *et al.*, 2009). The use of encapsulation technology, specifically inclusion complexes, using cyclodextrins (β-cyclodextrin and hydroxypropyl-β-cyclodextrin) allowed researchers to improve the biological properties of resveratrol (antioxidant and anticarcinogenic) as described by Lu and coworkers (Lu *et al.*, 2012; Lu *et al.*, 2009) (Table 8.2). Additionally, resveratrol concentration in an aqueous environment was improved by complexation with β-cyclodextrin and 6-*O*-α-maltosyl-β-cyclodextrin and, consequently, its antioxidant capacity. At the same time, cyclodextrins were capable of protecting the phenolic compound from rapid oxidation by entrapping it inside their cavities (Lucas-Abellán *et al.*, 2007).

8.5.4 Niosomes

Niosomes, or nonionic surfactant vesicles, are similar in physical structure to liposomes formed by phospholipids, and they can encapsulate hydrophilic bioactive compounds in the inner space and lipophilic bioactive compounds in the lipid bilayer (Tu *et al.*, 2014). These vesicles are commonly used to encapsulate both hydrophilic and lipophilic compounds for food, pharmaceutical, or cosmetic applications. In the study by Pando and coworkers (2013), resveratrol was protected in niosomes made of Span 60-cholesterol and Span 80-cholesterol (Matsuda and Arima, 1999) (Table 8.2). Niosomes were prepared using a system by a two-stage technique: mechanical agitation and sonication. Because cholesterol was used in the preparation of the niosomes and becauase cholesterol might not be suitable for use in functional foods because of potential adverse health effects, dodecanol was selected as a membrane stabilizer, because niosomes can be prepared with fatty alcohols instead of cholesterol (Pandita *et al.*, 2014).

8.6 Nanoencapsulation

Nanoparticle is derived from the Greek word *nano,* signifying "dwarf," and the technology dealing with these materials is called *nanotechnology.* Nanotechnology, according to the National Nanotechnology Initiative (NNI) and the U.S. National Science Foundation (NSF) is defined as the ability to understand, control, and manipulate matter at their individual atomic and molecular levels, as well as at the supermolecular level (ranging from 0.1 to 100 nm) of cluster molecules, in order to produce materials, devices, and systems with new properties and functions.

Nanotechnology has contributed significantly to the development of nanometric delivery systems, which allow encapsulation of bioactive materials in nanoparticles and thereby solve problems of deterioration during processing of food and increase activity by enhancing the mass transfer rate to the required active areas (Mogol *et al.*, 2013). Nanoencapsulation, defined as a technology to pack substances in miniature, making use of techniques such as nanocomposites, nanoemulsification, and nanostructuration, provides final product functionality that includes controlled release of the core. This technology protects sensitive bioactive food components against oxidation, enzymes, and other external factors before reaching the target.

A number of reports and reviews have identified the current and short-term projected applications of nanotechnologies for the food sector (Food Safety Authority of Ireland, 2008; Grobe *et al.*, 2008; Groves, 2008; Morris, 2008). The potential for food nanotechnology applications seems unlimited. There are already identified potential uses of nanotechnology in virtually every segment of the food industry, with four key focus areas (Martirosyan and Schneider, 2014): agriculture, food processing, food packaging, and nutrient supplements. Agricultural uses include pesticide, fertilizer, or vaccine delivery; animal and plant pathogen detection; and targeted genetic engineering. Food processing uses include encapsulation of flavor or odor enhancers, food textural or quality improvement, and new gelation or viscosifying agents. Food packaging uses include pathogen, gas or abuse sensors; anticounterfeiting devices; UV protection; and stronger, more impermeable polymer films. Nutrient supplements use nanotechnology to produce nutraceuticals with higher stability and bioavailability.

Application of nanotechnology in the food industry is the processing and formulation of food ingredients to form nanostructures that are claimed to offer improved taste, texture, and consistency (Weiss *et al.*, 2006) and to improve nutritional value, add functional ingredients, enhance bioavailability (International Union of Food Science & Technology, 2010), and allow mixing of incompatible ingredients in the food matrix (Hsieh and Ofori, 2007). Different types of functional nanostructures can be used as building blocks to create novel structures and introduce new functionalities into foods, such as nanoemulsions, nanoliposomes, nanofibers, and nanoparticles (Hsieh and Ofori, 2007; International Union of Food Science & Technology, 2010; Weiss *et al.*, 2006).

From a technological point of view, an efficient nanometric-size delivery system should benefit for the food industry with the following characteristics (McClements *et al.*, 2007):

- Food-grade ingredients: The delivery system should be formulated with food-grade, possibly all-natural, ingredients using solvent-free fabrication methods. In particular, one major challenge is to replace some of the polymers and surfactants used in the pharmaceuticals industry with food-grade alternatives (Acosta, 2009).
- Food incorporation: The delivery system should be able to incorporate the bioactive compounds into the food matrices with high physicochemical stability and minimal impact on the organoleptic properties of the product (Donsì *et al.*, 2007) .
- Protection against degradation: The delivery system should be able to protect the encapsulated bioactive compounds from interaction with other food ingredients, as well as from degradation due to temperature, light, and pH, during food manufacturing, storage, and preparation (McClements *et al.*, 2007) .
- Uptake and bioavailability: The delivery system should maximize the uptake of the encapsulated compounds upon consumption and their transport to the sites of action (Acosta, 2009). In addition, controlled release in response to specific environmental stimulus may be desirable (McClements *et al.*, 2007).
- Industrial scalability: The fabrication of the delivery system should be easily scalable to industrial production (Donsi *et al.*, 2010a; Donsi *et al.*, 2010b).

Currently, nanoencapsulated resveratrol studies are focused on drug development rather than on developing functional foods. Research efforts in the nanotechnology field to stabilize resveratrol and protect it from degradation, to increase its solubility, and to improve tumor selectivity have led to the emergence of novel formulations of the drug that have already revolutionized cancer therapy (Amri *et al.*, 2012; Lu *et al.*, 2009).

A lot of research exploits the use of food-grade nanodispersion such as liposomes, solid lipid nanoparticles, nanostructured lipid carriers, lipid-core nanocapsules, niosomes, polymeric nanoparticles, cyclodextrins, and nanoemulsions in delivering bioactive food components. The system has been classified as either solid or liquid, each of which provides a distinct advantage, depending on the compatibility of nanoparticle properties with that of the bioactive compounds and the intended application. The solid nanodelivery systems include lipid nanoparticles, nanostructured lipid carriers, and polymeric nanoparticles; liquid systems include liposomes, niosomes, and nanoemulsions.

8.6.1 Solid-based nanoparticle delivery systems

Properties of resveratrol nanoencapsulation are shown in Table 8.3.

Table 8.3 Properties of resveratrol nanoencapsulation.

Nanoencapsulation Technology	Encapsulation Method	Materials	Size (nm)	Encapsulation Efficiencies	Improved Characteristic	References
Solid-Based Nanoparticle Delivery Systems						
Solid lipid nanoparticles	Solvent diffusion–solvent evaporation method	Ethyl acetate solution containing stearic acid, Phospholipon® 90G and resveratrol. Surfactants (lecithin/poloxamer 188)	134	90%	Stability 4 °C (3 months)	Pandita *et al.* (2014)
Solid lipid nanoparticles	High-shear homogenization method ultrasound method	Cetyl palmitate and polysorbate 60	150–250	64% to 89%	Solubility, stability (2 months at room temperature)	Neves *et al.* (2013
Nanostructured lipid carriers	high shear homogenization method ultrasound method	Cetyl palmitate, polysorbate 60, and the liquid lipid miglyol-812	150–250	65% to 77%	Solubility, stability (2 months at room temperature)	Neves *et al.* (2013
Lipid-core nanocapsules	Precipitation of preformed polymer method	Poly(ε-caprolactone), grape seed oil, sorbitan monoestearate	200	100%	Increase photostability	Coradini *et al.* (2014)
Lipid-core nanocapsules	Interfacial deposition of the polymer	Poly(ε-caprolactone), capric/caprylic triglyceride and sorbitan monostearate	250	96%	Solubility, stability, neuroprotective	Frozza *et al.* (2013)
Polymeric nanoparticles (PNP)	Double emulsion and solvent evaporation	polyethylene glycol–poly lactic acid	150	78%	Anticarcinogenic	Guo *et al.* (2013)
Solid-Based Nanoparticle Delivery Systems						
Polymeric nanoparticles (PNP)	Liquid antisolvent precipitation	Zein coated with sodium caseinate	120	85% to 90%	Higher resveratrol concentration	Davidov-Pardo *et al.* (2015)
Polymeric nanoparticles (PNP)	Nanoprecipitation method	Poly(epsilon-caprolactone) (PCL) and poly(D,L-lactic-co-glycolic acid)-poly(ethylene glycol) conjugate (PLGA-PEG-COOH)	150	74% to 98%	Anticarcinogenic (prostate cancer chemoprevention, chemotherapy)	Sanna *et al.* (2013a)
Polymeric nanoparticles (PNP)	Resveratrol nanodispersion	Ethanol in water with hydroxypropylmethyl cellulose followed by spray drying	161		Stability, solubility, antioxidant	Zhang *et al.* (2013)
Polymeric nanoparticles (PNP)	Nano-precipitation method with minor modification	Poly-caprolactone (PCL) (hydrophobic core) and polyethyleneglycol (PEG) (hydrophilic core)	<100	89%	Antioxidant	Lu *et al.* (2009)

Cyclodextrins	Conventional inclusion complexation techniques	β-Cyclodextrin nanosponges	400–500		Solubility, stability	Ansari *et al.* (2011)
Cyclodextrins	Complexation using the freeze-drying method	Sulfobutylether-γ-cyclodextrin			Solubility, stability, anticarcinogenic (human breast cancer)	(86)Venuti *et al.* (2014)
Liquid-Based Nanoparticles Delivery Systems						
Liposomes			100–120	95%	Solubility, anticarcinogenic	Catania *et al.* (2013)
Liposomes	Thin film method	Resveratrol and Phospholipon 90G/ cholesterol; 1:20 w/w	100	90%	Antioxidant, stability (3 weeks)	Wang *et al.* (2011) Isailović *et al.* (2013)
	Proliposome method	Resveratrol and Phospholipon 90G; 1:20 w/w	100	90%	Antioxidant, stability (3 weeks)	
Niosomes	Thin film hydration method	Span 60 as surfactant	168	64%	Stability	Pando *et al.* (2015)
		Maisine 35-1 as surfactant	175	55%	Stability	
		Dodecanol as stabilizer	362	53%	Stability	
Nanoemulsions	Spontaneous emulsification method	10% oil phase (grape seed oil plus orange oil) and 10% surfactant (Tween 80). Orange oil–to–grape seed oil ratio of 1:1 (w/w)	100	90%	Stability	Davidov-Pardo and McClements (2015)
	High-pressure homogenization	Peanut oil–based emulsion	<200		Stability (4 weeks), solubility, antioxidant,	Donsi *et al.*, 2010a
Nanoemulsions	High-pressure homogenization	Peanut oil–based emulsion	235–128		Stability, bioavailability	Sessa *et al.* (2014)

8.6.1.1 Solid lipid nanoparticles

Solid lipid nanoparticles are particles consisting of a matrix made of solid lipid shell (Müller *et al.*, 2000). Solid lipid nanoparticles have attracted increasing scientific and commercial attention in pharmaceuticals and food sciences (Awad *et al.*, 2008; Gallarate *et al.*, 2009; Taylor *et al.*, 2007; Varshosaz *et al.*, 2010a; Varshosaz *et al.*, 2010b). There is great interest in solid lipid nanoparticles due to their advantages in enhancing the oral bioavailability of lipophilic compounds owing to their submicrometer size, ease of scale-up and manufacturing, use of physiological lipids, and controlled-release properties (Pandita *et al.*, 2011; Wong *et al.*, 2007). The research into encapsulating resveratrol into solid lipid nanoparticles could offer new opportunities to minimize the difficulties encountered in its delivery. In this regard, Teskac and Kristl (2010) developed solid lipid nanoparticles with resveratrol by a melt-emulsification process with glyceryl behenate, hydrogenated soybean lecithin, and poloxamer 188, for achieving sustained release of resveratrol (Table 8.3). In 2013, it was reported that the physical and chemical protection conferred to resveratrol by lipid nanoparticles could enhance the therapeutic effects of resveratrol by minimizing its instability *in vivo* and controlling its release profile (Neves *et al.*, 2013). The use of lipid systems is important because physiological and biodegradable lipids are hypothesized to enhance the oral absorption in the same way as the lipid components of normal food (Pandita *et al.*, 2014).

8.6.1.2 Nanostructured lipid carriers

Nanostructured lipid carriers are delivery systems for partially crystallized lipid particles (having mean radii of at most 100 nm) dispersed in an aqueous phase of emulsifier. The purpose of formulating nanostructured lipid carriers is to produce particles in which the oil is incorporated into the core of a solid lipid; this leads to a higher loading capacity and controlled bioactive compound release as the bioactive compound dissolves in the oil and simultaneously encapsulates in the solid lipid (Varshosaz *et al.*, 2010). nanostructured lipid carriers differ from solid lipid nanoparticles by the incorporation of a liquid lipid into their solid structure (Müller *et al.*, 2000). The lipid blend in nanostructured lipid carriers has slower polymorphic transition and low crystallinity index. Along with existing oil in the nanostructured lipid carrier core, the spherical shape of the particle might account for these improving properties (Jores *et al.*, 2004; Muller *et al.*, 2002). Nanostructured lipid carriers eliminate the limitation of poor water-solubility, chemical instability, and low bioavailability encountered during fortification of aqueous-based foods with nutraceutical ingredients. Thus, nanostructured lipid carriers can be a substitute for other nanocarriers and can be suitable for application in food and beverages (Tamjidi *et al.*, 2013). Specifically, Neves and colleagues (2013) observed that the physical and chemical protection conferred to resveratrol by these lipid nanoparticles (nanostructured lipid carriers and solid lipid nanoparticles) could enhance the therapeutic effects of resveratrol by minimizing its instability *in vivo* and controlling its release profile (Table 8.3) (Neves *et al.*, 2013).

8.6.1.3 Lipid-core nanocapsules

Lipid-core nanocapsules are a class of nanocapsules in which the oil core is formed by a dispersion of a liquid lipid and a solid lipid (sorbitan monostearate). This oil core is surrounded by a polymeric wall, and the particle–water interface is stabilized with polysorbate 80 (Pohlmann *et al.*, 2013). These colloidal systems can stabilize photolabile substances (Ourique *et al.*, 2010), control drug release (Fontana *et al.*, 2009), improve the effectiveness of the bioactive (Bernardi *et al.*, 2009a; Bernardi *et al.*, 2009b; Fontana *et al.*, 2011; Frozza *et al.*, 2013; Zanotto-Filho *et al.*, 2013), and increase the cerebral biodistribution of different substances (Bernardi *et al.*, 2009a; Frozza *et al.*, 2010). Lipid-core nanocapsules have been shown to improve the antioxidant effects of lipophilic compounds (Külkamp *et al.*, 2011). One research group showed that lipid-core nanocapsules increased the photostability of resveratrol (Detoni *et al.*, 2012) targeted to the brain tissue (Frozza *et al.*, 2010), improving its antiglioma activity (Figueiró *et al.*, 2013) and mitigating its deleterious effects against Ab1-42 in a model of Alzheimer's disease (Frozza *et al.*, 2013).

Coradini and colleagues (2014) showed that LCNs containing co-encapsulated resveratrol and curcumin were produced and showed consistent properties like a suitable nanomaterial. Nanoencapsulation increased the antioxidant activity and photostability of both resveratrol and curcumin (Table 8.3). The results showed that the strategy of co-encapsulating resveratrol and curcumin is a promising approach to improve the performance of medicines and functional foods used to prevent and treat diseases associated with oxidative stress (Coradini *et al.*, 2014).

8.6.1.4 Polymeric nanoparticles

Polymeric nanoparticles are frequently defined as solid, colloidal particles in the range 10 to 1000 nm (Couvreur, 1988; Vauthier and Couvreur, 2000). *Polymeric nanoparticle* is a collective term given for any type of polymer nanoparticle, but specifically for nanospheres and nanocapsules. Polymeric nanoparticles can be fabricated using antisolvent precipitation by decreasing the quality of the solvent in which the biopolymers are dissolved. In practice, this can be achieved by addition of a nonsolvent to induce supersaturation of the biopolymer, which provides the driving force for nucleation and subsequent particle growth (Joye and McClements, 2013). Additional components, such as polymers or surfactants, can be dissolved in the antisolvent phase to control particle formation and stability (Kim *et al.*, 2013; Zhang *et al.*, 2013). In addition, functional ingredients that coprecipitate with the biopolymer can be encapsulated by incorporating them in the original solvent. Davidov-Pardo and colleagues (2015) is showed that zein particles coated with sodium caseinate were the best system for encapsulating resveratrol (Table 8.3) (Davidov-Pardo *et al.*, 2015). Adverse effects such as crystal formation were not observed, so that biopolymer particles produced with antisolvent precipitation are a promising strategy to enrich functional foods with resveratrol. On the other hand, encapsulating drugs into polymeric nanoparticles protects them from degradation, enables sustained release, enhances intracellular penetration, and improves bioavailability (Davidov-Pardo *et al.*, 2015; Guo *et al.*, 2013; Lu *et al.*, 2009; Sanna *et al.*, 2013b).

8.6.1.5 Cyclodextrins

Cyclodextrins are cyclic oligosaccharides that are produced from starch and that possess a hydrophilic surface and hydrophobic inner cavity (Tiwari *et al.*, 2010). Cyclodextrins are typically between 1 and 2 nm in diameter and have a truncated shape that allows the entrapment of foreign molecules inside their inner cavity (Lu *et al.*, 2012). Commonly found natural cyclodextrins include α, β and γ, which contain 6, 7, and 8 glucopyranose units respectively (Tiwari *et al.*, 2010). Studies concerning resveratrol encapsulation in cyclodextrins have observed that cyclodextrin complexes greatly increased resveratrol's aqueous solubility, showing a roughly 5-log-fold increase for both the hydroxypropyl-β-cyclodextrin and hydroxypropyl-γ-cyclodextrin (Ansari *et al.*, 2011; Summerlin *et al.*, 2015; Venuti *et al.*, 2014). It was also found that hydroxypropyl-β-cyclodextrin increased the photostability of resveratrol more significantly then hydroxypropyl-γ-cyclodextrin. Also, in the study by Mukherjee's group (2011), the hydrogenated soy phosphatidyl choline complex of resveratrol was shown to improve the bioavailability and cardioprotective health benefit of resveratrol(Mukherjee *et al.*, 2011). The formulation showed 2.26 times higher bioavailability, good stability, and stronger antioxidant activity than that of nonencapsulated resveratrol.

8.6.2 Liquid-based nanoparticle delivery systems

8.6.2.1 Liposomes

Liposomes have been widely used in the food sector – in both research and industry – because they have many benefits, such as the possibility of large-scale production using natural ingredients and entrapment and release of water-soluble, lipid-soluble, and amphiphilic materials as well as targetability (Huwiler *et al.*, 2000; Mozafari *et al.*, 2008; Thompson *et al.*, 2006). The mechanism of liposome formation is based on the unfavorable interactions that occur between amphiphilic compounds (mainly phospholipids) and water molecules, where the polar head groups of phospholipids are subjected to the aqueous phases of the inner and outer media, and the hydrophobic hydrocarbon tails are associated into the bilayer and spherical core shell structures are formed (Goyal *et al.*, 2005; Jesorka and Orwar, 2008). Liposomes are microscopic vesicles with a diameter ranging from 25 nm to 1000 nm. Depending on their size, liposomes are known as small unilamellar vesicles (10–100 nm) or large unilamellar vesicles (100–3000 nm). If more than one bilayer is present, then they are referred as multilamellar vesicles. As a consequence of this alternating hydrophilic and hydrophobic structure, liposomes have the capacity to entrap compounds of different solubilities.

Liposomes can be produced using natural ingredients on an industrial scale (Mozafari and Khosravi-Darani, 2007). Another important advantage of liposomes (also known as lipid vesicles) is targetability. Lipid vesicles can be tailored to deliver and release their load in the target site inside and outside the body (Mozafari, 2006).

Liposomes have begun to gain in importance in food products (Mozafari *et al.*, 2008; Taylor *et al.*, 2005). Indeed, the ability of liposomes to solubilize compounds with scarce solubility in water, sequester compounds from potentially harmful media, and release incorporated molecules in a sustained and predictable way can be used in the food processing industry. Based on studies on liposomes for pharmaceutical and medical uses, food scientists have begun to use liposomes for controlled delivery of functional components such as proteins, enzymes, vitamins, antioxidants, and flavors (Catania *et al.*, 2013; Wang *et al.*, 2011).

Concerning resveratrol, in the pharmaceuticals sector has studied certain liposomal formulations, and it has observed very positive effects on certain cancers. Specifically, the liposomal formulation in co-delivery of curcumin and resveratrol showed a synergistic effect with respect to improved bioavailability and enhanced antitumor effect against prostate cancer (179). Isailovic and colleagues (2013) developed a study that provided evidence for food manufacturers and food scientists to make broader use of resveratrol-loaded liposomes that can add value and improve the quality of existing food products (Isailović *et al.*, 2013) (Table 8.3). It is reported that liposomes produced through the extrusion technique have advantages over those produced by sonication, because there is more-homogeneous distribution of liposomes and better entrapment of resveratrol. Liposomes are shown to be convenient carriers for resveratrol, because they are physically stable (for e weeks) and provide prolonged release of resveratrol.

8.6.2.2 Niosomes

Niosomes are vesicles formed by nonionic surfactants in aqueous media and, as liposomes, are bilayered structures. The main advantage of these vesicles, with respect to other encapsulation technologies, such as liposomes (Fang and Bhandari, 2010; Gibis *et al.*, 2014), is their low production cost, high stability, (Kopermsub *et al.*, 2011) and resultant ease of storage. Niosomes are chemically stable, can entrap both lipophilic and hydrophilic bioactive compounds either in an aqueous layer or in a vesicular membrane, and have low toxicity because they are nonionic. They are flexible in their structural constitution, offer improved bioactive compound availability and controlled delivery at a particular site, and are biocompatible, biodegradable, and nonimmunogenic. Niosomes range in size from 10 to 1000 nm. In the study of Pando and colleagues (2015), resveratrol-loaded niosomes with sorbitan monostearate (Span 60) or glyceryl monolinoleate (Maisine 35-1) as surfactants and dodecanol as stabilizer have demonstrated narrow size distribution, a small mean size, high resveratrol entrapment efficiency, and good stability (Table 8.3). In this report the resveratrol did not involve changes in the textural properties of regular yogurt, demonstrating that resveratrol-entrapped niosomes are suitable additives in these dairy products (Pando *et al.*, 2015).

8.6.2.3 Nanoemulsions

Nanoemulsions are nano-scale droplets of multiphase colloidal dispersions formed by dispersing one liquid in another immiscible liquid by physical share-induced rupturing (Liu *et al.*, 2006; Mason *et al.*, 2006; Meleson *et al.*, 2004; Russel *et al.*, 1989). Different size ranges have been reported in the literature for nanoemulsions: less than 100 nm (Guo *et al.*, 2007; Porras *et al.*, 2008; Shakeel and Ramadan, 2010), 10 to 100 nm (Talegaonkar *et al.*, 2010), 100 to 500 nm (Anton *et al.*, 2008; Constantinides *et al.*, 2008; Rossi and Leroux, 2006; Tadros *et al.*, 2004; Unger *et al.*, 2004), and 100 to 600 nm (Conxita *et al.*, 2002; Sakulku *et al.*, 2009). However, the most appropriate ones based on the definition of nanotechnology are those less than 100 nm and possessing different properties than ordinary emulsions. A feature of nanoemulsions is that the droplet sizes in nanoemulsions are much smaller than visible wavelengths; hence, most nanoemulsions appear optically transparent (McClements and Li, 2010; Shakeel and Ramadan, 2010). This is a very favorable feature of nanoemulsions for applying them as nutrient carriers in beverages.

In particular, emulsion-based delivery systems are a promising encapsulation technique because lipophilic bioactive components can be encapsulated within the hydrophobic core of the lipid droplets, where they may be protected from degradation during storage and then released after ingestion (McClements, 2012; McClements *et al.*, 2007). If the bioactive compound to be encapsulated is crystalline (such as resveratrol), it is necessary to ensure that it is used at a level below its saturation concentration in the carrier oil to avoid precipitation and sedimentation during storage (McClements, 2012). The two most common forms of emulsion-based delivery systems are nanoemulsions (radius 6–100 nm) and emulsions (radius >100 nm), which are both thermodynamically unstable systems but can be designed to have sufficient kinetic stability for many food applications.

Previous studies have shown that resveratrol can be encapsulated in either emulsions or nanoemulsions using various carrier oils, emulsifiers, and particle dimensions. Emulsions formed using both natural and synthetic emulsifiers have been shown to improve the stability of resveratrol (Donsì *et al.*, 2007; Sessa *et al.*, 2011).

Two approaches can be used to fabricate nanoemulsions: high-energy and low-energy approaches (Rao and McClements, 2012). High-energy methods use mechanical devices that generate intense disruptive forces to break the oil phase into tiny droplets that are then dispersed within the aqueous phase. Low-energy methods are based on the spontaneous formation of nano-sized oil droplets in surfactant–oil–water mixtures when the composition or temperature of the system is changed in a particular manner. Two approaches can be distinguished for preparing low-energy emulsions: phase-inversion and spontaneous-emulsification methods. The phase-inversion methods rely on the modification of the optimum curvature or solubility of the surfactant by changing the temperature (phase-inversion temperature) or composition (phase-inversion composition) of the system. The spontaneous-emulsification methods rely on the movement of surfactants from their original location in one phase into the other phase due to solubility preferences. This movement causes an increase in oil–water interfacial area, interfacial turbulence, and spontaneous formation of droplets (McClements, 2012). The main advantage of using low-energy methods over high-energy methods is the reduction in equipment and operating costs and the ease of implementation, whereas the main disadvantage is that they require considerably higher amounts of surfactant (Saberi *et al.*, 2013).

The encapsulation of bioactive compounds in nanoemulsion delivery systems has different advantages in comparison with traditional delivery systems: stabilization in aqueous systems (such as foodstuffs) of lipophilic bioactive compounds with scarce solubility in water, protection of bioactive compounds against degradation reactions with food constituents and minimization of the alteration of the food matrix, control of the release by engineering the dimension and composition of the capsules, and enhancement of cell uptake and bioavailability. In particular, the bioavailability of compounds encapsulated into emulsions is enhanced when emulsion droplets are of nanometric size (Acosta, 2009). Many authors have shown that reducing the particle size to values below cell size (500 nm) produces higher absorption of the active ingredient and higher particle uptake, by enhancing the mechanisms of passive transport through the intestinal walls (Luo *et al.*, 2006).

Davidov-Pardo and McClements (2015) observed that nanoemulsions formed by spontaneous emulsification offer a simple way to encapsulate resveratrol as a nutraceutical ingredient by combining byproducts from the wine industry, such as grape seed oil and grape skin extract (Table 8.3). These emulsions remained physically stable throughout storage at different temperatures and proved to be effective in protecting resveratrol against isomerization and degradation by UV light. Emulsions with a droplet size closer to the wavelength of UV light gave a higher resveratrol protection (Davidov-Pardo and McClements, 2015).

Donsi and colleagues (2011) showed that nanoemulsion-based delivery systems can be efficiently used in the encapsulation of bioactives, improving their water dispersability, protecting them from degradation, and preserving the antioxidant activity (Table 8.3). Encapsulation of resveratrol (0.01% wt) in peanut oil–based nanoemulsions improved its stability, as shown by the significant reduction of the chemical degradation of *trans*-resveratrol to *cis*-resveratrol. The nanoencapsulation in oil-in-water nanoemulsions-based delivery systems represents an effective approach for incorporating bioactive compounds, such as resveratrol, in foods (Donsi *et al.*, 2011).

Sessa and colleagues (2011) showed that oil-in-water nanoemulsions produced by a combined use of lipophilic and hydrophilic emulsifiers not only significantly improved resveratrol's dispersibility in an aqueous phase but also protected resveratrol from chemical degradation (Table 8.3). The nanoemulsions also better preserved the antioxidant activity of resveratrol during the digestion process. Sessa's group (2011) suggested that bioactive compounds such as resveratrol that have low water solubility and are prone to chemical and biological degradation can be encapsulated into specially formulated food-grade nanoemulsion-based delivery systems to increase their stability and bioavailability (Sessa *et al.*, 2011).

The protection of bioactive compounds against degradation and interaction with food ingredients occurs through encapsulation in nanometric delivery systems. For this reason, an efficient nanodelivery system must be stable in the food matrices over long periods of time. However, some of the conditions that a nanoemulsion encounters during processing (e.g., heating, high-shear mixing) are not conducive to stability.

Research has historically focused mainly on the physical aspects of emulsion stability in foods. Nevertheless, many types of chemical reactions can have adverse effects on the quality of food emulsions, including lipid oxidation, hydrolysis, flavor or color degradation, and bioactive degradation due to a chemical interaction of the nutraceutical compound with food components.

Unencapsulated resveratrol is poorly absorbed and quickly metabolized once the food has been ingested and, therefore, it is prevented from reaching the target organs in its active form. Nanometric-size delivery systems can contribute to increasing the bioavailability of bioactive compounds by protecting them during the digestive processes, as well as improving their uptake in the gastrointestinal tract and enhancing transport to the target sites.

8.7 Conclusions

Resveratrol is a molecule that has many limitations to its direct use as a bioactive compound in the development of functional foods. It is therefore necessary to use encapsulation techniques to protect the resveratrol and to provide the necessary features to use it as a functional ingredient. The encapsulation type to be used in the development of functional ingredients is very important. Therefore selecting an appropriate delivery system for a particular application is key to getting a functional ingredient with the desired characteristics. This selection depends on a number of factors.

First, it should be possible to prepare the delivery system from food-grade ingredients using a robust, reliable, and inexpensive manufacturing operation. Second, the delivery system should not adversely affect the quality attributes of the product (such as appearance, texture, and flavor) and it should remain stable throughout the expected shelf life of the product. Third, the delivery system should have high encapsulation and retention efficiencies. Fourth, the delivery system should be capable of protecting and releasing resveratrol within the gastrointestinal tract to ensure high oral bioavailability. Each type of delivery system has its own advantages and disadvantages that make it more or less suitable for different applications. In developing a functional food using resveratrol, it is necessary to know very well the physical and chemical properties, the food matrix, the processing of the food, the storage and the transport methods, and where in the body the resveratrol will act.

Future research could focus on combining encapsulation techniques to achieve a greater effect on increasing the solubility, stability, and bioavailability of resveratrol, as well as a low interaction with the food matrix. Combinations of techniques may also improve the properties of the capsules, as well as increasing the amount of resveratrol that can be loaded into them. Finally, further work is needed to explore the incorporation of different types of resveratrol delivery systems into food products. It is important to evaluate the impact of food matrices on the stability of capsules and resveratrol and the effect of the capsules on the physicochemical and sensory properties of the food product. Also it is necessary to evaluate the beneficial effects of resveratrol after ingestion of the food. Let us not forget that in order to develop a functional food ingredient, its production process has to be low cost. This is important when it comes to selecting the encapsulation technique and the materials to obtain a functional ingredient in the food industry.

References

Acosta, E. (2009). Bioavailability of nanoparticles in nutrient and nutraceutical delivery. *Current Opinion in Colloid & Interface Science* 14(1): 3–15.

Ali Khan, W., Ahmad, J., and Srivastava, P. K. (2014). Functional Food Products and Their Role in Health and Prevention of Disease. *International Journal of Life Sciences Biotechnology and Pharma Research* 3(2): 27–34.

Allan, K. E., Lenehan, C. E., and Ellis, A. V. (2009). UV light stability of α-cyclodextrin/resveratrol host–guest complexes and isomer stability at varying pH. *Australian Journal of Chemistry* 62(8): 921–926.

Al-Sheraji, S. H., Ismail, A., Manap, M. Y., Mustafa, S., Yusof, R.M., and Hassan, F. A. (2013). Prebiotics as functional foods: A review. *Journal of Functional Foods* 5(4): 1542–1553.

Aluyen, J. K., Ton, Q. N., Tran, T., Yang, A. E., Gottlieb, H. B., and Bellanger, R.A. (2012). Resveratrol: Potential as anticancer agent. *Journal of Dietary Supplements* 9(1): 45–56.

Amri, A., Chaumeil, J. C., Sfar, S., and Charrueau, C. (2012). Administration of resveratrol: What formulation solutions to bioavailability limitations? *Journal of Controlled Release* 158(2): 182–193.

Ansari, K., Vavia, P., Trotta, F., and Cavalli, R. (2011). Cyclodextrin-based nanosponges for delivery of resveratrol: *In vitro* characterisation, stability, cytotoxicity and permeation study. *AAPS PharmSciTech* 12(1): 279–286.

Anton, N., Benoit, J. P., and Saulnier, P. (2008). Design and production of nanoparticles formulated from nano-emulsion templates-a review. *Journal of Controlled Release* 128(3): 185–199.

Arvanitoyannis, I. S., and Van Houwelingen-Koukaliaroglou, M. (2005). Functional foods: A survey of health claims, pros and cons, and current legislation. *Critical Reviews in Food Science and Nutrition* 45(5): 385–404.

Aserin, A. (2008). *Multiple Emulsions: Technology and Applications*. Hoboken: Wiley-Interscience.

Ashwell, M. (2002). *Concepts of Functional Foods*. Brussels: ILSI - International LIfe Sciences Institute.

Assmann, G., Buono, P., Daniele, A., Della Valle, E., Farinaro, E., *et al.* (2014). Functional foods and cardiometabolic diseases: International Task Force for Prevention of Cardiometabolic Diseases. *Nutrition, Metabolism and Cardiovascular Diseases* 24(12): 1272–1300.

Augustin, M. A., Abeywardena, M. Y., Patten, G., Head, R., Lockett, T., *et al.* (2011). Effects of microencapsulation on the gastrointestinal transit and tissue distribution of a bioactive mixture of fish oil, tributyrin and resveratrol. *Journal of Functional Foods* 3(1): 25–37.

Augustin, M. A., and Hemar, Y. (2009). Nano- and micro-structured assemblies for encapsulation of food ingredients. *Chemical Society Reviews* 38(4): 902–912.

Augustin, M. A., Sanguansri, L., and Lockett, T. (2013). Nano- and micro-encapsulated systems for enhancing the delivery of resveratrol. *Annals of the New York Academy of Sciences* 1290(1): 107–112.

Awad, T., Helgason, T., Kristbergsson, K., Decker, E., Weiss, J., and McClements, D. J. (2008). Effect of cooling and heating rates on polymorphic transformations and gelation of tripalmitin solid lipid nanoparticle (SLN) suspensions. *Food Biophysics* 3(2): 155–162.

Bernardi, A., Braganhol, E., Jäger, E., Figueiró, F., Edelweiss, M. I., *et al.* (2009a). Indomethacin-loaded nanocapsules treatment reduces *in vivo* glioblastoma growth in a rat glioma model. *Cancer Letters* 281(1): 53–63.

Bernardi, A., Zilberstein, A., Jäger, E., Campos, M. M., Morrone, F. B., *et al.* (2009b). Effects of indomethacin-loaded nanocapsules in experimental models of inflammation in rats. *British Journal of Pharmacology* 158(4): 1104–1111.

Bertelli, A. A., Giovannini, L., Giannessi, D., Migliori, M., Bernini, W., *et al.* (1995). Antiplatelet activity of synthetic and natural resveratrol in red wine. *International Journal of Tissue Reactions* 17(1): 1–3.

Bhavnani, B. R. (2003). Estrogens and menopause: Pharmacology of conjugated equine estrogens and their potential role in the prevention of neurodegenerative diseases such as Alzheimer's. *Journal of Steroid Biochemistry and Molecular Biology* 85(2–5): 473–482.

Bigliardi, B., and Galati, F. (2003). Innovation trends in the food industry: The case of functional foods. *Trends in Food Science & Technology* 31(2): 118–129.

Borgogna, M., Bellich, B., Zorzin, L., Lapasin, R., and Cesàro, A. (2010). Food microencapsulation of bioactive compounds: Rheological and thermal characterisation of non-conventional gelling system. *Food Chemistry* 122(2): 416–423.

Brown, V. A. , Patel, K. R., Viskaduraki, M., Crowell, J. A., Perloff, M., *et al.* (2010). Repeat dose study of the cancer chemopreventive agent resveratrol in healthy volunteers: Safety, pharmacokinetics, and effect on the insulin-like growth factor axis. *Cancer Research* 70(22): 9003–9011.

Burdock, G. A., Carabin, I. G., and Griffiths, J. C. (2006). The importance of GRAS to the functional food and nutraceutical industries. *Toxicology.* 221: 17–27.

Burns, J., Yokota, T., Ashihara, H., Lean, M. E. J., and Crozier, A. (2002). Plant foods and herbal sources of resveratrol. *Journal of Agricultural and Food Chemistry* 50(11): 3337–3340.

Catania, A., Barrajón-Catalán, E., Nicolosi, S., Cicirata, F., and Micol, V. (2013). Immunoliposome encapsulation increases cytotoxic activity and selectivity of curcumin and resveratrol against HER2 overexpressing human breast cancer cells. *Breast Cancer Research and Treatment* 141(1): 55–65.

Chávarri, M., Marañón, I., and Villarán, M. C. (2012). *Encapsulation Technology to Protect Probiotic Bacteria*. Rijeka, Croatia: InTech Open Access Publisher.

Chen, L., Remondetto, G. E., and Subirade, M. (2006). Food protein based materials as nutraceutical delivery systems. *Trends in Food Science & Technology* 17(5): 272–283.

Chung, M. I., Teng, C. M., Cheng, K. L., Ko, F. N., and Lin, C. N. (1992). An antiplatelet principle of *Veratrum formosanum*. *Planta Medica* 58(3): 274–276.

Constantinides, P. P., Chaubal, M. V., and Shorr, R. (2008). Advances in lipid nanodispersions for parenteral drug delivery and targeting. *Advanced Drug Delivery Reviews* 60(6): 757–767.

Conxita, S., Paqui, I., Jordi, E., Garcia-Celma, M. J., Nuria, U., *et al.* (2002). Nano-Emulsions. Adsorption and Aggregation of Surfactants in Solution. In: *Surfactant Science*, pp. 525–554. Boca Raton, FL: CRC Press.

Coradini, K., Lima, F. O., Oliveira, C. M., Chaves, P. S., Athayde, M. L, *et al.* (2014). Co-encapsulation of resveratrol and curcumin in lipid-core nanocapsules improves their in vitro antioxidant effects. *European Journal of Pharmaceutics and Biopharmaceutics* 88(1): 178–185.

Cottart, C.-H., Nivet-Antoine, V., Laguillier-Morizot, C., and Beaudeux, J.-L. (2010). Resveratrol bioavailability and toxicity in humans. *Molecular Nutrition & Food Research* 54(1): 7–16.

Couvreur, P. (1988). Polyalkylcyanoacrylates as colloidal drug carriers. *Critical Reviews in Therapeutic Drug Carrier Systems* 5(1): 1–20.

da Rocha Lindner, G., Khalil, N. M., and Mainardes, R. M. (2013). Resveratrol-loaded polymeric nanoparticles: Validation of an HPLC-PDA method to determine the drug entrapment and evaluation of its antioxidant activity. *The Scientific World Journal* 2013: 9.

Davidov-Pardo, G., Joye, I.J., McClements, D. J. (2015). Encapsulation of resveratrol in biopolymer particles produced using liquid antisolvent precipitation. Part 1: Preparation and characterization. *Food Hydrocolloids* 45(0): 309–316.

Davidov-Pardo, G., and McClements, D. J. (2014). Resveratrol encapsulation: Designing delivery systems to overcome solubility, stability and bioavailability issues. *Trends in Food Science & Technology* 38(2): 88–103.

Davidov-Pardo, G., and McClements, D. J. (2015). Nutraceutical delivery systems: Resveratrol encapsulation in grape seed oil nanoemulsions formed by spontaneous emulsification. *Food Chemistry* 167: 205–212.

Davis, M. E., and Brewster, M. E. (2004). Cyclodextrin-based pharmaceutics: past, present and future. *Nature Reviews Drug Discovery* 3(12): 1023–1035.

Desai, K. G. H., and Park, H. J. (2005). Recent developments in microencapsulation of food ingredients. *Drying Technology* 23(7): 1361–1394.

Detoni, C. B., Souto, G. D., da Silva, A. L. M., Pohlmann, A. R., and Guterres, S. S. (2012). Photostability and skin penetration of different e-resveratrol-loaded supramolecular structures. *Photochemistry and Photobiology* 88(4): 913–921.

de Vos, P., Faas, M. M., Spasojevic, M., and Sikkema, J. (2010). Encapsulation for preservation of functionality and targeted delivery of bioactive food components. *International Dairy Journal* 20(4): 292–302.

Donsi, F., Senatore, B., Huang, Q., and Ferrari, G. (2010a). Development of novel pea protein–based nanoemulsions for delivery of nutraceuticals. *Journal of Agricultural and Food Chemistry* 58(19): 10653–10660.

Donsì, F., Sessa, M., Mediouni, H., Mgaidi, A., and Ferrari, G. (2011). Encapsulation of bioactive compounds in nanoemulsion- based delivery systems. *Procedia Food Science* 1(0): 1666–1671.

Donsì, F., Wang, Y., Li, J., and Huang, Q. (2010b). Preparation of curcumin sub-micrometer dispersions by high-pressure homogenization. *Journal of Agricultural and Food Chemistry* 58(5): 2848–2853.

Drusch, S., and Mannino, S. (2009). Patent-based review on industrial approaches for the microencapsulation of oils rich in polyunsaturated fatty acids. *Trends in Food Science & Technology* 20(6–7): 237–244.

Fang, Z., and Bhandari, B. (2010). Encapsulation of polyphenols – a review. *Trends in Food Science & Technology* 21(10): 510–523.

Fern, E. B. (2007). Marketing of functional foods: A point of view of the industry. International Developments in Science & Health Claims, ILSI International Symposium on Functional Foods in Europe, Brussels.

Figueiró, F., Bernardi, A., Frozza, R. L., Terroso, T., Zanotto-Filho, A., *et al.* (2013). Resveratrol-loaded lipid-core nanocapsules treatment reduces *in vitro* and *in vivo* glioma growth. *Journal of Biomedical Nanotechnology* 9(3): 516–526.

Folmer, B. M., Barron, D., Hughes, E., Miguet, L., Sanchez, B., *et al.* (2009). Monocomponent hexa- and dodecaethylene glycol succinyl-tocopherol esters: Self-assembly structures, cellular uptake and sensitivity to enzyme hydrolysis. *Biochemical Pharmacology* 78(12): 1464–1474.

Fontana, M. C., Coradini, K., Guterres, S. S., Pohlmann, A. R., and Beck, R. C. R. (2009). Nanoencapsulation as a way to control the release and to increase the photostability of clobetasol propionate: Influence of the nanostructured system. *Journal of Biomedical Nanotechnology* 5(3): 254–263.

Fontana, M. C., Rezer, J. F. P., Coradini, K., Leal, D. B. R., and Beck, R. C. R. (2011). Improved efficacy in the treatment of contact dermatitis in rats by a dermatological nanomedicine containing clobetasol propionate. *European Journal of Pharmaceutics and Biopharmaceutics* 79(2): 241–249.

Food Safety Authority of Ireland. (2008). *The Relevance for Food Safety of Applications of Nanotechnology in the Food and Feed Industries*. Dublin: Food Safety Authority of Ireland.

Frankel, E. N., Waterhouse, A. L., and Kinsella, J. E. (1993). Inhibition of human LDL oxidation by resveratrol. *Lancet* 341(8852): 1103–1104.

Frémont, L., Belguendouz, L., and Delpal, S. (1999). Antioxidant activity of resveratrol and alcohol-free wine polyphenols related to LDL oxidation and polyunsaturated fatty acids. *Life Sciences* 64(26): 2511–2521.

Frozza, R. L., Bernardi, A., Hoppe, J. B., Meneghetti, A. B., Matte, A., *et al.* (2013). Neuroprotective effects of resveratrol against Aβ administration in rats are improved by lipid-core nanocapsules. *Molecular Neurobiology* 47(3): 1066–1080.

Frozza, R. L., Bernardi, A., Paese, K., Hoppe, J. B., da Silva T., *et al.* (2010). Characterization of *trans*-resveratrol-loaded lipid-core nanocapsules and tissue distribution studies in rats. *Journal of Biomedical Nanotechnology* 6(6): 694–703.

Gallarate, M., Trotta, M., Battaglia, L., and Chirio, D. (2009). Preparation of solid lipid nanoparticles from W/O/W emulsions: Preliminary studies on insulin encapsulation. *Journal of Microencapsulation* 26(5): 394–402.

Gharsallaoui, A., Roudaut, G., Chambin, O., Voilley, A., and Saurel, R. (2007). Applications of spray-drying in microencapsulation of food ingredients: An overview. *Food Research International* 40(9): 1107–1121.

Gibbs, B. F., Kermasha, S., Alli, I., and Mulligan, C. N. (1999). Encapsulation in the food industry: A review. *International Journal of Food Sciences and Nutrition* 50(3): 213–224.

Gibis, M., Zeeb, B., and Weiss, J. (2014). Formation, characterization, and stability of encapsulated hibiscus extract in multilayered liposomes. *Food Hydrocolloids* 38: 28–39.

Goyal, P., Goyal, K., Vijaya Kumar, S. G., Singh, A., Katare, O. P., and Mishra, D. N. (2005). Liposomal drug delivery systems–clinical applications. *Acta Pharmaceutica* (Zagreb, Croatia). 55(1): 1–25.

Grajek, W., Olejnik, A., and Sip, A. (2005). Probiotics, prebiotics and antioxidants as functional foods: A review. *Acta Biochimica Polonica* 52: 665–671.

Grobe, A., Renn, O., and Jaeger, A. (2008). *Risk Governance of Nanotechnology Applications in Food and Cosmetics*. Geneva: International Risk Governance Council.

Groves, K. (2008). Potential benefits of micro and nano technology for the food industry: Does size matter? *New Food Magazine* 4: 49–52.

Guo, W., Li, A., Jia, Z., Yuan, Y., Dai, H., and Li, H. (2013). Transferrin modified PEG-PLA-resveratrol conjugates: *In vitro* and *in vivo* studies for glioma. *European Journal of Pharmacology* 718(1–3): 41–47.

Guo, H., Wilking, J. N., Liang, D., Mason, T. G., Harden, J. L., and Leheny, R. L. (2007). Slow, nondiffusive dynamics in concentrated nanoemulsions. *Physical Review E* 75(4): 041401.

Gürbüz, O., Göçmen, D., Dağdelen F., Gürsoy, M., Aydin, S., *et al.* (2007). Determination of *flavan-3-ols* and *trans*-resveratrol in grapes and wine using HPLC with fluorescence detection. *Food Chemistry* 100(2): 518–525.

Hilliam, M. (1998). The market for functional foods. *International Dairy Journal* 8: 349–353.

Howitz, K. T., Bitterman, K. J., Cohen, H. Y., Lamming, D. W., Lavu, S., *et al.* (2003). Small molecule activators of sirtuins extend *Saccharomyces cerevisiae* lifespan. *Nature* 425(6954): 191–196.

Hsieh, Y. H., and Ofori, J. A. (2007). Innovations in food technology for health. *Asia Pacific Journal of Clinical Nutrition* 16 Suppl 1: 65–73.

Hung, C.-F., Chen, J.-K., Liao, M.-H., Lo, H.-M., and Fang, J.-Y. (2006). Development and evaluation of emulsion–liposome blends for resveratrol delivery. *Journal of Nanoscience and Nanotechnology*. 6(9–1): 2950–2958.

Hung, L. M., Chen, J. K., Huang, S. S., Lee, R. S., and Su, M. J. (2000). Cardioprotective effect of resveratrol, a natural antioxidant derived from grapes. *Cardiovascular Research* 47(3): 549–555.

Huwiler, A., Kolter, T., Pfeilschifter, J., and Sandhoff, K. (2000). Physiology and pathophysiology of sphingolipid metabolism and signaling. *Biochimica et Biophysica Acta* 1485(2–3): 63–99.

International Life Sciences Institute. (1999). Scientific concepts of functional foods in Europe: Consensus document. *British Journal of Nutrition* 81: S1–S28.

International Union of Food Science & Technology (IUFoST). (2010). Nanotechnology and Food. IUFoST Scientific Information Bulletin. PDF available at http://iufost.org/sites/default/files/docs/IUF.SIB.NanotechnologyandFoodupdate.pdf

Isailović, B. D., Kostić, I. T., Zvonar, A., Đorđević, V. B., Gašperlin, M., *et al.* (2013). Resveratrol loaded liposomes produced by different techniques. *Innovative Food Science & Emerging Technologies* 19: 181–189.

Jesorka, A., and Orwar, O. (2008). Liposomes: Technologies and analytical applications. *Annual Review of Analytical Chemistry* (Palo Alto, Calif). 1: 801–832.

Jores, K., Mehnert, W., Drechsler, M., Bunjes, H., Johann, C., and Mader, K. (2004). Investigations on the structure of solid lipid nanoparticles (SLN) and oil-loaded solid lipid nanoparticles by photon correlation spectroscopy, field-flow fractionation and transmission electron microscopy. *Journal of Controlled Release: Official Journal of the Controlled Release Society* 95(2): 217–227.

Joye, I. J., and McClements, D. J. (2013). Production of nanoparticles by anti-solvent precipitation for use in food systems. *Trends in Food Science & Technology* 34(2): 109–123.

Khan, R. S., Grigor, J., Winger R., and Win, A. (2013). Functional food product development – Opportunities and challenges for food manufacturers. *Trends in Food Science & Technology* 30(1): 27–37.

Kim, S. T., Park, K. H., Oh, S. C., Seo, J. H, Kim, J. S., *et al.* (2013). Chemotherapy in patients older than or equal to 75 years with advanced non-small cell lung cancer. *Cancer Research and Treatment* 44(1): 37–42.

Kolouchová-Hanzlíková, I., Melzoch, K., Filip, V, and Šmidrkal, J. (2004). Rapid method for resveratrol determination by HPLC with electrochemical and UV detections in wines. *Food Chemistry* 87(1): 151–158.

Kopermsub, P., Mayen, V., and Warin, C. (2011). Potential use of niosomes for encapsulation of nisin and EDTA and their antibacterial activity enhancement. *Food Research International* 44(2): 605–612.

Kotilainen, L., Rajalahti, R., Ragasa, C., and Pehu, E. (2006). Health enhancing foods: Opportunities for strengthening the sector in developing countries. Agriculture and Rural Development Discussion Paper 30.

Kristl, J., Teskač, K., Caddeo, C., Abramović, Z., and Šentjurc, M. (2009). Improvements of cellular stress response on resveratrol in liposomes. *European Journal of Pharmaceutics and Biopharmaceutics* 73(2): 253–259.

Külkamp, I. C., Rabelo, B. D., Berlitz, S. J., Isoppo, M., Bianchin, M. D., *et al.* (2011). Nanoencapsulation improves the *in vitro* antioxidant activity of lipoic acid. *Journal of Biomedical Nanotechnology* 7(4): 598–607.

Kumpugdee-Vollrath, M. (2012). Solid state characterization of *trans* resveratrol complexes with different cyclodextrins. *Journal of the Asian Association of Schools of Pharmacy* 1(2): 125–136.

Lai, C.-S., Wu, J.-C., and Pan, M.-H. (2015). Molecular mechanism on functional food bioactives for anti-obesity. *Current Opinion in Food Science* 2: 9–13.

Landete, J. M. (2011). Updated knowledge about polyphenols: Functions, bioavailability, metabolism, and health. *Critical Reviews in Food Science and Nutrition* 52(10): 936–948.

Leonard, N. B. (2000). Stability Testing of Nutraceuticals and Functional Foods. Handbook of Nutraceuticals and Functional Foods. In: *Modern Nutrition*. CRC Press; 2000.

Lesmes, U., and McClements, D. J. (2009). Structure–function relationships to guide rational design and fabrication of particulate food delivery systems. *Trends in Food Science & Technology* 20(10): 448–457.

Li, H., Xu, X., Liu, M., Sun, D, Li, L. (2010). Microcalorimetric and spectrographic studies on host–guest interactions of α-, β-, γ- and Mβ-cyclodextrin with resveratrol. *Thermochimica Acta* 510(1–2): 168–172.

Li, X., Li, H., Liu, M., Li, G., Li, L., and Sun, D. (2011). From guest to ligand – A study on the competing interactions of antitumor drug resveratrol with β-cyclodextrin and bovine serum albumin. *Thermochimica Acta* 521(1–2): 74–79.

Liu, W., Sun, D., Li, C., Liu, Q., and Xu, J. (2006). Formation and stability of paraffin oil-in-water nano-emulsions prepared by the emulsion inversion point method. *Journal of Colloid and Interface Science* 303(2): 557–563.

López-Hernández, J., Paseiro-Losada, P., Sanches-Silva, A., and Lage-Yusty, M. (2007). Study of the changes of trans-resveratrol caused by ultraviolet light and determination of *trans*- and *cis*-resveratrol in Spanish white wines. *European Food Research Technology* 225(5–6): 789–796.

Lu, X., Ji, C., Xu, H., Li, X., Ding, H., *et al.* (2009). Resveratrol-loaded polymeric micelles protect cells from Aβ-induced oxidative stress. *International Journal of Pharmaceutics* 375(1–2): 89–96.

Lu, Z., Chen, R., Fu, R., Xiong, J., and Hu, Y. (2012). Cytotoxicity and inhibition of lipid peroxidation activity of resveratrol/cyclodextrin inclusion complexes. *Journal of Inclusion Phenomena and Macrocyclic Chemistry* 73(1–4): 313–320.

Lu, Z., Cheng, B., Hu, Y., Zhang, Y., and Zou, G. (2009). Complexation of resveratrol with cyclodextrins: Solubility and antioxidant activity. *Food Chemistry* 113(1): 17–20.

Lucas-Abellán, C., Fortea, I., López-Nicolás, J. M., and Núñez-Delicado, E. (2007). Cyclodextrins as resveratrol carrier system. *Food Chemistry* 104(1): 39–44.

Luo, Y., Chen, D., Ren, L., Zhao, X., Qin, J. (2006). Solid lipid nanoparticles for enhancing vinpocetine's oral bioavailability. *Journal of Controlled Release* 114(1): 53–59.

Lyons, M. M., Yu, C., Toma, R. B., Cho, S. Y., Reiboldt, W., *et al.* (2003). Resveratrol in raw and baked blueberries and bilberries. *Journal of Agricultural and Food Chemistry* 51(20): 5867–5870.

Manach, C., Scalbert, A., Morand, C., Rémésy, C., and Jiménez, L. (2004). Polyphenols: Food sources and bioavailability. *American Journal of Clinical Nutrition* 79(5): 727–747.

Martirosyan, A., and Schneider, Y. J. (2014). Engineered nanomaterials in food: Implications for food safety and consumer health. *International Journal of Environmental Research and Public Health* 11(6): 5720–5750.

Mason, T. G., Wilking, J. N., Meleson, K., Chang, C. B., and Graves, S. M. (2006). Nanoemulsions: Formation, structure, and physical properties. *Journal of Physics: Condensed Matter* 18(41): R635.

Matos, M., Gutiérrez, G., Coca, J., and Pazos, C. (2014). Preparation of water-in-oil-in-water (W1/O/W2) double emulsions containing *trans*-resveratrol. *Colloids and Surfaces A: Physicochemical and Engineering Aspects* 442: 69–79.

Matsuda, H., and Arima, H. (1999). Cyclodextrins in transdermal and rectal delivery. *Advanced Drug Delivery Reviews* 36(1): 81–99.

McClements, D. J. (2012). Crystals and crystallization in oil-in-water emulsions: Implications for emulsion-based delivery systems. *Advances in Colloid and Interface Science* 174: 1–30.

McClements, D. J., Decker, E. A., Park, Y. (2009). Controlling lipid bioavailability through physicochemical and structural approaches. *Critical Reviews in Food Science and Nutrition* 49(1): 48–67.

McClements, D. J., Decker, E. A., Park, Y., and Weiss, J. (2009). Structural design principles for delivery of bioactive components in nutraceuticals and functional foods. *Critical Reviews in Food Science and Nutrition* 49(6): 577–606.

McClements, D. J., Decker, E. A., and Weiss, J. (2007). Emulsion-based delivery systems for lipophilic bioactive components. *Journal of Food Science* 72(8): R109–R124.

McClements, D. J., and Li, Y. (2010). Structured emulsion-based delivery systems: Controlling the digestion and release of lipophilic food components. *Advances in Colloid and Interface Science* 159(2): 213–228.

Meleson, K., Graves, S., and Mason, T. G. (2004). Formation of concentrated nanoemulsions by extreme shear. *Soft Materials* 2(2–3): 109–123.

Menrad, K. (2004). Innovations in the food industry in Germany. *Research Policy* 33(6–7): 845–878.

Menrad, K. (2003). Market and marketing of functional food in Europe. *Journal of Food Engineering* 56: 181–188.

Mogol, B. A., Gökmen, V., and Shimoni, E. (2013). Nano-encapsulation improves thermal stability of bioactive compounds Omega fatty acids and silymarin in bread. *Agro Food Industry* 24(3): 62–65.

Morris, V. (2008). Nanotechnology in the food industry. *New Food Magazine* 4: 53–55.

Montsko, G., Nikfardjam, M. S. P., Szabo, Z., Boddi, K., Lorand, T., *et al.* (2008). Determination of products derived from trans-resveratrol UV photoisomerisation by means of HPLC–APCI–MS. *Journal of Photochemistry and Photobiology A: Chemistry* 196(1): 44–50.

Mozafari, M. R. (2006). *Nanocarrier Technologies: Frontiers of Nanotherapy.* Dordrecht: SpringerLink.

Mozafari, M. R., Johnson, C., Hatziantoniou, S., and Demetzos, C. (2008). Nanoliposomes and their applications in food nanotechnology. *Journal of Liposome Research* 18(4): 309–327.

Mozafari, M. R., and Khosravi-Darani, K. (2007). An Overview of Liposome-Derived Nanocarrier Technologies. In: *Nanomaterials and Nanosystems for Biomedical Applications*, pp. 113–123. M. R. Mozafari, ed. Dordrecht: Springer-Verlag.

Mukherjee, K., Venkatesh, M., Venkatesh, P., Saha, B. P., and Mukherjee, P. K. (2011). Effect of soy phosphatidyl choline on the bioavailability and nutritional health benefits of resveratrol. *Food Research International* 44(4): 1088–1093.

Müller, R. H., Dingler, A., Schneppe, T., and Gohla, S. (2000). Large Scale Production of Solid Lipid Nanoparticles (SLN) and Nanosuspensions. In: *Handbook of Pharmaceutical Controlled Release Technology*, pp. 377–392. I. D. L. Wise, ed. New York: CRC Press.

Müller, R. H., Mäder, K., and Gohla, S. (2000). Solid lipid nanoparticles (SLN) for controlled drug delivery – a review of the state of the art. *European Journal of Pharmaceutics and Biopharmaceutics* 50(1): 161–177.

Muller, R. H., Radtke, M., and Wissing, S. A. (2002). Nanostructured lipid matrices for improved microencapsulation of drugs. *International Journal of Pharmaceutics* 242(1-2): 121–128.

Munin, A., and Edwards-Lévy, F. (2011). Encapsulation of natural polyphenolic compounds; A review. *Pharmaceutics* 3(4): 793.

Narayanan, N. K., Nargi, D., Randolph, C., Narayanan, B. A. (2009). Liposome encapsulation of curcumin and resveratrol in combination reduces prostate cancer incidence in PTEN knock-out mice. *International Journal of Cancer* 125(1): 1–8.

Ndiaye, M., Kumar, R., and Ahmad, N. (2011). Resveratrol in cancer management: Where are we and where we go from here? *Annals of the New York Academy of Sciences* 1215(1): 144–149.

Nedovic, V., Kalusevic, A., Manojlovic, V., Levic, S., and Bugarski, B. (2011). An overview of encapsulation technologies for food applications. *Procedia Food Science* 1: 1806–1815.

Neves, A. R., Lucio, M., Lima, J. L., and Reis, S. (2012). Resveratrol in medicinal chemistry: A critical review of its pharmacokinetics, drug-delivery, and membrane interactions. *Current Medicinal Chemistry* 19(11): 1663–1681.

Neves, A. R., Lucio, M., Martins, S., Lima, J. L., and Reis, S. (2013). Novel resveratrol nanodelivery systems based on lipid nanoparticles to enhance its oral bioavailability. *International Journal of Nanomedicine* 8: 177–187.

Niva, M. (2007). "All foods affect health": Understandings of functional foods and healthy eating among health-oriented Finns. *Appetite* 48(3): 384–393.

Ourique, A. F., Azoubel, S., Ferreira, C.V., Silva, C.B., Marchiori, M. C. L., *et al.* (2010). Lipid-core nanocapsules as a nanomedicine for parenteral administration of tretinoin: Development and *in vitro* antitumor activity on human myeloid leukaemia cells. *Journal of Biomedical Nanotechnology* 6(3): 214–223.

Pace-Asciak, C. R., Hahn, S., Diamandis, E. P., Soleas, G., Goldberg, D. M. (1995). The red wine phenolics *trans*-resveratrol and quercetin block human platelet aggregation and eicosanoid synthesis: Implications for protection against coronary heart disease. *Clinica Chimica Acta* 235(2): 207–219.

Palzer, S. (2009). Food structures for nutrition, health and wellness. *Trends in Food Science & Technology* 20(5): 194–200.

Pandita, D., Ahuja, A., Lather, V., Benjamin, B., Dutta, T., *et al.* (2011). Development of lipid-based nanoparticles for enhancing the oral bioavailability of paclitaxel. *AAPS PharmSciTech* 12(2): 712–722.

Pandita, D., Kumar, S., Poonia, N., and Lather, V. (2014). Solid lipid nanoparticles enhance oral bioavailability of resveratrol, a natural polyphenol. *Food Research International* 62: 1165–1174.

Pando, D., Beltrán, M., Gerone, I., Matos, M., and Pazos, C. (2015). Resveratrol entrapped niosomes as yoghurt additive. *Food Chemistry* 170: 281–287.

Pando, D., Gutiérrez, G., Coca, J., and Pazos, C. (2013). Preparation and characterization of niosomes containing resveratrol. *Journal of Food Engineering* 117(2): 227–234.

Peng, H., Xiong, H., Li, J., Xie, M., Liu, Y., *et al.* (2010). Vanillin cross-linked chitosan microspheres for controlled release of resveratrol. *Food Chemistry* 121(1): 23–28.

Pinho, E., Grootveld, M., Soares, G., and Henriques, M. (2014). Cyclodextrins as encapsulation agents for plant bioactive compounds. *Carbohydrate Polymers* 101: 121–135.

Pinto, M. del C., García-Barrado, J. A., and Macías, P. (2003). Oxidation of resveratrol catalyzed by soybean lipoxygenase. *Journal of Agricultural and Food Chemistry* 51(6): 1653–1657.

Pohlmann, A. R., Fonseca, F. N., Paese, K., Detoni, C. B., Coradini, K., *et al.* (2013). Poly(ε-caprolactone) microcapsules and nanocapsules in drug delivery. *Expert Opinion on Drug Delivery* 10(5): 623–638.

Porras, M., Solans, C., González, C., Gutiérrez, J. M. (2008). Properties of water-in-oil (W/O) nano-emulsions prepared by a low-energy emulsification method. *Colloids and Surfaces A: Physicochemical and Engineering Aspects* 324(1–3): 181–188.

Poshadri, A., and Kuna, A. (2010). Microencapsulation technology: A review. *Journal of Research Angrau* 38(1):86–102.

Pravst, I. (2012). Functional Foods in Europe: A Focus on Health Claims. In: *Scientific, Health and Social Aspects of the Food Industry*, pp. 165–208. B. Valdez, ed. Rijeka, Croatia: InTech. .

Rao, J., and McClements, D. J. (2012). Food-grade microemulsions and nanoemulsions: Role of oil phase composition on formation and stability. *Food Hydrocolloids* 29(2): 326–334.

Rius, C., Abu-Taha, M., Hermenegildo, C., Piqueras, L., Cerda-Nicolas, J. M., *et al.* (2010). *Trans*-but not *cis*-resveratrol impairs angiotensin-II–mediated vascular inflammation through inhibition of NF-κB activation and peroxisome proliferator–activated receptor-γ upregulation. *Journal of immunology* (Baltimore, Md : 1950) 185(6): 3718–3727.

Roberfroid MB. (2002). Functional food: Concepts and application to inulin and oligofructose. *British Journal of Nutrition* 87: S139–S143.

Rodriguez, R. A., Lahoz, I. R., Faza, O. N., Cid, M. M., and Lopez, C. S. (2012). Theoretical and experimental exploration of the photochemistry of resveratrol: Beyond the simple double bond isomerization. *Organic & Biomolecular Chemistry* 10(46): 9175–9182.

Rossi, D., Guerrini, A., Bruni, R., Brognara, E., Borgatti, M., *et al.* (2012). *trans*-Resveratrol in nutraceuticals: Issues in retail quality and effectiveness. *Molecules* 17(10): 12393.

Rossi, J., and Leroux, J.-C. (2006). Principles in the Development of Intravenous Lipid Emulsions. In: *Role of Lipid Excipients in Modifying Oral and Parenteral Drug Delivery*, pp. 88–123. Hoboken: John Wiley & Sons.

Rotches-Ribalta, M., Andres-Lacueva, C., Estruch, R., Escribano, E., and Urpi-Sarda, M. (2012). Pharmacokinetics of resveratrol metabolic profile in healthy humans after moderate consumption of red wine and grape extract tablets. *Pharmacological Research* 66(5): 375–382.

Russel, W. B., Saville, D. A., Schowalter, W. R. (1989). *Colloidal Dispersions*. Cambridge: Cambridge University Press.

Saberi, A. H., Fang, Y., and McClements, D. J. (2013). Fabrication of vitamin E–enriched nanoemulsions: Factors affecting particle size using spontaneous emulsification. *Journal of Colloid and Interface Science* 391: 95–102.

Sagalowicz, L., and Leser, M. E. (2010). Delivery systems for liquid food products. *Current Opinion in Colloid & Interface Science* 15(1–2): 61–72.

Saiko, P., Szakmary, A., Jaeger, W., and Szekeres, T. (2008). Resveratrol and its analogs: Defense against cancer, coronary disease and neurodegenerative maladies or just a fad? *Mutation Research/Reviews in Mutation Research* 658(1–2): 68–94.

Sakulku, U., Nuchuchua, O., Uawongyart, N., Puttipipatkhachorn, S., Soottitantawat, A., and Ruktanonchai, U. (2009). Characterization and mosquito repellent activity of citronella oil nanoemulsion. *International Journal of Pharmaceutics* 372(1–2): 105–111.

Sanna, V., Roggio, A. M., Pala, N., Marceddu, S., Lubinu, G., *et al.* (2015). Effect of chitosan concentration on PLGA microcapsules for controlled release and stability of resveratrol. *International Journal of Biological Macromolecules* 72(0): 531–536.

Sanna, V., Siddiqui, I. A., Sechi, M., and Mukhtar, H. (2013a). Nanoformulation of natural products for prevention and therapy of prostate cancer. *Cancer Letters* 334(1): 142–151.

Sanna, V., Siddiqui, I. A., Sechi, M., and Mukhtar, H. (2013b). Resveratrol-loaded nanoparticles based on poly(epsilon-caprolactone) and poly(D,L-lactic-co-glycolic acid)–poly(ethylene glycol) blend for prostate cancer treatment. *Molecular Pharmaceutics* 10(10): 3871–3881.

Santos, A. C., Veiga, F., and Ribeiro, A. J. (2011). New delivery systems to improve the bioavailability of resveratrol. *Expert Opinion on Drug Delivery* 8(8): 973–990.

Sapino, S., Carlotti, M. E., Caron, G., Ugazio, E., and Cavalli, R. (2009). *In silico* design, photostability and biological properties of the complex resveratrol/hydroxypropyl-β-cyclodextrin. *Journal of Inclusion Phenomena and Macrocyclic Chemistry* 63(1-2): 171–180.

SciFinder. (2013). Resveratrol CAS 501–36–0. Washington, D.C.: American Chemical Society.

Schmidt, B. M., Erdman, J. W., and Lila, M. A. (2005). Effects of food processing on blueberry antiproliferation and antioxidant activity. *Journal of Food Science* 70(6): S389–S394.

Sessa, M., Balestrieri, M. L., Ferrari, G., Servillo, L., Castaldo, D., *et al.* (2014). Bioavailability of encapsulated resveratrol into nanoemulsion-based delivery systems. *Food Chemistry* 147: 42–50.

Sessa, M., Tsao, R., Liu, R., Ferrari, G., and Donsi, F. (2011). Evaluation of the stability and antioxidant activity of nanoencapsulated resveratrol during *in vitro* digestion. J Agric Food Chem. 2011;59(23):12352-60.

Shakeel, F., and Ramadan, W. (2010). Transdermal delivery of anticancer drug caffeine from water-in-oil nanoemulsions. *Colloids and surfaces B, Biointerfaces* 75(1): 356–362.

Shulman, M., Cohen, M., Soto-Gutierrez, A., Yagi, H., Wang, H., *et al.* (2011). Enhancement of naringenin bioavailability by complexation with hydroxypropyl-beta-cyclodextrin. [corrected]. *PloS ONE* 6(4): e18033.

Siró, I., Kápolna, E., Kápolna, B., and Lugasi, A. (2008). Functional food. Product development, marketing and consumer acceptance—A review. *Appetite* 51(3): 456–467.

Spence, J. T. (2006). Challenges related to the composition of functional foods. *Journal of Food Composition and Analysis* 19: S4–S6.

Summerlin, N., Soo, E., Thakur, S., Qu, Z., Jambhrunkar, S., and Popat, A. (2015). Resveratrol nanoformulations: Challenges and opportunities. *International Journal of Pharmaceutics* 479(2): 282–290.

Tadros, T., Izquierdo, P., Esquena, J., and Solans, C. (2004). Formation and stability of nanoemulsions. *Advances in Colloid and Interface Science* 108–109:303–318.

Talegaonkar, S., Mustafa, G., Akhter, S., and Iqbal, Z. I. (2010). Design and development of oral oil-in-water nanoemulsion formulation bearing atorvastatin: *In vitro* assessment. *Journal of Dispersion Science and Technology* 31(5): 690–701.

Tamayo-Esquivel, D., Ganem-Quintanar, A., Martinez, A. L., Navarrete-Rodriguez, M., Rodriguez-Romo, S., and Quintanar-Guerrero, D. (2006). Evaluation of the enhanced oral effect of omapatrilat–monolein nanoparticles prepared by the emulsification–diffusion method. *Journal of Nanoscience and Nanotechnology* 6(9–10): 3134–3138.

Tamjidi, F., Shahedi, M., Varshosaz, J., and Nasirpour, A. (2013). Nanostructured lipid carriers (NLC): A potential delivery system for bioactive food molecules. *Innovative Food Science & Emerging Technologies* 19: 29–43.

Taylor, T. M., Davidson, P. M., Bruce, B. D., and Weiss, J. (2005). Liposomal nanocapsules in food science and agriculture. *Critical Reviews in Food Science and Nutrition* 45(7–8): 587–605.

Taylor, T. M., Gaysinsky, S., Davidson, P. M., Bruce, B., and Weiss, J. (2007). Characterization of antimicrobial-bearing liposomes by ζ-potential, vesicle size, and encapsulation efficiency. *Food Biophysics* 2(1): 1–9.

Thies, C. (2005). A Survey of Microencapsulation Processes. In: *Microencapsulation*, pp. 1–20. I. S. Benita, ed. New York: Marcel Dekker.

Thompson, A. K., Hindmarsh, J. P., Haisman, D., Rades, T., and Singh, H. (2006). Comparison of the structure and properties of liposomes prepared from milk fat globule membrane and soy phospholipids. *Journal of Agricultural and Food Chemistry* 54(10): 3704–3711.

Tiwari, G., Tiwari, R., and Rai, A. K. (2010). Studies on development of controlled delivery of combination drug(s) to periodontal pocket. *Indian Journal of Dental Research* 21(1): 72–83.

Trela, B. C., and Waterhouse, A. L. (1996). Resveratrol: Isomeric molar absorptivities and stability. *Journal of Agricultural and Food Chemistry* 44(5): 1253–1257.

Tu, Y. S., Sun, D. M., Zhang, J. J., Jiang, Z. Q., Chen, Y. X., *et al.* (2014). Preparation and characterisation of andrographolide niosomes and its anti-hepatocellular carcinoma activity. *Journal of Microencapsulation* 31(4): 307–316.

Unger, E. C., Porter, T., Culp, W., Labell, R., Matsunaga, T., Zutshi, R. (2004). Therapeutic applications of lipid-coated microbubbles. *Advanced Drug Delivery Reviews* 56(9): 1291–1314.

Valenzano, D. R., Terzibasi, E., Genade, T., Cattaneo, A., Domenici, L., and Cellerino, A. (2006). Resveratrol prolongs lifespan and retards the onset of age-related markers in a short-lived vertebrate. *Current Biology* 16(3): 296–300.

Vang, O., Ahmad, N., Baile, C. A., Baur, J. A., Brown, K., *et al.* (2011). What is new for an old molecule? Systematic review and recommendations on the use of resveratrol. *PloS ONE* 6(6): e19881.

Varshosaz, J., Eskandari, S., and Tabakhian, M. (2010). Production and optimization of valproic acid nanostructured lipid carriers by the Taguchi design. *Pharmaceutical Development and Technology* 15(1): 89–96.

Varshosaz, J., Ghaffari, S., Khoshayand, M. R., Atyabi, F., Azarmi, S., and Kobarfard, F. (2010a). Development and optimization of solid lipid nanoparticles of amikacin by central composite design. *Journal of Liposome Research* 20(2): 97–104.

Varshosaz, J., Minayian, M., and Moazen, E. (2010b). Enhancement of oral bioavailability of pentoxifylline by solid lipid nanoparticles. *Journal of Liposome Research* 20(2): 115–123.

Vauthier, C., and Couvreur, P. (2000). Development of Polysaccharide Nanoparticles as Novel Drug Carrier Systems. In: *Handbook of Pharmaceutical Controlled Release Technology*, pp. 413–429. D. L. Wise, ed. New York: Marcel Dekker.

Venuti, V., Cannavà, C., Cristiano, M. C., Fresta, M., Majolino, D., *et al.* (2014). A characterization study of resveratrol/sulfobutyl ether-β-cyclodextrin inclusion complex and *in vitro* anticancer activity. *Colloids and Surfaces B: Biointerfaces* 115: 22–28.

Veršič, R. J. (2014). The Economics of Microencapsulation in the Food Industry. In: *Microencapsulation in the Food Industry*, pp. 409–417. A. G. Gaonkar, N. Vasisht, A. R. Khare, and R. Sobel, eds. San Diego: Academic Press.

Walle, T. (2011). Bioavailability of resveratrol. *Annals of the New York Academy of Sciences* 1215(1): 9–15.

Walle, T., Hsieh, F., DeLegge, M. H., Oatis, J. E., and Walle, U. K. (2004). High absorption but very low bioavailability of oral resveratrol in humans. *Drug Metabolism and Disposition* 32(12): 1377–1382.

Wang, J., Ho, L., Zhao, Z., Seror, I., Humala, N., *et al.* (2006). Moderate consumption of Cabernet Sauvignon attenuates Aβ neuropathology in a mouse model of Alzheimer's disease. *FASEB Journal* 20(13): 2313–2320.

Wang, X.-X., Li, Y.-B., Yao, H.-J., Ju, R.-J., Zhang, Y., *et al.* (2011). The use of mitochondrial targeting resveratrol liposomes modified with a dequalinium polyethylene glycol-distearoylphosphatidyl ethanolamine conjugate to induce apoptosis in resistant lung cancer cells. *Biomaterials* 32(24): 5673–5687.

Weiss, J., Takhistov, P., and McClements, D. J. (2006). Functional materials in food nanotechnology. *Journal of Food Science* 71(9): R107–R116.

Wong, H. L., Bendayan, R., Rauth, A. M., Li, Y., and Wu, X. Y. (2007). Chemotherapy with anticancer drugs encapsulated in solid lipid nanoparticles. *Advanced Drug Delivery Reviews* 59(6): 491–504.

Yu, C., Shin, Y., Chow, A., Li, Y., Kosmeder, J., *et al.* (2002). Human, rat, and mouse metabolism of resveratrol. *Pharmaceutical Research* 19(12): 1907–1914.

Zanotto-Filho, A., Coradini, K., Braganhol, E., Schröder, R., de Oliveira, C. M., *et al.* (2013). Curcumin-loaded lipid-core nanocapsules as a strategy to improve pharmacological efficacy of curcumin in glioma treatment. *European Journal of Pharmaceutics and Biopharmaceutics* 83(2): 156–167.

Zhang, X.-P., Le, Y., Wang, J.-X., Zhao, H., and Chen, J.-F. (2013). Resveratrol nanodispersion with high stability and dissolution rate. *LWT – Food Science and Technology* 50(2): 622–628.

Zink, D. L. (1997). The impact of consumer demands and trends on food processing. *Emerging Infectious Diseases* 3(4): 467–469.

Zuidam, N., and Heinrich, E. (2010). Encapsulation of Aroma, pp. 127–160. In: *Encapsulation Technologies for Active Food Ingredients and Food Processing*. N. J. Zuidam and V. Nedovic, eds. New York: Springer.

CHAPTER 9

Nutraceutical compounds encapsulated by extrusion–spheronization

Thi Trinh Lan Nguyen, Nicolas Anton, and Thierry F. Vandamme
Université de Strasbourg, Faculté de Pharmacie, Laboratoire de Conception et d'Application de Biomolécules, 74 Route du Rhin -B.P.60024- 67401, Illkirch Cedex, France

9.1 Extrusion–spheronization process application for nutraceuticals

9.1.1 Pellets

Pellets are defined as spherical or nearly spherical, free-flowing particles with a narrow size distribution, varying between 500 and 1500 μm for pharmaceutical applications (Ghebre-Sellassie, 1989). Pellets manufactured in the pharmaceuticals industry are commonly filled into hard gelatin capsules but can also be compressed to tablets (Conine and Hadley, 1970; Ghanam and Kleinebudde, 2011; Hosseini *et al.*, 2013; Malinowski and Smith, 1975; Mehta *et al.*, 2012; Millili and Schwartz, 1990).

Pelletized dosage forms date back to the 1950s, when the first product was introduced to the market. Since then, these dosage forms have gained considerable popularity because of their distinct advantages, such as ease of capsule filling because of better flow properties of the spherical pellets; enhancement of drug dissolution; ease of coating; sustained, controlled, or site-specific delivery of the drug from coated pellets; uniform packing; even distribution in the gastrointestinal (GI) tract; and less GI irritation (Trivedi *et al.*, 2007).

Pellets as a drug-delivery system offer not only therapeutic advantages such as less irritation of the GI tract and a lowered risk of side effects due to dose dumping (Bechgaard and Hegermann Nielsen, 1978) but also technological advantages, for example, better flow properties, less-friable dosage form, narrow particle size distribution, ease of coating, and uniform packing (Reynolds, 1970).

Pellets are an excellent tool for numerous applications. Pellets can be coated with sustained-release and enteric film coatings to achieve unique release

New Polymers for Encapsulation of Nutraceutical Compounds, First Edition.
Edited by Jorge Carlos Ruiz Ruiz and Maira Rubi Segura Campos.

profiles or multiple release rates in a single dosage unit by mixing pellets that are coated with different film coatings (Haaser *et al.*, 2013; Dekyndt *et al.*, 2015; Xu *et al.*, 2015; Palugan *et al.*, 2015).

Pellets also offer the ability to mix multiple active ingredients or incompatible active ingredients in a single capsule. Multiple-units are single-dose forms that disintegrate into several parts after ingestion. Hard gelatin capsules are particularly suitable for their development and manufacture. Multiple-units might consist of a single pellet, homogeneous granules, or a combination of several pellets and granules with various substances and different release characteristics. It is even possible to include a number of dosage forms – such as tablets, pellets, capsules, powders, and granules – within a single formulation. In this way, incompatibilities and interaction among the different drug substances in combination products can be prevented (Stegemann, 2002).

The invention by Zerbe *et al.* (2007) provides an innovative solution to the problem of preventing and/or reducing interactions between a calcium nutrient and an iron nutrient present in a single dosing form by isolating the calcium nutrient in an enterically coated particle, granule, or pellet. An enterically coated particle, granule, or pellet containing a calcium nutrient allows an iron nutrient to be formulated in an immediate-release portion of a dosage form, while release of the calcium nutrient is delayed until the enterically coated particle, granule, or pellet reaches the higher pH region (>5.5 pH) of the GI tract (i.e., the upper part of the intestine). This controlled or delayed release of the calcium nutrient prevents or reduces simultaneous presence of the iron and calcium nutrients, thereby reducing or eliminating interactions between the two nutrients that would otherwise reduce bioavailability and absorption.

Ebube (2006) invented a method to produce pellets including a mixture of multiple active pharmaceutical ingredients (guaifenesin, dextromethorphan HBr, and pseudoephedrine HCl) with optional inactive additives that display a uniform distribution of the multiple active ingredients within each pellet that can be formed into a solid dosing form. The amount of active ingredients in the mixture may vary, according to the desired composition of the solid dosing form. One advantage of the invention is that it allows higher concentration of active ingredients in the solid form due to higher concentration of active ingredients in the pellets produced according to the methods and processes provided herein. The daily dose may be included in a single delivery unit or may be divided into multiple delivery units. Dividing the daily dose among multiple delivery units may be desirable if a tablet is used, for example, to provide a hard gelatin capsule size that is convenient to swallow. If multiple delivery units are used, they may be administered at one time or administered at intervals during the dosing period (typically a day), if desired. Accordingly it should be understood that the amounts of the active ingredients are for a dose that may be delivered in one unit or multiple delivery units.

Pelletized dosing forms can be prepared by a number of techniques, including drug layering on nonpareil sugar or microcrystalline cellulose beads, spray-drying, spray-congealing, rotogranulation, hot-melt extrusion, and spheronization of low-melting materials or extrusion–spheronization of a wet mass (Vervaet *et al.*, 1995).

9.1.2 General description of the extrusion–spheronization process (wet-mass extrusion)

Conine and Hadley (1970) were the first to describe the production of pellets via extrusion–spheronization in the pharmaceuticals industry, and Reynolds (1970) elaborated this work through the further description of the equipment and process mechanisms. Extrusion–spheronization is a multistep process consisting of the consecutive stages shown in Figure 9.1.

The extrusion–spheronization process typically involves a specific sequence of steps (Figure 9.2). The characteristics and quality of the final pellets produced by the extrusion–spheronization process depend on the physicochemical properties of the active pharmaceutical ingredient and excipients and on process variables. Specifically, the physicochemical properties of the active pharmaceutical

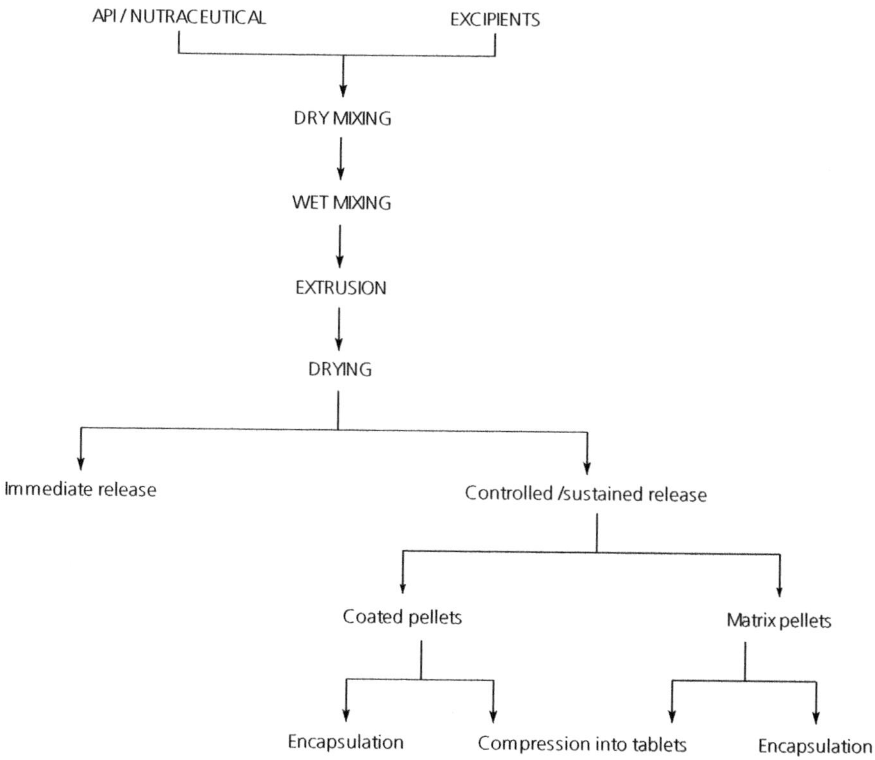

Figure 9.1 The extrusion–spheronization process (wet-mass extrusion).

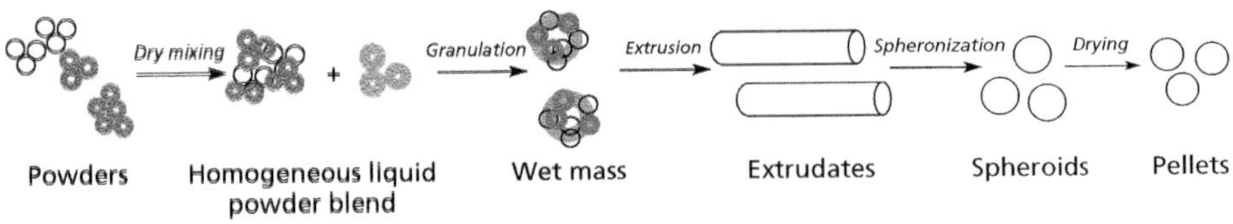

Figure 9.2 Schematic overview of the steps involved in an extrusion–spheronization process.

ingredient and excipients that affect the types of pellets produced by the process include particle size and surface area, moisture sorption capacity, polymorphism of the active pharmaceutical ingredient, aqueous solubility, and density. The process variables that affect the quality of the pellets include mixing time and speed, type and amount of binder and/or solvent added to wet the powder mixture, type of extruder, diameter of the orifice and thickness of the die or screen, rate of extrusion, spheronization time, speed, load, plate design, and drying time and rate (Hellén, 1993a,b). The main steps of the process are

1 Dry mixing of ingredients to achieve homogeneous powder dispersion
2 Wet massing to produce a sufficiently plastic wet mass
3 Extrusion to form rod-shaped particles of uniform diameter
4 Spheronization to round off these rods into spherical particles
5 Drying to achieve the desired final moisture content
6 Screening (optional) to achieve the desired narrow size distribution

The disadvantages of the extrusion–spheronization process are that it is a multistep, labor-intensive, and time-consuming batch process. Each step in the process has its own variables that have major effects on the quality of the final product. Consequently, it is necessary to optimize the processing parameters for each formulation. Furthermore, the process requires the use of a relatively large amount of water compared to the traditional granulation process, uniform distribution of the water in the wetted mass, and appropriate drying conditions, which might not be suitable for moisture- and heat-sensitive drugs (Trivedi *et al.*, 2007).

9.1.3 Process and equipment

9.1.3.1 Dry mixing and wet granulation

A uniform blend has to be obtained before wet granulation can take place, because it affects the pellets' content uniformity. An uneven distribution can also result in local overwetting during granulation for materials with large differences in size and solubility properties (Parikh, 2009). Dry mixing and wet granulation are usually carried out in the same equipment (e.g., planetary mixer, high-shear mixer, sigma-blade mixer).

9.1.3.2 Extrusion

During extrusion, the plastic wet mass is forced through a die and shaped into cylindrical particles with a uniform diameter. The resulting extrudate's diameter is determined by the diameter of the die, and its length depends upon the properties of the wet mass and the extruder type. A variety of extruder types have been developed and can be divided into three classes based on their feed mechanism (i.e., the way the wet mass is transported through the extrusion zone): screw-feed extruders, gravity-feed extruders, and piston-feed extruders, shown in Figure 9.3.

According to Reynolds (1970) and Rowe (1985), an axial-screw extruder produces a denser material than a radial-screw extruder. The latter has a higher output but also produces greater heat during the processing. Pellet quality depends

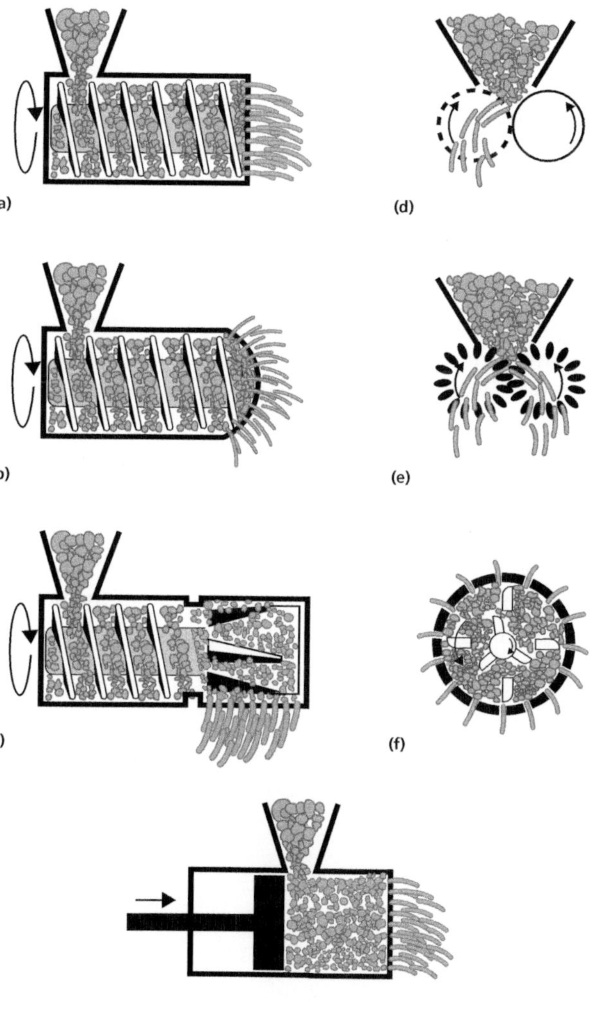

Figure 9.3 Schematic overview of the extruder types applied in extrusion–spheronization. Screw feed extruders with axial **(a)**, dome **(b)**, and radial **(c)** type; gravity-feed extruders with cylinder **(d)**, gear **(e)**, and radial **(f)** type; and piston-feed ram extruders **(g)**. (Erkoboni D.F., 2003).

on the thickness of the screen and the diameter of the perforations (Hellén *et al.*,1992). A thinner screen produces a rough and loosely bound extrudate, whereas a thicker screen forms smooth and well-bound extrudate because of the higher densification of the wet mass. Similarly, the diameter of the perforations determines the size of pellets: A larger diameter in the perforations will produce pellets with a larger diameter under similar processing conditions (Hellén, 1993b).

A number of studies compare the extrusion and spheronization behavior of wet powder masses processed by a ram extruder and a cylinder extruder (Fielden *et al.*, 1992b), between the extrusion forces and sphere quality of a gravity-feed extruder and a ram extruder (Baert *et al.*, 1992), and between a gravity-feed extruder and a twin-screw extruder (Baert *et al.*, 1993).

9.1.3.3 Spheronization

A spheronizer consists of a bowl with fixed sidewalls and a bottom plate or disk that rotates at a high speed (Figure 9.4). The spheronizer is filled with extrudates, and due to frictional forces generated by particle–particle and particle–equipment interaction, the extrudates are initially broken into smaller cylinders and then rounded into spheres. To enhance the forces generated as particles move across its surface, the bottom plate generally exhibits a grooved surface (cross-hatched pattern or radial pattern). Different manufacturers produce different types of plates. Most spheronizer plates have grooved surfaces, which are designed to increase the frictional forces (Vervaet *et al.*, 1995).

Pellet quality also depends on spheronizer load, which affects the particle size distribution, bulk, and tap density of the final pellets. The increase in the spheronizer speed and a low spheronizer load will result in wider particle size distribution with less yield of pellets, whereas it increases with extended spheronization time at a higher spheronizer load. Hellén *et al.* (1992) reported that the bulk and tap density increased and the size of the pellets decreased with an increasing spheronizer load.

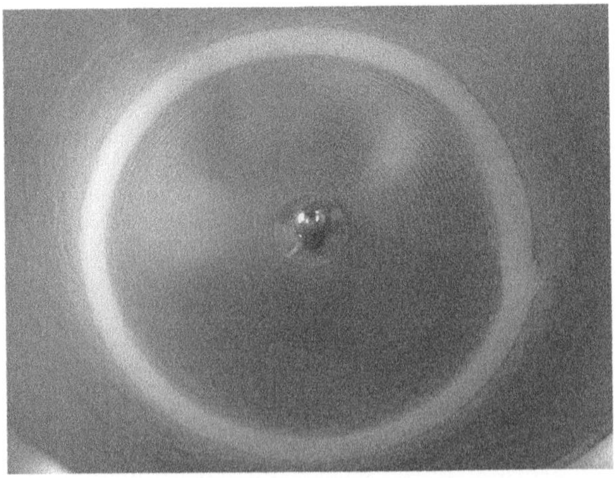

Figure 9.4 Photograph (plan view) of spheronizer plate in motion.

Four different spheronizer friction plate patterns (cross-hatch, radial, striated-edge, pyramidal cross-hatch patterns) have been used (Figure 9.5) (Michie *et al.*, 2012).

The transformation from a cylindrical extrudate in a spherical particle occurs in various stages, and two models have been proposed to describe this process (Figure 9.5a and b). According to Rowe (1985) (Figure 9.6a), the cylinders are rounded off at the edges, followed by the formation of dumbbell-shaped particles, ellipsoids, and finally spheres. The model proposed by Baert and Remon (1993) (Figure 9.6b) suggests that the cylinders are rounded off at the edges but are additionally bent, resulting in the formation of a rope-shaped particle. Next, a dumbbell with a twisted middle is formed, initiating particle breakage into two

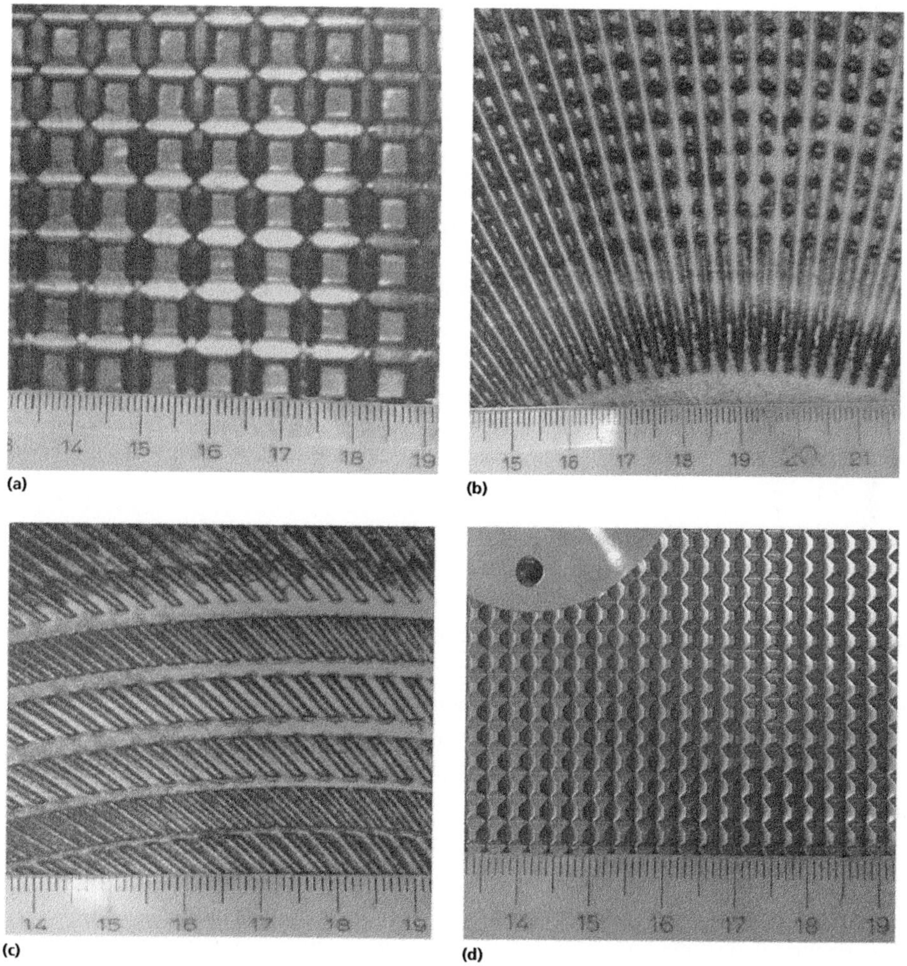

Figure 9.5 Friction plate design. **(a)** Cross-hatch pattern, **(b)** radial pattern, **(c)** striated edge pattern, **(d)** cross-hatched friction plate (pyramidal elements on a square pattern, spacing 1.40 mm, height 0.86 mm, and width at top 0.50 mm).

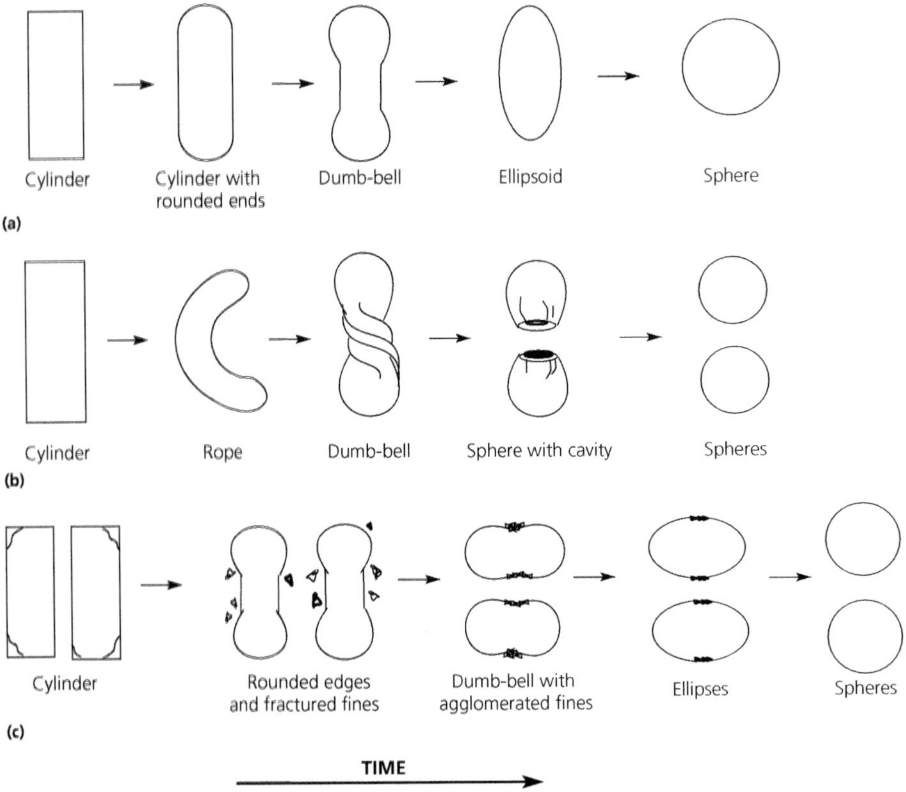

Figure 9.6 Schematic presentation of the different pellet formation stages during spheronization according to Rowe (1985) **(a)**, Baert and Remon (1993) **(b)**, and Koester and Thommes (2010) **(c)**.

spherical particles with a cavity on their flat side. Further rounding in the spheronizer creates completely spherical particles. Koester and Thommes (2010) reported that these generally adopted pelletization mechanisms need to be extended to account for the material transfer between pellet particles (Figure 6c). In addition to plastic deformation, these authors also observed a material transfer between pellet particles for different formulations. Herewith, regional distinctions in the amount of mass transfer and an influence of the water content were observed.

The duration of spheronization is usually 2 to 10 minutes (Gamlen, 1985), and a rotational speed between 200 and 400 rpm of the friction plate is optimum to obtain a highly spherical pellet (West, 1988).

9.1.3.4 Drying

The spherical particles are then dried at room temperature or at an elevated temperature (in an oven, a fluidized bed, or a microwave oven) until the desired residual moisture level is achieved. Because the different process steps are influenced by a number of interrelated process and formulation variables, the extrusion–spheronization process requires the necessary control to obtain the required pellet quality.

Wet pellets are mostly dried in an oven or fluid bed, although microwave and freeze-drying have been also used to study the influence of drying method on pellet properties. The main differences between oven and fluid-bed drying are the rate of granulation liquid evaporation and the way the material is handled during drying: During oven drying in a static bed, liquid evaporates from the material over a longer time, whereas during fluid-bed drying, the turbulent motion of dried material in a heated air stream promotes significantly faster drying (Lieberman and Rankell, 1970). Several authors have studied the influence of different drying techniques on pellet characteristics (Airaksinen *et al.*, 2004; Bashaiwoldu *et al.*, 2004; Bataille *et al.*, 1993; Kleinebudde, 1994; Römer, M., *et al.*, 2007; Sousa *et al.*, 1996; Wlosnewski *et al.*, 2010).

9.1.3.5 Screening

Screening may be necessary to achieve the desired size distribution, and for this purpose sieves are used. In case of pellets prepared by extrusion–spheronization, screening is essentially required after manufacture, in order to avoid pellets having high size distribution. (Koo *et al.*, 2001).

9.1.4 Formulation

Selection of suitable excipients for any formulation is one of the major tasks during formulation development. In a multistep process, the quality of the final product depends on the quality of intermediate products obtained at the end of each step, and that depends significantly on the type of the excipients used. The formulation must have certain qualities in order to produce extrudates that can be spheronized into appropriate particle-size pellets with desired surface characteristics. The next section describes various excipients that have been used to prepare pellets using the extrusion–spheronization process (Trivedi *et al.*, 2007).

9.1.4.1 Microcrystalline cellulose as a spheronization aid

Microcrystalline cellulose (MCC) is the most commonly used spheronizing aid in a formulation undergoing extrusion–spheronization. It is available in different grades and particle sizes. Of all the different brands and grades of MCC, Avicel PH 101 or Emcocel 50 have been the most widely used. MCC helps in the formation of spheres because of its unique properties. Like other cellulosic materials, MCC is a filamentous material with a large surface area, high internal porosity, and high moisture-retaining property (Shah *et al.*, 1995).

MCC is the gold standard extrusion–spheronization aid based on its good binding properties, which provide cohesiveness to a wetted mass containing MCC. Furthermore, it is able to absorb and retain a large quantity of water due to its large surface area and high internal porosity (Sonaglio *et al.*, 1995), thus facilitating extrusion, improving wetted mass plasticity, and enhancing spheronization.

Moreover, by controlling the movement of water through the plastic mass, it prevents phase separation during extrusion or spheronisation. Due to these properties, MCC-based pellets produced via extrusion–spheronization have a good sphericity, low friability, high density, and smooth surface.

MCC's capacity to retain very large quantities of water internally means that wet masses made with MCCs have rheological properties that are very suitable for extrusion–spheronization (Fielden *et al.*, 1992a).

9.1.4.2 Alternative excipients for microcrystalline cellulose

To date, MCC has been considered the gold standard for extrusion–spheronization. However, several investigators have attempted to replace MCC as a spheronizing agent, but with limited success. For example, Agrawal and colleagues (2004) studied the effect of formulation and process variables on the physical properties of pellets prepared with varying concentrations of chitosan, ethyl cellulose, and hydroxypropyl methylcellulose (HPMC), without using MCC. Results of the study indicated that process variables such as spheronizer and extruder speed, and formulation variables such as chitosan, HPMC, and water content, significantly affected the physical properties of the pellets. Pellet size decreased with an increase in chitosan content. Glyceryl monostearate (GMS) has also been used as an appropriate replacement for MCC for producing spherical pellets, using the extrusion–spheronization process in two studies (Bashaiwoldu *et al.*, 2004; Basit *et al.*, 1999). Other excipients that have been used to prepare spherical pellets include hydroxypropyl cellulose (Kleinebudde, 1994), starch–dextrin blend (Prieto, 2005), K-carrageenan (Ghanam and Kleinebudde, 2011; Koester and Thommes, 2010), HPMC, hydroxyethyl cellulose (HEC) (with isopropanol as a solvent) (Chatlapalli and Rohera, 1998), powdered cellulose (Alvarez *et al.*, 2003), and isomalt (Antal *et al.*, 2013).

9.1.4.3 Use of other excipients in the extrusion–spheronization process

Other excipients, such as water-soluble/swellable polymers (e.g., polyvinylpyrrolidone, hydroxypropyl methylcellulose, polyethylene oxide), ionic polymers (e.g., carboxypolymethylene, chitosan, eudragit), hydrophobic/water-insoluble polymer (e.g., ethylcellulose), waxes (e.g., glyceryl monostearate, carnuba wax), disintegrants (e.g., croscarmellose sodium, sodium starch glycolate, crospovidone), and polysaccharides (e.g., starch, dextrin), are also added to formulations containing MCC in order to attain the desired drug-release characteristics from the pellets (Trivedi *et al.*, 2007).

Excipients used in combination with microcrystalline cellulose (MCC) to improve pellet disintegration and/or drug release from MCC-based pellets include fillers and surfactants.

Fillers are the excipients used to form the bulk of the material. in the process of pelletization, 70% to 80% of the excipient is formed by fillers. Generally, microcrystalline cellulose is used for this purpose. Other fillers are lactose, dicalcium diphosphate, mannitol, starch and derivatives, glucose, and β-cyclodextrine.

Surfactants are added to the liquid to improve wettability by lowering the interfacial tension between the liquid and drug particles. Examples include sodium lauryl sulfate, polyethylene glycol, polysorbate 80, glyceryl and sorbitan mono-oleate, sorbitan mono-palmitate, glycerol monostearate, and self-emulsifying systems (Dukić *et al.*, 2009).

The types and concentrations of specific excipients incorporated in the formulations depend on the specific need and the desired drug-release rates from the pellets. For example, in spite of the large surface area of pellets, which provides faster absorption from this dosing form, poorly soluble drugs might require superdisintegrants to compensate for the delay in drug dissolution due to the high density of pellets (Souto *et al.*, 2005).

9.1.5 Evaluation of pellets

A number of techniques are used to evaluate the physical properties of pellets prepared by the extrusion–spheronization process (Box 9.1) (Trivedi *et al.*, 2007).

Particle size distribution of the pellets is one of the most important physical properties that must be controlled during the manufacturing process, because most of the pelletized dosage forms are eventually either coated or filled into capsules. Ideally, a narrow particle-size distribution is desired, because a wider distribution can cause problems during coating and capsule-filling operations. Particle-size distribution is generally determined using sieve analysis. However, image analysis techniques are also often used.

Determination of bulk and tapped densities of the pellets provide an idea of their packing characteristics. The bulk and tapped-density values help to determine the size of the capsules that could be used to fill the pellets. Bulk and tapped density is generally determined using a tap densitometer.

Because the pellets are either filled into a capsule before or after coating or compressed into tablets, they should be spherical in order to exhibit good flow characteristics. Pellets produced by the extrusion–spheronization process are not always perfectly spherical. Some of the factors that could affect the sphericity of pellets include the properties of the wet mass, the amount of MCC used as the spheronizing agent, the type and amount of binder, the length and diameter of the extrudates, the spheronization speed and time, and the design of the base plate in the spheronizer (Trivedi *et al.*, 2007).

Sphericity is determined by a number of techniques, as outlined in Box 9.1. Determination of the aspect ratio after image analysis is one of the two-dimensional techniques that is often used to determine the sphericity of the pellets. Other two-dimensional methods, such as one-plane critical stability (OPCS), shape-factor analysis, and three-dimensional methods, such as Heywood's shape coefficient and perimetric shape factor analysis, have also been used to determine sphericity of the pellets. The pros and cons of the two- and

Box 9.1 Evaluation methods for determining pellet properties

Properties

Particle Size
Sieve analysis

Particle Size Distribution
Image analysis

Density
Bulk density
Tapped density

Sphericity or Roundness
Two-Dimensional Methods
Image analysis (aspect ratio)
OPCS (one-plane critical stability)
Shape factor (eR)

Three-Dimensional Methods
Heywood's shape coefficient
Perimetric shape factor

Flow Property
Angle of repose
Dynamic flow
Carr's index
Hausner's ratio

Porosity
Surface-area analysis
Porosimetry
True and bulk densities

Surface Roughness
Microscopic method (SEM-scanning electron microscopy)

Strength of Pellets
Friability
Crushing strength

Drug Release
Dissolution

three-dimensional methods for determining the sphericity of pellets have been well documented by Eriksson and colleagues (1997).

Flow properties of the pellets can be determined by a number of static and dynamic techniques such as the angle of repose and dynamic flow. The angle of repose is a static method, whereas the dynamic flow method determines the flow rate of the pellets through an appropriate orifice. The size and shape of the orifice used during the dynamic flow test is determined by the size or diameter of the capsule or by the size of the die cavity if the pellets are going to be compressed into tablets. Other static methods that have also been used to calculate the flow characteristics of the pellets include determining Carr's index using bulk and tapped-density values, and determining Hausner's ratio, which is the ratio of the tap volume to the bulk volume of the pellets.

Porosity and surface roughness are important pellet characteristics that must be controlled during the manufacturing operation, particularly if the pellets are to be coated or compressed into tablets.

Pellets that are highly porous may also have a rough surface. During a fluid-bed coating operation, pellets with rough surfaces can generate fine particles in the coating chamber because the pellets are fluidized, thus resulting in uneven coating. In addition, the rough pellets may also have poor flow characteristics, which could result in weight variation due to uneven filling of the capsules or the die cavity during tableting. Scanning electron microscopy (SEM) is a powerful technique to determine the surface roughness of the pellets. However, it is only a qualitative technique. A surface area analysis technique can also be used to calculate the porosity of the pellets using an appropriate gas. Interpellet porosity can be calculated from the true and bulk density values. The true density evaluates the porosity of the pellets and can be determined by an air compression pycnometer or helium pycnometer (Boutell *et al.*, 2002; Sousa *et al.*,1992; Sousa *et al.*, 2002).

It is important to know the strength and friability of the pellets, because soft or friable pellets can break apart during further processing, such as capsule filling, coating, or tableting operations. Friability of the pellets is determined by a friability tester or a crushing strength apparatus.

The pellet size distribution, shape, friability, density, porosity, flow properties, and dissolution behavior are generally evaluated to assess the pellet quality (Box 9.2 (Podczeck and Newton, 2014; Podczeck *et al.*, 1999; Sousa *et al.*, 2002; Vervaet *et al.*, 1995).

9.2 Nanoemulsions for nutraceutical applications

9.2.1 Introduction

Nanotechnology is an emerging technology that holds potential to transform the food industry (Huang *et al.*, 2010; Luykx *et al.*, 2008). Nanotechnology involves research, technology development, and control of structures within sizes from 1 to 100 nm (Quintanilla-Carvajal *et al.*, 2010). Materials at the nanometer scale (10^{-9} m) and the development of technology to manipulate or assemble such materials can provide commercial, technological, and scientific opportunities for the industry (Huang *et al.*, 2010). The application of nanotechnology to the food field may allow the modification of many macro-scale characteristics of food, such as texture, taste, other sensory attributes, coloring strength, processability, and stability during shelf life, leading to a great number of new products. Nanotechnology can

Box 9.2 Desirable properties of pellets

Uncoated pellets have
- Uniform spherical shape
- Uniform size
- Good flow properties
- Reproducible packing (into hard gelatin capsules)
- High strength
- Low friability
- Low dust
- Smooth surface
- Ease of coating

And once coated they
- Maintain all of the above properties, and
- Have desired drug-release characteristics

Adapted from Aulton, M. E., and Summers, M. P. (2013)

also improve the water solubility, thermal stability, and oral bioavailability of functional compounds (Huang *et al.*, 2010; McClements *et al.*, 2009).

Nanoemulsions are defined as the structures having typical droplet diameters of 20 to 200 nm (Solans *et al.*, 2005). The term *nanoemulsion* was first used by Nakajima and colleagues (1993); other terms have also been used, including *miniemulsion* (El-Aasser and Sudol, 2004), *submicron emulsion* (Amselem and Friedman, 1998), and ultrafine emulsion (Nakajima, 1997). Solans *et al.* (2005) recommend the term *nanoemulsion* because it clearly describes that droplets are at nano-level and it differs completely from the term *microemulsion*.

Nanoemulsions are superior to conventional emulsions because they have a transparent or semitranslucent appearance and smaller droplet size, they are stable against sedimentation and creaming, and they tend to increase bioavailability (Shakeel *et al.*, 2008; Solans and Solé, 2012; Wang *et al.*, 2008; Zhang, 2011). In addition to their high colloidal stability, nanoemulsions need less than 10% surface-active agent in preparation stages; this rate is 20% or higher in microemulsions. Furthermore, because nanoemulsions provide a wide surface area, they allow active components to be penetrated quickly (Laouini *et al.*, 2012). Due to their long-term stability under storage and an improved high bioavailability, they have attained particular interest as delivery systems for bioactive substances such as carotenoids, phytosterols, polyunsaturated fatty acids, goryzanol, lipophilic vitamins, and numerous other compounds.

Contrary to thermodynamically stable microemulsions, nanoemulsions are unstable systems that might be exposed to environmental degradation (Solans and Solé, 2012). The formation and manufacturing control of nanoemulsions require high shear forces to be applied to cope with surface tension of droplets

(Mason *et al.*, 2006). Because nanoemulsions are non-equilibrium systems, they cannot be formed spontaneously, and typically energy input from a mechanical device is required (Zhang, 2011). Thus, in general, high-energy methods are used for preparing nanoemulsions: high-pressure homogenizers (Sanguansri and Augustin, 2006; Solans *et al.*, 2005; Zhang, 2011), microfluidizers (Dalgleish *et al.*, 1997; Guraya and James, 2002; Jafari *et al.* 2006, 2007; Kwon *et al.*, 2002; Swientek, 1990; Thompson and Singh, 2006), and ultrasonic generators (Chandrapala *et al.*, 2012; Ghosh *et al.*, 2013; Li and Chiang, 2012; Sanguansri and Augustin, 2006; Xia *et al.*, 2001). There have also been a number of studies applying low-energy methods for production of nanoemulsions, by using the chemical potential of the components under special conditions (Acosta, 2009; Calderó, *et al.*, 2011; Rao and McClements, 2010; Solans and Solé, 2012).

Nanoemulsions have become increasingly important in food industry as an innovative approach in carrying functional agents like fatty acids, polyphenols, vitamins, natural colorants, antimicrobials, some micronutrients, and flavors (Laouini *et al.*, 2012; Mao *et al.*, 2009; McClements and Rao, 2011; Rao *et al.*, 2011; Seikikawa and Watanabe, 2008; Zhang, 2011). Oil-in-water nanoemulsions are being investigated, and their role in such polymerization reactions as nanoreactors has been searched (Solans *et al.*, 2005). In previous studies, oil-in-water nanoemulsion systems have been used as a carrier and combiner in food in order to encapsulate ω-3 fatty acids in yogurt (Chee *et al.*, 2005) and ice cream (Chee *et al.*, 2007). Therefore, it could be concluded that oil-in-water nanoemulsions offer a good potential in food applications, especially for encapsulation of lipophilic compounds. It is necessary to understand basic physicochemical characteristics of food nanoemulsions in order to provide key information to increase the applicability of nanoemulsions in foods and to guide better formulations (Zhang, 2011).

9.2.2 Method

9.2.2.1 High-energy approaches

The formation of nanoemulsions by high-energy methods is governed by the selected composition (i.e., surfactants and functional compounds) and by the quantity of energy applied. Therefore, nanoemulsions produced through high-energy methods present a natural predisposition to preserve the form of the nanoemulsion against formulation modification, such as addition of monomer, surfactant, or co-surfactant (Anton *et al.*, 2008).

The mechanical processes generating nanoemulsions can be divided into three major groups based on the devices used: high-pressure homogenization, ultrasound, and high-speed rotor/stator devices (Anton *et al.*, 2008; Sanguansri and Augustin 2006). In these high-energy approaches, most of the energy provided is dissipated in the form of heat. Although this idea is generally known, only very few authors report energy calculations in their publications.

In high-pressure homogenization, the mixture is subjected to very high pressures and is pumped through a restrictive valve. The very high shear stress causes the formation of very fine emulsion droplets (Quintanilla-Carvajal *et al.*, 2010; Sanguansri and Augustin, 2006). In the ultrasound process, two immiscible liquids are submitted to high-frequency sound waves in the presence of a surfactant, and emulsion droplets are formed by cavitation. This causes intense shock waves in the surrounding liquid, and the formation of liquid jets at high speed is responsible for the formation of emulsion droplets. However, this technology has not yet been proved as efficient for industrial-scale applications (Fielden and Hsu, 1999; Quintanilla-Carvajal *et al.*, 2010; Sanguansri and Augustin, 2006). High-speed rotor/stator devices (such as Ultra-Turrax), when compared with the other high-energy approaches, do not provide a good dispersion in terms of droplet sizes, and the energy provided is mostly dissipated, generating heat (Anton *et al.*, 2008; Walstra, 1993).

9.2.2.2 Low-energy approaches

In low-energy approaches, nanoemulsions are obtained as a result of phase transitions produced during the emulsification process, which is generally carried out at constant temperature while changing the composition (Usón *et al.* 2004) or at constant composition while changing the temperature (Izquierdo *et al.* 2001; Morales *et al.* 2003). The methods used more often are membrane emulsification, spontaneous emulsification, solvent displacement, emulsion inversion point, and phase inversion point.

Membrane emulsification is a low-energy process that requires less surfactant (compared with high-energy methods) and produces emulsions with a narrow size distribution range. This method involves formation of a dispersed phase (droplets) through a membrane into a continuous phase. This method has as limitation the low flux of the dispersed phase through the membrane, this being an issue during scale-up (Sanguansri and Augustin, 2006).

Spontaneous emulsification occurs when an organic phase and an aqueous phase are mixed. The organic phase is a homogeneous solution of oil, lipophilic surfactant, and water-miscible solvent, and the aqueous phase consists of water and hydrophilic surfactant (Bouchemal *et al.*, 2004). The spontaneous features of this method result from the initial nonequilibrium states of two bulk liquids when they are brought into contact without stirring. It is only under specific conditions that spontaneous emulsification occurs. Spontaneous emulsification is produced by different mechanisms (e.g., diffusion of solutes between two phases, interfacial turbulence, surface tension gradient, dispersion mechanism, condensation mechanism) that seem to be affected by the systems' compositions and their physicochemical characteristics, such as the physical properties of the oily phase and nature of the surfactants (Bouchemal *et al.*, 2004). This process itself increases entropy and thus decreases the Gibbs free energy of the system (Anton *et al.*, 2008).

Solvent displacement consists of mixing a water-miscible organic solvent containing lipophilic functional compounds in an aqueous phase containing an emulsifier. The rapid diffusion of the organic solvent in the aqueous phase promotes the formation of nanoemulsions, enabling their preparation in one step at low-energy input with high yield of encapsulation. Finally, the organic solvent is removed from the nanodispersion under reduced pressure. The use of this technique is limited to water-miscible solvents (Chu *et al.*, 2007; Yin *et al.*, 2009).

The emulsion inversion point method consists in varying the composition of the system at a constant temperature. The structures are formed through a progressive dilution with water or oil to create kinetically stable nanoemulsions (Anton *et al.*, 2008; Sadtler *et al.*, 2010).

The phase inversion point method uses the specific ability of surfactants (nonionic) to alter their affinities to water and oil as a function of temperature at a fixed composition (Shinoda and Saito, 1968, 1969). It consists in suddenly breaking up the microemulsions maintained at the phase inversion point by a rapid cooling (Izquierdo *et al.*, 2001; Izquierdo *et al.*, 2004; Sadurní *et al.*, 2005) or by a dilution in water or oil (Anton *et al.*, 2007, 2008). The nanoemulsions immediately formed are kinetically stable and can be considered irreversible. This process is relatively simple, prevents the encapsulated drug from being degraded during processing, consumes low amounts of energy, and allows an easy industrial scale-up (Anton *et al.*, 2008).

9.2.3 Materials used in nanoemulsions production

In general, the oil-in-water nanosized emulsion should be formulated with compatible vehicles and additives. The components of internal and external phases of nanosized emulsion should be chosen to confer enhanced solubility and stability to the incorporated lipophilic drug. In addition, the selected excipients should also preferably be chosen to favorably influence the biofate or therapeutic index of the incorporated drug following administration via parenteral, ocular, percutaneous, and nasal routes. This section is a comprehensive presentation of the general considerations concerning excipient selection and their optimum concentrations. Common excipients used for formulation of oil-in-water nanosized emulsions are listed in Box 9.3 (Tamilvanan *et al.*, 2010).

9.3 Nano-size nutraceutical emulsion encapsulated by extrusion–spheronization

9.3.1 Objective of experimental design

Encapsulation is a process to entrap active agents within a carrier material, and it is a useful tool to improve delivery of bioactive molecules and living cells into foods. Encapsulation may be defined as a process to entrap one substance or

Box 9.3 Excipients used for formulation of oil-in-water nanosized emulsions

Oils

- Castor oil
- Corn oil
- Glycerin monostearate
- Lanolin
- Paraffin light
- Medium-chain monoglycerides
- Medium-chain triglycerides
- Paraffin oil
- Petroleum jelly (Vaseline)
- Sesame oil
- Soybean oil
- Squalene

Emulsifiers

- Cholesterol
- Cremophor RH
- Miranol C_2 M and MHT
- Phospholipids (Lipoid)
- Poloxamer 407
- Poloxamer 188
- Polysorbate 80 and 20 (Tween 80 and 20)
- Transcutol P
- Tyloxapol TPGS

Cationic lipids and polysaccharide

- Chitosan
- Oleylamine
- Stearylamine

Miscellaneous

- EDTA
- Glycerin
- Methylparaben
- Propylparaben
- Sorbitol
- Thiomersal
- α-Tocopherol
- Xylitol

EDTA, ethylenediaminetetraacetic acid; TPGS, α-tocopheryl polyethylene glycol succinate many substances within other excipients, thereby producing particles with diameters of a few nanometers to a few millimeters.

Encapsulation may be defined as a process to entrap one substance (active agent) within another substance (wall material). The encapsulated substance, the active agent, can be called the core, fill, active, internal, or payload phase. The substance that is encapsulating is often called the coating, membrane, shell, capsule, carrier material, external phase, or matrix (Fang and Bhandari, 2010; Wandrey *et al.*, 2009).

In the food industry, the encapsulation process can be applied for a variety of reasons; a list of these is shown in Box 9.4. Encapsulation is a useful tool to improve delivery of bioactive molecules (e.g., antioxidants, minerals, vitamins, phytosterols, lutein, fatty acids, lycopene) and living cells (e.g., probiotics) into foods (Vos *et al.*, 2010; Wandrey *et al.*, 2009). In most cases, encapsulation refers to a technology in which the bioactive components are completely enveloped, covered, and protected by a physical barrier, without any protrusion of the bioactive components (Vos *et al.*, 2010). Also, encapsulation has been defined as a technology of packaging solids, liquids, or gaseous materials in small capsules that release their contents at controlled rates over prolonged periods and under specific conditions (Frost and Sullivan, 2005). Produced particles usually have diameters of a few nanometers to a few millimeters (Wandrey *et al.*, 2009).

Box 9.4 Benefits of microencapsulated ingredients

The possible benefits of microencapsulated ingredients in the food industry include the following:

- Superior handling of the active agent (e.g., conversion of liquid active agent into a powder, which might be dust free and/or free flowing and might have a more neutral smell)
- Immobility of active agent in food-processing systems
- Improved stability in final product and during processing (i.e., less evaporation of volatile active agent and/or no degradation or reaction with other components in the food product such as oxygen or water)
- Improved safety (e.g., reduced flammability of volatiles like aroma, no concentrated volatile oil handling)
- Creation of visible and textural effects (visual cues)
- Adjustable properties of active components (particle size, structure, oil-soluble or water-soluble, color)
- Off-taste masking
- Controlled release (differentiation, release by the right stimulus)

Such benefits should overcome the following possible negatives:

- Additional costs
- Increased complexity of production process and/or supply chain
- Undesirable consumer perception (visual or touch) of the encapsulates in food products
- Stability challenges of encapsulates during processing and storage of the food product

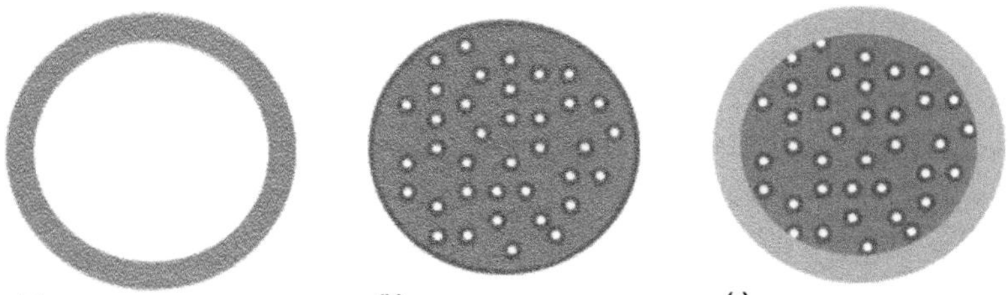

Figure 9.7 Reservoir type **(a)**, matrix type **(b)**, and coated matrix type **(c)** encapsulates.

Two main types of encapsulates may be distinguished: the reservoir type and the matrix type (Figure 9.7). The reservoir type has a shell around the active agent. This type is also called capsule, single-core, monocore, or core-shell type. Application of pressure can lead to breakage of the reservoir type of encapsulates and thus to the release of its contents. Poly- or multiple-core type of encapsulates with several reservoir chambers in one particle also exist. The active agent in the matrix type is much more dispersed over the carrier material; it can be in the form of relatively small droplets or it can be more homogeneously distributed over the encapsulate.

Active agents in the matrix type of encapsulates are in general also present at the surface (unless they have an additional coating; see Figure 9.7), in contrast to those in the reservoir type. For simplification, Figure 9.7 shows only spherical encapsulates, but they can also be cylindrical, oval, or an irregular shape. The last is a combination of the first two. In the figure, the active is indicated in white, and the carrier material is in gray. The bioactive or nutraceutical in the matrix type of encapsulates might be in the form of tiny droplets or is dispersed at the molecular level throughout the particle. Encapsulates might also be defined by their particle size, such as nanoparticles, microcapsules, or microreservoirs.

The possible benefits of microencapsulated ingredients in the food industry are listed in Box 9.4. Such benefits should overcome the possible drawbacks, such as additional costs, increased complexity of the production process and/or supply chain, undesirable perception by the consumer (visual or touch) of the encapsulates in the food product, and stability challenges of encapsulates during processing and storage of the food product.

Because of these possible drawbacks, encapsulates should generally not be seen as a first option when designing food formulations. Only when other, simple options fail may one consider encapsulation. Nevertheless, because encapsulates facilitate formulations of food products that are healthier, tastier, and more convenient, the demand for encapsulation has been growing (Frost and Sullivan, 2005).

Nutraceuticals are a large variety of products that include vitamin and mineral supplements (either single or in combinations), bioactive food substances, specific parts of plants, herbal supplements, specially formulated foods such as cereals, yogurt, soups, and beverages, and even genetically modified foods.

Nutraceuticals are products derived from food sources that provide extra health benefits in addition to the basic nutritional value. Depending on the jurisdiction and regulation, products may claim to prevent chronic diseases, improve health, delay the aging process, increase life expectancy, and support specific diets. Vitamins are categorized into fat-soluble vitamins and water-soluble vitamins. The fat-soluble vitamins are A, D, E, and K, and many cannot be formulated as aqueous preparations because these would have bioavailability problems and hence reduce patient compliance.

Like the fat-soluble vitamins, many chemical entities and nutraceuticals are poorly water-soluble and show high lipophilicity. It is difficult to formulate them into oral preparations because their low aqueous solubility ultimately affects bioavailability. To enhance the bioavailability of such drug compounds, encapsulation by extrusion–spheronization is the reliable drug-delivery system.

9.3.2 Daily dosage of nutraceuticals

Daily dosages of some nutraceuticals are recommended by the U.S. National Institutes of Health. These are listed in Table 9.1.

Recommended intakes of nutrients vary by age and sex and are known as recommended dietary allowances (RDAs) and adequate intakes (AIs). However, one value for each nutrient, known as the daily value (dV), is selected for the labels of dietary supplements and foods. A daily value is often, but not always, similar to the RDA or AI for that nutrient. Some daily values have been developed by the U.S. Food and Drug Administration (FDA) to help consumers determine the level of various nutrients in a standard serving of food in relation to their approximate requirement for it. The label actually

Table 9.1 U.S. National institutes of health recommendations for daily dosages of some nutraceuticals.

Nutraceutical	Daily Dosage from Dietary Supplement
Vitamin A palmitate	900 μg RAE (retinol activity equivalents)
Vitamin B_{12}	2.8 μg
β-Carotene	6 mg/day
Vitamin C	90–125 mg
Cholecalciferol (D_3)	600 IU (15 μg); >70 years 800 IU (20 μg)
DL-α-tocopherol acetate (liquid)	15 mg (22.4 IU) = 22.4 mg α-tocopherol acetate
Folic acid	200 μg
Lini oleum virginale (virgin linseed oil)	457.5 mg
Linoleic acid	0.8 g
Oleic acid	21.5 mg

U.S. National Institutes of Health, Office of Dietary Supplements (2016a,b,c; 2011).

provides the "% Daily Value" so that one can see how much (what percentage) of a serving of the product contributes to reaching the daily value.

Daily dosages of nutritional supplements are different depending on age, sex, and health, and during acute or chronic diseases such as hypertension, diabetes, cardiovascular disease, weight management, and bone and joint diseases.

For example, we can use nutraceuticals in diabetes management. A vitamin E derivative has been shown to improve insulin action, reduce resistance, improve glucose control, and reduce glycosylation of proteins. Optimal dosages are unclear, but 200 to 400 IU of a mixture of tocopherols and tocotrienols are recommended. Vitamin C (ascorbic acid) reduces glycosylation of proteins and reduces sorbitol accumulation but was found not to have any direct effect on glucose. Folate and vitamin B_{12} (cyanocobalamin) have no significant effects on glucose metabolism; however, both are noted to improve symptoms of diabetic peripheral neuropathy (Pathak, 2010).

9.3.3 Material and methods to prepare nano-size nutraceutical emulsions encapsulated by extrusion–spheronization

9.3.3.1 Materials and methods

9.3.3.1.1 Materials

Vitamin A palmitate, vitamin B_{12}, cholecalciferol (D_3), microcrystalline cellulose (Avicel PH-101), lactose monohydrate, and silica colloidal anhydrous were purchased from Fagron (France). DL-α-Tocopherol acetate (liquid) was purchased from Fluka. Folic acid was purchased from Sigma-Aldrich. Talc was purchased from Cooper (France). Sodium starch glycolate was obtained from Avebe (Holland). Cremophor ELP (polyoxiethylated-35 castor oil, hydrophilic–lipophilic [HLP] balance approximately 12–14) and Kollidon 25 were provided by BASF (Ludwigshafen, Germany). Labrafil M1944CS (oleoyl macrogol-6 glycerides) was purchased from Gattefossé (France). Advantia Preferred HS 245008CR01 (ISP technologies Inc.), Pharmacoat 606 was purchased from Seppic (France).

Finally, ultrapure water was obtained using the MilliQ filtration system (Millipore, Saint-Quentin-en-Yvelines, France). The composition of pellets is shown in Table 9.2.

9.3.3.1.2 Preparation of emulsions

The blend was prepared by mixing Cremophor ELP in Labrafil M1944CS with fat-soluble vitamins in different formulations of nanoemulsions, with optimized proportions measured by using a Mastersizer (Droplet size <200 nm). Water-soluble vitamins were dissolved in an adequate amount of water. Folic acid was dissolved in an adequate amount of buffer pH 6.8 and 7.5.

9.3.3.1.3 Extrusion and spheronization

Powders were blended in different proportions and wetted by emulsions in a mortar. Water was gradually added for 3 minutes, and then the plastic mass was

Table 9.2 Composition of pellets.

Ingredient (g)	F1	F2	F3	F4	F5	F6	F7	F8
Vitamin A palmitate	0.09	—	—	—	—	—	—	0.09
Vitamin B_{12}	—	0.00028	—	—	—	—	—	0.00028
Cholecalciferol (D_3)	—	—	0.006	—	—	—	—	0.006
DL-α-Tocopherol acetate	—	—	—	1.5	—	—	—	1.5
Folic acid	—	—	—	—	0.02	0.02	0.02	0.02
Microcrystalline cellulose	35	35	35	35	35	35	35	35
Lactose	10	10	10	10	10	10	10	10
PVP 25	5	5	5	5	5	5	5	5
Talc	1	1	1	1	1	1	1	1
Sodium starch glycolate	2.5	2.5	2.5	2.5	2.5	2.5	2.5	2.5
Cremophor ELP	1.8	3	3	3	—	—	1.8	9
Labrafil M1944 CS	1.2	2	2	2	—	—	1.2	6
Phosphate buffer solution pH 6.8	—	—	—	—	40	—	—	—
Phosphate buffer solution pH 7.5	—	—	—	—	—	40	35	—
Water	45	40	40	40	—	—	—	26

mixed for a further 3 minutes. During granulation, the material was repeatedly scraped from the mixing bowl walls to ensure uniform water distribution. The wet mass was extruded at an extrusion speed of 20 rpm using a single-screw extruder (Variable Density Extrusion Caleva 120 [UK] for the laboratory) equipped with axial extrusion in a single benchtop unit (extrusion screen thickness: 1.2 mm; perforation diameter: 1 mm). The extrudates were spheronized for 6 minutes at 1200 rpm in a spheronizer with a cross-hatched friction plate (Caleva Model 15, Caleva, Sturminster Newton, Dorset, UK). The pellets were dried in the ventilated oven (Memmert, Schwabach, Germany) at 45 °C for 12 hours. The pellets were stored in sealed bags.

9.3.3.1.4 Moisture content of pellets

Moisture content was measured by heating about 3 g accurately weighed samples at 105 ° C, on a Sartorius MA100 Infrared Moisture Analyser. The weight was monitored every 30 seconds, and measurement was stopped when the weight loss between two successive measurements was less than 0.01 g.

9.3.3.1.5 Size distribution

Size distribution of pellets was vibrated by a set of standard sieves (DIN/ISO3310-1, Retch, Germany) with 0.25-, 0.5-, 0.71-, 1.0-, and 1.4-mm aperture, for determining size distribution. Fraction of the sieve was calculated taking into account the percentage of pellets remaining on each sieve. The subsequent tests were carried out on the modal size fraction (710–1400 μm).

9.3.3.1.6 Pellet bulk and tapped density

Pellets were poured lightly into a graduated 25-mL cylinder and leveled. The pellets were tapped for 5 minutes and then observed. Pellet bulk density (ρ_b) was calculated as the ratio of the weight of the pellets to the volume of the cylinder before tapping. Pellet tapped density (ρ_t) was calculated as the ratio of the weight of the pellets to its volume after tapping. The Hausner ratio (H_R) was calculated according to equation 9.1:

$$H_R = \frac{\rho_t}{\rho_b} \tag{9.1}$$

9.3.3.1.7 Pellet friability

Pellet friability was measured in a friability test for 4 minutes at 25 rpm with Pharma Test PTF E apparatus (Hamburg, Germany). Friability was used to tumble 10 g of pellets between 1000 µm and 1400 µm. At the end of the test, the mass retained on the sieve 710 µm was weighed and the abrasion resistance was calculated as the percentage loss of mass between initial and final weights of each pellet batch. Each batch was analyzed in triplicate.

9.3.3.1.8 Disintegration

The disintegration time of pellets 1000–1400 µm in diameter was determined in a modified reciprocating cylinder USP Apparatus 3 (Bio-Dis RRT9, G.B. Caleva, Sturminster Newton, UK). The cylinders were fitted at the bottom with 420-µm nylon grids and were immersed in wider thermostated glass vessels filled with deionized water, in order to avoid exit and turbulence. Standard tablet disintegration disks of increased diameter equal to the internal cylinder diameter were used so as to enable smooth sliding inside the cylinder during testing (disk moving in the opposite direction to the cylinder movement) and apply light pressure to the pellets against the grid upon reaching the bottom of the cylinder after a dip. Thirty milligrams of pellets were tested at a temperature of 37 ± 0.5 °C and cylinder dip rate of 30 dpm until no pellets were left in the cylinder. The results represent means of three determinations.

9.3.3.1.9 Size distribution and polydispersity

Size distribution and polydispersity of the nanoemulsions were assessed by dynamic light scattering using a Malvern Nano ZS instrument (Malvern, Orsay, France). A helium neon laser (4 mW) was operated at 633 nm, with the scattering angle fixed at 173 degrees and the temperature maintained at 25 °C. The polydispersity index is a measure of the broadness of the size distribution derived from the cumulative analysis of dynamic light scattering.

To observe the droplet size and size distribution, 250 µL of an emulsion was added to 300 mL of distilled water in a 500-mL beaker. A glass rod was used to induce gentle agitation in the mixture. The droplet size and size distribution of the resultant emulsion were examined using a Malvern Mastersizer 2000 laser diffraction particle analyzer.

9.3.3.1.10 Reconstitution study

The pellets (100 mg) were dispersed in 10 mL of deionized water by shaking for about 1 minute. The solution was filtered through Whatman filter paper (Cat No 1001 090). Of the resulting solution, 1 mL was placed in a test tube and allowed to stand for a few minutes and characterized for mean particle size and distribution by dynamic laser scattering.

9.3.3.1.11 Dissolution tests

Dissolution tests were performed on uncoated pellets containing 1 mg of folic acid using the reciprocating-cylinder method (USP apparatus 3) at 15 dpm in 230 mL of pH 1.2 at 37 ± 0.5 °C. Samples (5 mL) were withdrawn at regular time intervals (5, 10, 20, 30, 45, 60 min) and filtered using a Whatman filter paper (Cat No 1001 090). An equal volume of the respective dissolution medium was added to maintain the volume constant. Folic acid content of the samples was analyzed by Shimadzu UV Spectrophotometer at 297.8 nm. All measurements were performed in triplicate from three independent samples.

9.3.3.2 Results and discussion

9.3.3.2.1 Influence of nutraceutical, oil, and surfactant ratios on droplet size and size distribution

The optimum emulsion formulation is shown in Table 9.3.

A mix of Cremophor ELP plus Labrafil M1944CS was prepared with a ratio of 2:1.33 (SOR 60) and nutraceuticals were added little by little until the droplet size of the emulsion reached a diameter less than 250 nm.

Depending on recommended daily intakes of each vitamin, one can determine the optimum quantity of oil and surfactant for preparing a nanoemulsion to produce a batch of pellets.

The effect of oil, surfactant, and co-surfactant concentrations on the extrusion–spheronization process was important because they were used as wetting liquids for the preparation of experimental pellet batches. The relative quantities of oil/surfactant and water had an effect on the amount of liquid and oil/surfactant that could be incorporated into the powder, as well as the extrusion force, median diameter, spread size, disintegration time, tensile strength, and surface roughness.

The maximum quantity of the oil/surfactant combination studied that can be incorporated was 28% of the dry pellet weight (formulation F8).

The size and weight distribution of sieved pellets (100 g) are presented in Table 9.4. They indicate that a pellet yield (710–1400 μm fraction) of higher than 90% could be obtained. This shows that the addition of a binder (Kollidon 25) was necessary to obtain an acceptable yield because the binder increased the

Table 9.3 Optimum emulsion formulation.

Nutraceutical	Amount of Nutraceutical (%)	Cremophor ELP (%)	Labrafil M1944 CS (%)	Droplet Size	Polydispersity index (PDI)
Non-nutraceutical	0	60	40	23.86 ± 0.128	0.043 ± 0.013
Vitamin A palmitate	24.28	47.35	28.37	158.5 ± 5.667	0.395 ± 0.023
Cholecalciferol (D_3)	8.85	54.45	36.69	27.05 ± 0.4119	0.052 ± 0.009
DL-α-Tocopherol acetate	59.85	25.29	14.86	221.5 ± 7.17	0.320 ± 0.014

Table 9.4 Results of size distribution, flowability of pellets, friability of pellets.

Formula	Size Distribution (%)			Flowability of Pellets			Friability (%)
	1.4–1 mm	1–0.71 mm	0.71–0.5 mm	D Tapped (g/cm³)	D Bulk (g/cm³)	Hausner's Ratio	
F1	30.77	69.23	0.00	0.55	0.53	1.04	0.01
F2	59.80	37.14	3.06	0.61	0.55	1.11	0.04
F3	42.96	52.00	5.04	0.51	0.49	1.04	0.03
F4	28.26	67.11	4.63	0.55	0.50	1.11	0.01
F5	31.46	68.21	0.33	0.52	0.51	1.02	0.02
F6	32.54	67.0	0.46	0.52	0.51	1.02	0.03
F7	13.93	79.29	6.78	0.47	0.46	1.02	0.03
F8	31.20	61.20	7.60	0.49	0.47	1.04	0.01

mechanical strength of wet extrudates, and consequently fewer fine particles were formed during spheronization.

Study of particle size distribution data (Table 9.4) reveals that the size distribution becomes narrow. This might be due to the uniformity in the length of extrudates that were formed when compositions containing oil and surfactant were extruded. This size distribution was not affected significantly by the addition of oil and surfactant.

Results of the investigation of flow properties indicate that all the formulations possess good flow properties (Table 9.4). The pellets from all the batches are not friable at all.

9.3.3.2.2 Disintegration of pellets

The time taken for complete disintegration of pellets prepared with oil and surfactant was 5 to 10 minutes, and pellets prepared without oil and surfactant (formulation F5 + F6) were more than 60 minutes in water, respectively. Pellets containing the surfactant and oil were observed to disintegrate during the dissolution test, whereas those without surfactant did not. As expected, disintegration time decreases as the concentration of oil and surfactant is reduced (Figure 9.8).

9.3.3.2.3 Reconstitution study

The results of reconstitution studies of different formulations of nanoemulsion pellets are presented in Table 9.5, measured by a Malvern Zetasizer to determine their droplet size and polydispersity index (PDI). Overall, all formulations showed small mean droplet sizes between 30 nm and 166 nm. It can be seen from the table that the droplet sizes decreased with an increase in the oil concentration. All the formulations showed low PDI in a range between 0.160 and 0.484.

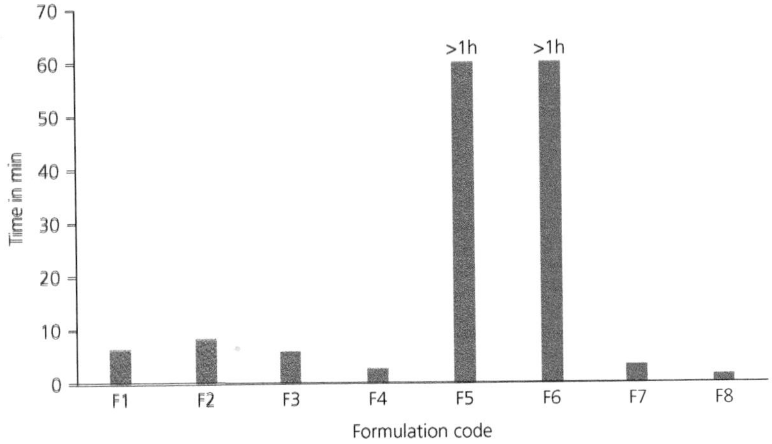

Figure 9.8 Disintegration time of various formulations.

Table 9.5 Droplet size and polydispersity index measurement of nanoemulsion release from pellets.

Formula	After Production		3 Months of Storage at Room Temperature	
	Droplet size (nm)	**Polydispersity index (PDI)**	**Droplet size (nm)**	**Polydispersity index (PDI)**
F1	129.3±0.7506	0.306±0.038	136.8±1.762	0.411±0.060
F2	35.92±0.8062	0.351±0.011	39.78±0.7104	0.323±0.005
F3	40.22±0.7707	0.484±0.011	30.04±0.589	0.379±0.010
F4	165.6±1.572	0.160±0.017	113.3±3.553	0.194±0.015
F5	—	—	—	—
F6	—	—	—	—
F7	91.97±3.744	0.465±0.046	57.85±1.597	0.199±0.007
F8	76.04±1.490	0.385±0.001	68.14±0.3436	0.378±0.012

There was a slightly significant increase in the droplet size of the nanoemulsion after 3 months of storage at room temperature.

9.3.3.2.4 Drug release from pellets

The effect of addition of oil and surfactant on the improvement of dissolution rate of acid folic is illustrated in Figure 9.9. Formulation F7 showed a significant increase in the dissolution rate of the drug: About 80% of folic acid was released within 20 minutes, and 100% of folic acid was released after 60 minutes, whereas F5 and F6 showed 60% release within 60 minutes.

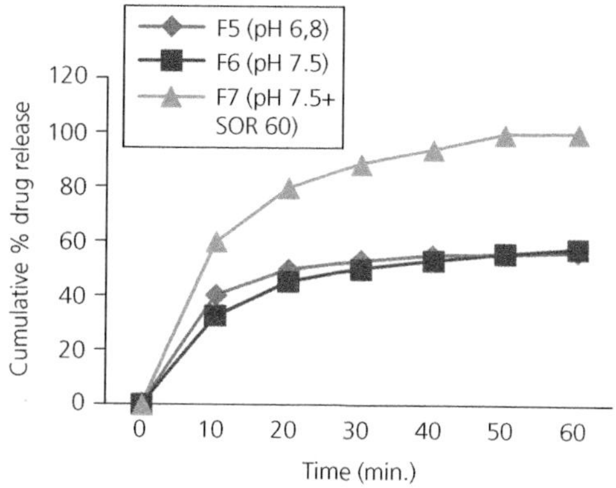

Figure 9.9 Percentage of folic acid released from pellet formulations prepared from mixtures of solutions of folic acid dissolved in phosphate buffer solution with pH 6.8 (F5), pH 7.5 (F6), and pH 7.5 + SOR 60 (F7).

9.4 Conclusion

The results have established that it is possible to prepare pellets by extrusion/spheronization from the individual nutraceutical or multiple nutraceuticals (pellets F8). Pellets should contain at least 28% of a mixture of oil and surfactant to ensure the droplet size in the nanoemulsion is less than 150 nm.

Thus, the work demonstrates that the choice of type and quantity of the surfactant used in the formulation of nanoemulsions contained in pellets has an important influence on their production and performance.

References

Acosta, E. (2009). Bioavailability of nanoparticles in nutrient and nutraceutical delivery. *Current Opinion in Colloid Interface Science* 14: 3–15.

Agrawal, A. M., Howard, M. A., and Neau, S. H. (2004). Extruded and spheronized beads containing no microcrystalline cellulose: Influence of formulation and process variables. *Pharmaceutical Development and Technology* 9: 197–217.

Airaksinen, S., Karjalainen, M., Räsänen, E., Rantanen, J., and Yliruusi, J. (2004). Comparison of the effects of two drying methods on polymorphism of theophylline. *International Journal of Pharmaceutics* 276: 129–141.

Alvarez, L., Concheiro, A., Gomez-Amoza, J. L., Souto, C., and Martinez-Pacheco, R. (2003). Powdered cellulose as excipient for extrusion–spheronization pellets of a cohesive hydrophobic drug. *European Journal of Pharmaceutics and Biopharmaceutics* 55: 291–295.

Amselem, S., and Friedman, D. (1998). Submicron Emulsions as Drug Carriers for Topical Administration. In: *Submicron Emulsions in Drug Targeting and Delivery*. 9th ed., pp. 153–173. S. Benita, ed. London: Harwood Academic Publishers.

Antal, I., Kállai, N., Luhn, O., Bernard, J., Nagy, Z. K., *et al.* (2013). Supramolecular elucidation of the quality attributes of microcrystalline cellulose and isomalt composite pellet cores. *Journal of Pharmaceutical and Biomedical Analysis* 84: 124–128.

Anton, N., Gayet, P., Benoit, J.-P., and Saulnier, P. (2007). Nanoemulsions and nanocapsules by the PIT method: An investigation on the role of the temperature cycling on the emulsion phase inversion. *International Journal of Pharmaceutics* 344(1–2): 44–52.

Anton, N., Benoit, J.-P., and Saulnier, P. (2008). Design and production of nanoparticles formulated from nano-emulsion templates—A review. *Journal of Controlled Release* 128(3): 185–199.

Aulton, M. E., and Summers, M. P. (2013). Powders, Granules and Granulation. In: *Aulton's Pharmaceutics: The Design and Manufacture of Medicines*, 4th edition, pp. 465–486. M. E. Aulton and K. M. G. Taylor, eds. Philadelphia: Churchill Livingstone.

Baert, L., and Remon, J. P. (1993). Influence of amount of granulation liquid on the drug release rate from pellets made by extrusion spheronisation. *International Journal of Pharmaceutics* 95: 135–141.

Baert, L., Remon, J. P., Elbers, J. A. C., and Van Bommel, E. M. G. (1993). Comparison between a gravity feed extruder and a twin screw extruder. *International Journal of Pharmaceutics* 99: 7–12.

Baert, L., Remon, J. P., Knight, P., and Newton, J. M. (1992). A comparison between the extrusion forces and sphere quality of a gravity feed extruder and a ram extruder. *International Journal of Pharmaceutics* 86: 187–192.

Baert, L., Vermeersch, H., Remon, J. P., Smeyers-Verbeke, J., and Massart, D. L. (1993). Study of parameters important in the spheronization process. *International Journal of Pharmaceutics* 96: 225–229.

Bashaiwoldu, A. B. B., Podczeck, F., and Newton, M. (2004). A study on the effect of drying techniques on the mechanical properties of pellets and compacted pellets. *European Journal of Pharmaceutical Sciences* 21: 119–129.

Basit, A. W., Newton, J. M., and Lacey, L. F. (1999). Formulation of ranitidine pellets by extrusion spheronization with little or no microcrystalline cellulose. *Pharmaceutical Development and Technology* 4: 499–505.

Bataille, B., Ligarski, K., Jacob, M., Thomas, C., and Duru, C. (1993). Study of the influence of spheronization and drying conditions on the physico-mechanical properties of neutral spheroids containing Avicel PH 101 and lactose. *Drug Development Industrial Pharmacy* 19: 653–671.

Bechgaard, H., and Nielsen, G.H. (1978). Controlled-release multiple-units and single-unit doses. A literature review. *Drug Development Industrial Pharmacy* 4(1): 53–67.

Bouchemal, K., Briançon, S., Perrier, E., and Fessi, H. (2004). Nanoemulsion formulation using spontaneous emulsification: Solvent, oil and surfactant optimisation. *International Journal of Pharmaceutics* 280(1–2): 241–251.

Boutell, S., Newton, J. M., Bloor, J. R., and Hayes, G. (2002).The influence of liquid binder on the liquid mobility and preparation of spherical granules by the process of extrusion/spheronization. *International Journal of Pharmaceutics* 238: 61–76.

Calderó, G., García-Celma, M. J., and Solans, C. (2011). Formation of polymeric nano-emulsions by a low-energy method and their use for nanoparticle preparation. *Journal of Colloid and Interface Science* 353: 406–411.

Chandrapala, J., Oliver, C., Kentish, S., and Ashokkumar, M. (2012). Ultrasonics in food processing. *Ultrasonics Sonochemistry* 19: 975–983.

Chatlapalli, R., and Rohera, B. D. (1998). Physical characterization of HPMC and HEC and investigation of their use as pelletization aids. *International Journal of Pharmaceutics* 161: 179–193.

Chee, C. P., Djordjevic, D., Faraji, H., Decker, E. A., Hollender, R., *et al.* (2007). Sensory properties of vanilla and strawberry flavored ice cream supplemented with omega-3 fatty acids. *Milchwissenschaft* 62: 66–69.

Chee, C. P., Gallaher, J. J., Djordjevic, D., Faraji, H., McClements, D. J., *et al.* (2005). Chemical and sensory analysis of strawberry flavoured yogurt supplemented with an algae oil emulsion. *Journal of Dairy Research* 72: 311–316.

Chu, B.-S., Ichikawa, S., Kanafusa, S., Nakajima, M. (2007). Preparation of protein-stabilized β-carotene nanodispersions by emulsification–evaporation method. *Journal of the American Oil Chemists' Society* 84(11): 1053–1062.

Conine, J. W., and Hadley, H. R. (1970). Preparation of small solid pharmaceutical spheres. *Drug and Cosmetic Industry* 106: 38–41.

Dalgleish, D. G., West, S. J., and Hallett, F. R. (1997). The characterization of small emulsion droplets made from milk proteins and triglyceride oil. *Colloids and Surfaces A: Physicochemical and Engineering Aspects* 123: 145–53.

DeFelice, S. L. (1995). The nutraceutical revolution, its impact on food industry. *Trends in Food Science and Technology* 6: 59–61.

Dekyndt, B., Verin, J., Neut, C., Siepmann, F., and Siepmann, J. (2015). How to easily provide zero order release of freely soluble drugs from coated pellets. *International Journal of Pharmaceutics* 478: 31–38.

Dukić, R., Mens, A., Adriaensens, P., Foreman, P., Gelan, J. P., *et al.* (2009). Production of pellets via extrusion–spheronization without the incorporation of microcrystalline cellulose: A critical review. *European Journal of Pharmaceutics and Biopharmaceutics* 71: 38–46.

Ebube, N. (2006). Simultaneous encapsulation technique for use in pharmaceutical compositions. United States Patent Application Publication, 20060068011A1.

El-Aasser, M. S., and Sudol, E. D. (2004). Miniemulsions: Overview of research and applications. *Journal of Coatings Technology and Research* 1: 21–31.

Eriksson, M., Alderborn, G., Nyström, C., Podczeck, F., and Newton, J. M. (1997). Comparison between and evaluation of some methods for the assessment of the sphericity of pellets. *International Journal of Pharmaceutics* 148(2): 149–154.

Erkoboni, D. F. (2003). Extrusion/Spheronization. In: *Pharmaceutical Extrusion Technology*, vol. 133, pp. 277–322. I. Ghebre-Sellassie and C. Martin, eds. New York: Marcel Dekker.

Fang, Z., and Bhandari, B. (2010). Encapsulation of polyphenols – a review. *Trends in Food Science and Technology* 21: 510–523.

Food and Agriculture Organization/World Health Organization (FAO/WHO). (2015). Expert meeting on the application of nanotechnologies in the food and agriculture sectors: Potential food safety implications. Rome: Food and Agriculture Organization/World Health Organization.

Fielden, K. E., Newton, J. M., and Rowe, R. C. (1992a). The influence of lactose particle size on spheronization of extrudate processed by a ram extruder. *International Journal of Pharmaceutics* 81: 205–212.

Fielden, K. E., Newton, J. M., and Rowe, R. C. (1992b). A comparison of the extrusion and spheronization behaviour of wet powder masses processed by a ram extruder and a cylinder extruder. *International Journal of Pharmaceutics* 81: 225–233.

Fielden, K. E., Newton, J. M., and Rowe, R. C. (1995). The influence of lactose particle size on spheronization of extrudate processed by a ram extruder. *International Journal of Pharmaceutics* 81: 205–224.

Frost & Sullivan Research Service. (2005). *Opportunities in the Microencapsulated Food Ingredients Market.*London.http://www.frost.com/prod/servlet/report-brochure.pag?id=B716-01-00-00-00

Gamlen, M.J. (1985). Pellet manufacture for controlled release. *Manufacturing Chemist* 56: 55–59.

Gao, Y., Hong, Y., Xian, J., Lin, X., Shen, L., *et al.* (2013). A protocol for the classification of wet mass in extrusion–spheronization. *European Journal of Pharmaceutics and Biopharmaceutics* 85: 996–1005.

Ghanam, D., and Kleinebudde, P. (2011). Suitability of κ-carrageenan pellets for the formulation of multiparticulate tablets with modified release. *International Journal of Pharmaceutics* 409(1–2): 9–18.

Ghebre-Sellassie, I., and Knoch, A. (2002). Pelletization Techniques. In: *Encyclopedia of Pharmaceutical Technology*, 2nd ed. vol. 3, pp. 2067–2080. J. Swarbrick and J. C. Boylan, eds. New York: Marcel Dekker.

Ghebre-Sellassie, I. (1989): Pellets: A General Overview. In: *Pharmaceutical Pelletization Technology*, pp. 1–13. New York: Marcel Dekker.

Ghosh, V., Mukherjee, A., and Chandrasekaran, N. (2013). Ultrasonic emulsification of food-grade nanoemulsion formulation and evaluation of its bactericidal activity. *Ultrasonics Sonochemistry* 20: 338–344.

Guraya, H.S., and James, C. (2002). Deagglomeration of rice starch–protein aggregates by high pressure homogenization. *Starch* 54(3–4): 108–116.

Haaser, M., Karrout, Y., Velghe, C., Cuppok, Y., Gordon, K.C., *et al.* (2013). Application of terahertz pulsed imaging to analyse film coating characteristics of sustained-release coated pellets. *International Journal of Pharmaceutics* 457: 521–526.

Hellén, L., Ritala, M., Yliruusi, J., Palmroos, P, and Kristoffersson, E. (1992). Process variables of the radial screen extruder. Part II. Size and distribution of pellets. *PharmTech International Biophysics* 4: 50–57.

Hellén, L., Yliruusi, J., and Kristoffersson, E. (1993a). Process variables of instant granulator and spheroniser: II. Size and size distributions of pellets. *International Journal of Pharmaceutics* 96: 205–216.

Hellén, L., Yliruusi, J., Merkku, P., and Kristoffersson, E. (1993b). Process variables of instant granulator and spheroniser: I. Physical properties of granules, extrudate and pellets. *International Journal of Pharmaceutics* 96: 197–204.

Hosseini, A., Körber, M., and Bodmeier, R. (2013). Direct compression of cushion-layered ethyl cellulose-coated extended release pellets into rapidly disintegrating tablets without changes in the release profile. *International Journal of Pharmaceutics* 457(2): 503–509.

Hu, X., Lin, C., Chen, D., Zhang, J., Liu, Z., *et al.* (2012). Sirolimus solid self-microemulsifying pellets: Formulation development, characterization and bioavailability evaluation. *International Journal of Pharmaceutics* 438: 123–133.

Huang, Q., Yu, H., and Ru, Q. (2010). Bioavailability and delivery of nutraceuticals using nanotechnology. *Journal of Food Science* 75(1): R50–R57.

Iyer, R.M. (2006). Scale-up of Extrusion and Spheronization. In: *Pharmaceutical Process Scale-Up*, pp. 325–369. M. Levin, ed. New York: Taylor & Francis.

Izquierdo, P., Esquena, J., Tadros, T. F., Dederen, C., Garcia, M. J., and Azemar, N. (2001). Formation and stability of nanoemulsions prepared using the phase inversion temperature method. *Langmuir* 18(1): 26–30.

Izquierdo, P., Esquena, J., Tadros, T. F., Dederen, J. C., Feng, J., and Garcia-Celma, M. J. (2004). Phase behavior and nanoemulsion formation by the phase inversion temperature method. *Langmuir* 20(16): 6594–6598.

Jafari, S. M., He, Y., and Bhandari, B. (2006). Nano-emulsion production by sonication and microfluidization – a comparison. *International Journal of Food Properties* 9: 475–485.

Jafari, S. M., He, Y., and Bhandari, B. (2007). Optimization of nano-emulsions production by microfluidization. *European Food Research and Technology* 225: 773–741.

Kleinebudde, P. (1994). Shrinking and swelling properties of pellets containing microcrystalline cellulose and low substituted hydroxypropyl cellulose: I. Shrinking properties. *International Journal of Pharmaceutics* 109(3): 209–219.

Koester, M., and Thommes, M. (2010). New insights into the pelletization mechanism by extrusion/spheronization. *AAPS PharmSciTech* 11: 1549–1551.

Koo, O. M. Y, and Heng, P. W. S. (2001). The influence of microcrystalline cellulose grade on shape and shape distributions of pellets produced by extrusion–spheronization. *Chemical and Pharmaceutical Bulletin* 49: 1383–1387.

Kwon, S. S., Nam, Y. S., Lee, J. S., Ku, B. S., Han, S. H., *et al.* (2002). Preparation and characterization of coenzyme Q_{10}–loaded PMMA nanoparticles by a new emulsification process based on microfluidization. *Colloids and Surfaces A: Physicochemical and Engineering Aspects* 210: 95–104.

Laouini, A., Fessi, H., and Charcosset, C. (2012). Membrane emulsification: A promising alternative for vitamin E encapsulation within nano-emulsion. *Journal of Membrane Science* 423–424: 85–96.

Li, P., and Chiang, B. (2012). Process optimization and stability of d-limonene-in-water nanoemulsions prepared by ultrasonic emulsification using response surface methodology. *Ultrasonics Sonochemistry* 19: 192–197.

Lustig-Gustafsson, C., Kaur Johal, H., Podczeck, F., and Newton, J. M. (1999).The influence of water content and drug solubility on the formulation of pellets by extrusion and spheronisation. *European Journal of Pharmaceutical Sciences* 8: 147–152.

Luykx, D. M. A. M., Peters, R. J. B., van Ruth, S. M., and Bouwmeester, H. (2008). A review of analytical methods for the identification and characterization of nano delivery systems in food. *Journal of Agricultural and Food Chemistry* 56(18): 8231–8247.

Maa, Y. F., and Hsu, C. C. (1999). Performance of sonication and microfluidization for liquid–liquid emulsification. *Pharmaceutical Development and Technology* 4(2): 233–240.

Malinowski, H. J., and Smith, W. E. (1975). Use of factorial design to evaluate granulations prepared by spheronization. *Journal of Pharmaceutical Science* 64: 1688–1692.

Mantanus, J., Ziémons, E., Lebrun, P., Rozet, E., Klinkenberg, R., *et al.* (2009). Moisture content determination of pharmaceutical pellets by near infrared spectroscopy: Method development and validation. *Analytica Chimica Acta* 642: 186–192.

Mao, L., Xu, D., Yang, J., Yuan, F., Gao, Y., and Zhao, J. (2009). Effects of small and large molecule emulsifiers on the characteristics of β-carotene nanoemulsions prepared by high pressure homogenization. *Food Technology and Biotechnology* 47: 336–342.

Mason, T., Wilking, J., Meleson, K., Chang, C., and Graves, S. (2006). Nanoemulsions: Formation, structure, and physical properties. *Journal of Physics – Condensed Matter* 18: 635–666.

McClements, D. J., Decker, E. A., Park, Y., and Weiss, J. (2009). Structural design principles for delivery of bioactive components in nutraceuticals and functional foods. *Critical Reviews in Food Science and Nutrition* 49(6): 577–606.

McClements, D. J., and Rao, J. (2011). Food-grade nanoemulsions: Formulation, fabrication, properties, performance, biological fate, and potential toxicity. *Critical Reviews in Food Science and Nutrition* 51: 285–330.

Mehta, S., De Beer, T., Remona, J. P., and Vervaet, C. (2012). Effect of disintegrants on the properties of multiparticulate tablets comprising starch pellets and excipient granules. *International Journal of Pharmaceutics* 422: 310–317.

Michie, H., Podczeck, F., and Newton, J. M. (2012). The influence of plate design on the properties of pellets produced by extrusion and spheronization. *International Journal of Pharmaceutics* 434(1–2): 175–182.

Millili, G. P., and Schwartz, B. (1990). The strength of microcrystalline cellulose pellets: The effect of granulating with water-ethanol mixtures. *Drug Development and Industrial Pharmacy* 16: 1411–1426.

Morales, D., Gutiérrez. J. M., García-Celma, M. J., and Solans, Y. C. (2003). A study of the relation between bicontinuous micro-emulsions and oil/water nano-emulsion formation. *Langmuir* 19(18): 7196–7200.

Nakajima, H. (1997). Microemulsions in Cosmetics. In: *Industrial Applications of Microemulsions*, pp. 175–197. C. Solans and H. Kunieda, eds. New York: Marcel Dekker.

Nakajima, H., Tomomasa, S., and Okabe, M. (1993). Preparation of nanoemulsions. *Proceedings First World Congress on Emulsions*, 19–22 October 1993, Paris, France.

Palugan, L., Cerea, M., Zema, L., Gazzaniga, A., and Maroni, A. (2015). Coated pellets for oral colon delivery. *Journal of Drug Delivery Science and Technology* 25: 1–15.

Parikh, D. M. (2009). *Handbook of Pharmaceutical Granulation Technology*, 3rd ed. New York: Informa Healthcare.

Pathak, Y. V. (2010) *Handbook of Nutraceuticals. Volume 1: Ingredients, Formulations, and Applications*. Boca Raton, FL: CRC Press.

Piorkowski, D. T., and McClements, D. J. (2014). Beverage emulsions: Recent developments in formulation, production, and applications. *Food Hydrocolloids* 42: 5–41.

Podczeck F. (2008). A novel aid for the preparation of pellets by extrusion/spheronization. *Pharmaceutical Technology Europe* 20: 26–31.

Podczeck, F., and Newton, J. M. (2014). Influence of the standing time of the extrudate and speed of rotation of the spheroniser plate on the properties of pellets produced by extrusion and spheronization. *Advanced Powder Technology* 25: 659–665.

Podczeck, F., Rahman, S. R., and Newton J. M. (1999). Evaluation of a standardised procedure to assess the shape of pellets using image analysis. *International Journal of Pharmaceutics* 192: 123–138.

Prieto, S. M., Mendez, J. B., and Oreto Espinar, F. J. (2005). Starch–dextrin mixtures as base excipients for extrusion spheronization pellets. *European Journal of Pharmaceutics and Biopharmaceutics* 59: 511–521.

Quintanilla-Carvajal, M., Camacho-Díaz, B., Meraz-Torres, L., Chanona-Pérez, J., Alamilla-Beltrán, L., and Jimenéz-Aparicio, A. (2010). Nanoencapsulation: A new trend in food engineering processing. *Food Engineering Reviews* 2(1): 39–50.

Rao, J. J., and McClements, D. J. (2010). Stabilization of phase inversion temperature nanoemulsions by surfactant displacement. *Journal of Agricultural and Food Chemistry* 58: 7059–7066.

Reynolds, A. D. 1970. A new technique for the production of spherical particles. *Manufacturing Chemist and Aerosol News* 44: 40–44.

Römer, M., Heinämäki, J., Miroshnyk, I., Sandler, N., Rantanen, J., and Yliruusi, J. (2007). Phase transformations of erythromycin A dihydrate during pelletisation and drying. *European Journal of Pharmaceutics and Biopharmaceutics* 67: 246–252.

Rowe, R.C. (1985). Spheronization: A novel pill-making process? *Pharmacy International* 6: 119–123.

Sadtler, V., Rondon-Gonzalez, M., Acrement, A., Choplin, L., and Marie, E. (2010). PEO-covered nanoparticles by emulsion inversion point (EIP) method. *Macromolecular Rapid Communications* 31(11): 998–1002.

Sadurní, N., Solans, C., Azemar, N., and García-Celma, M. J. (2005). Studies on the formation of O/W nano-emulsions, by low-energy emulsification methods, suitable for pharmaceutical applications. *European Journal of Pharmaceutical Sciences* 26(5): 438–445.

Sanguansri, P., and Augustin, M. A. (2006). Nanoscale materials development – a food industry perspective. *Trends in Food Science and Technology* 17: 547–556.

Seikikawa, K., and Watanabe, M. (2008). Transparent emulsified composition for use in beverages. Givaudan SA, Publication number WO2008/055374.

Shah, R. D., Kabadi, M., Pope, D. G., and Augsburger, L. L. (1995). Physico-mechanical characterization of the extrusion–spheronization process. Part II: Rheological determinants for successful extrusion and spheronization. *Pharmaceutical Research* 12(4): 496–507.

Shakeel, F., Baboota, S., Ahuja, A., Ali, J., and Shafiq, S. (2008). Accelerated stability testing of celecoxib nanoemulsion containing Cremophor-EL. *African Journal of Pharmacy and Pharmacology* 2: 179–183.

Shinoda, K., and Saito, H. (1968). The effect of temperature on the phase equilibria and the types of dispersions of the ternary system composed of water, cyclohexane, and nonionic surfactant. *Journal of Colloid and Interface Science* 26(1): 70–74.

Shinoda, K., and Saito, H. (1969). The stability of o/w type emulsions as a function of temperature and the HLB of emulsifiers: the emulsification by pit-method. *Journal of Colloid and Interface Science* 30(1): 258–263.

Solans, C., Izquierdo, P., Nolla, J., Azemar, N., and Garcia-Celma, M. J. (2005). Nanoemulsions. *Current Opinion in Colloid Interface Science* 10: 102–110.

Solans, C., and Solé, I. (2012). Nano-emulsions: Formation by low-energy methods. *Current Opinion in Colloid and Interface Science* 17: 246–254.

Sonaglio, D., Bataille, B., Ortigosa, C., and Jacob, M. (1995). Factorial design in the feasibility of producing Microcel MC 101 pellets by extrusion/spheronisation. *International Journal of Pharmaceutics* 115: 53–60.

Sousa, J. J., Sousa, A., Podczeck, F., and Newton, J. M. (1992). Influence of process conditions on drug release from pellets. *International Journal of Pharmaceutics* 144: 159–169.

Sousa, J. J., Sousa, A., Podczeck, F., and Newton, J. M. (2002). Factors influencing the physical characteristics of pellets obtained by extrusion–spheronization. *International Journal of Pharmaceutics* 232: 91–106.

Souto, C., Rodriguez, A., Parajes, S., and Martinez-Pacheco, R. (2005). A comparative study of the utility of two superdisintegrants in microcrystalline cellulose pellets prepared by extrusion–spheronization. *European Journal of Pharmaceutics and Biopharmaceutics* 61(1–2): 94–99.

Stegemann, S. (2002). Hard gelatin capsules today– and tomorrow. *Capsugel Library,* 13.

Swientek, R. J. (1990). Microfluidizing technology enhances emulsion stability. *Food Processing* 152–153.

Tamilvanan, S., Senthilkumar, R. S., Baskar, R., and Sekharan, T. R. (2010). Manufacturing techniques and excipients used during the formulation of oil-in-water type nanosized emulsions for medical applications. *Journal of Excipients and Food Chemistry* (1): 11–29.

Thompson, A. K., and Singh, H. (2006). Preparation of liposomes from milk fat globule membrane phospholipids using a microfluidizer. *Journal Dairy Science* 89: 410–419.

Trivedi, N. R., Rajan, M. G., Johnson, J. R., and Shukla, A. J. (2007). Pharmaceutical approaches to preparing pelletized dosage forms using the extrusion–spheronisation process. *Critical Reviews in Therapeutic Drug Carrier Systems* 24: 1–40.

U.S. National Institutes of Health, Office of Dietary Supplements. (2016a). Folate. http://ods.od.nih.gov/factsheets/Folate-HealthProfessional/

U.S. National Institutes of Health, Office of Dietary Supplements. (2016b). Vitamin D. http://ods.od.nih.gov/factsheets/VitaminD-HealthProfessional/

U.S. National Institutes of Health, Office of Dietary Supplements. (2016c). Vitamin E. http://ods.od.nih.gov/factsheets/VitaminE-HealthProfessional/

U.S. National Institutes of Health, Office of Dietary Supplements. (2011). Vitamin B12. http://ods.od.nih.gov/factsheets/VitaminB12-Consumer/

Usón, N., Garcia, M. J., and Solans, C. (2004). Formation of water-in- oil (W/O) nanoemulsions in a water/mixed non-ionic surfactant/oil systems prepared by a low-energy emulsification method. *Colloids and Surfaces A: Physicochemical and Engineering Aspects* 250(1–3): 415–421.

Vervaet, C., Baert, L., and Remon, J. P. (1995). Extrusion–spheronisation: A literature review. *International Journal of Pharmaceutics* 116: 131–146.

Vos, P., Faas, M. M., Spasojevic, M., and Sikkema, J. (2010). Review: Encapsulation for preservation of functionality and targeted delivery of bioactive food components. *International Dairy Journal* 20: 292-302.

Walstra, P. (1993). Principles of emulsion formation. *Chemical Engineering Science* 48(2): 333–349.

Wandrey, C., Bartkowiak, A., Harding, S. E. (2009). Materials for Encapsulation In: *Encapsulation Technologies for Food Active Ingredients and Food Processing*, pp. 31–100. N. J. Zuidam and V. A. Nedovic, eds. Dordrecht: Springer.

Wang, X., Jiang, Y., Wang, Y., Huang, M., Ho, C. T., and Huang, Q. (2008). Enhancing anti-inflammation activity of curcumin through O/W nanoemulsions. *Food Chemistry* 108: 419–424.

West, A.J., and Rowe, R.C., (1988). Production spheronisers ten years on. *Manufacturing Chemist* 59: 79–80.

Wlosnewski, J. C., Kumpugdee-Vollrath, M., and Sriamornsak, P. (2010). Effect of drying technique and disintegrant on physical properties and drug release behaviour of microcrystalline cellulose-based pellets prepared by extrusion/spheronization. *Chemical Engineering Research and Design* 88: 100–108.

Xia, H., Zhang, C., and Wang, Q. (2001). Study on ultrasonic induced encapsulating emulsion polymerization in the presence of nanoparticles. *Journal of Applied Polymer Science* 80: 1130–1139.

Xu, M., Liew, C. V., and Heng, P. W. S. (2015). Evaluation of the coat quality of sustained release pellets by individual pellet dissolution methodology. *International Journal of Pharmaceutics* 478: 318–327.

Yin, L. J., Chu, B. S., Kobayashi, I., and Nakajima, M. (2009). Performance of selected emulsifiers and their combinations in the preparation of β-carotene nanodispersions. *Food Hydrocolloids* 23(6): 1617–1622.

Zerbe, H. G., Paiement, N., and and Ispas-Szabo, P. (2007). Multi-vitamin and mineral supplement. United States Patent Application Publication, 20070128272A1.

Zhang, J. (2011). *Novel emulsion-based delivery systems*. PhD Dissertation, University of Minnesota, USA.

CHAPTER 10

Biopolymeric archetypes for the oral delivery of nutraceuticals

Mershen Govender, Miles C. Braithwaite, Pradeep Kumar, Yahya E. Choonara, and Viness Pillay

Wits Advanced Drug Delivery Platform Research Unit, Department of Pharmacy and Pharmacology, School of Therapeutic Sciences, Faculty of Health Sciences, University of the Witwatersrand, Johannesburg, 7 York Road, Parktown, 2193, South Africa

10.1 Introduction

There is an increasing need to deliver bioactives such as vitamins, minerals, probiotics, and other nutraceuticals to overcome both acute and chronic diseases such as diabetes, hypertension, malnutrition, and cancer (Mun *et al.*, 2015). Various functional oral delivery systems exist including monolithic matrix-based systems such as tablets, capsules, hydrogels, and films to micro- or nanoencapsulated particulate systems in the form of microparticles, nanoparticles, and bead-like conformations. This chapter focuses on these broad, widely employed nutraceutical formulations and delivery approaches, with emphasis on the ability of the respective systems to provide bioactive protection from the harsh physiological environment. Biopolymeric archetypes discussed in detail include carbohydrate-based hydrogels and protein films cross-linked with pharmaceutical excipients. Additionally, the use of natural products in the enteric coating of pharmaceutical agents is discussed with an in-depth evaluation of the functionality of biopolymers in the nutraceuticals industry. Various delivery mechanisms being employed to package nutrients, vitamins, minerals, and even herbal macromolecules are explained and their role in improving the physiological functionality of nutraceuticals (through enhanced solubility, permeability, and targeted release) is emphasized. The applicability of specialized biopolymers being employed for encapsulation including proteins and polysaccharides is highlighted with respect to protected nutraceutical delivery that not only improves the physicochemical properties of nutraceuticals but also masks strong flavors, potentiates pharmacodynamic effects, and minimizes interactions.

New Polymers for Encapsulation of Nutraceutical Compounds, First Edition.
Edited by Jorge Carlos Ruiz Ruiz and Maira Rubi Segura Campos.

10.2 Monolithic matrix-based systems

Many natural bioactive molecules show high lipophilicity, resulting in an increased permeability into the hydrophobic cell membrane, thereby allowing greater drug efficiency and targeting (Josef *et al.*, 2010). This lipophilicity, however, often results in a decreased dissolution of the bioactive in aqueous media. The result of this decreased water solubility is therefore a significant obstacle in nutraceutical delivery, because a decreased bioavailability results in decreased bioactives reaching the systemic circulation in addition to a decreased stability of the product (Wankhade *et al.*, 2014; Mun *et al.*, 2015). The first part of this chapter provides a critical evaluation of monolithic oral delivery systems using direct compression of the polymer matrix in addition to hydrogel formulations, films, and coatings, and the effectiveness of these delivery systems for the enhanced delivery of nutraceutical products is emphasized.

10.2.1 Compressed tablet systems

Compressed delivery systems such as tablets and capsules provide a rapid or controlled drug release formulated often through an uncomplicated, cost-effective production process. This method is also applicable to nutraceutical products where the natural bioactives are incorporated with various pharmaceutical excipients to overcome the therapeutic issue of decreased bioavailability, ensuring therapeutic effectiveness to the patient. Tablet formulations can often include numerous additional steps prior to compaction, such as dry and wet granulation. A study undertaken by Sultana *et al.* (2014) detailed the formulation and evaluation of an immediate-release nutraceutical multivitamin antioxidant tablet. The tablet system was formulated by wet granulation and coated prior to evaluation. Stability analysis of the system showed that the tablet system was stable for 24 months under storage conditions, indicating that compression systems such as tablets in combination with formulation enhancements such as coatings can protect the bioactives against environmental factors such as humidity and photodegradation.

Tablets, which are not commonly used for probiotic delivery, have also been noted to be effective delivery systems for this viable bioactive (Govender *et al.*, 2015; Villena *et al.* 2015). Succinylated β-lactoglobulin has been shown to be a novel functional tablet excipient for the protection of probiotic bacteria against the harsh gastric environment (Poulin *et al.*, 2011). Evaluation of the direct compressed tablets showed that grafting of the β-lactoglobulin with carboxylic acid groups allowed the survival of up to 10^8 and 10^7 colony-forming units (CFU) after 1 hour and 2 hours in gastric media, respectively. These tablets were also determined to be stable under refrigerated conditions for 3 months, highlighting the possibility of succinylated β-lactoglobulin to be effectively used as a probiotic carrier.

Nutraceuticals are often used as formulation excipients to exert a nutritional benefit in addition to a production effect. One such example is calcium lactate, which is a source of calcium but also serves as a filler–binder in tablet formulations, in addition to having good solubility and bioavailability (Bolhuis *et al.*, 2001). Two modifications of the calcium lactate structure by Bolhuis and coworkers (2001), calcium lactate trihydrate and calcium lactate pentahydrate, were evaluated. With regard to compaction and flow, calcium lactate pentahydrate has greater compactive and flow properties when compared to calcium lactate trihydrate. From this study it can be concluded that directly compressible calcium lactate can be considered an effective excipient in manufacturing pharmaceutical and nutraceutical tablets.

10.2.2 Hydrogels

Hydrogels are defined as an infinite water-absorptive three-dimensional polymeric network made of hydrophilic matrices cross-linked through covalent bonds, van der Waals interactions, hydrogen bonding, or physical entanglements (Chen *et al.*, 2006). Advancements in hydrogels research have resulted in the increased delivery of bioactive nutraceuticals in simulated release media. These hydrogels are often freeze-dried into powder and placed into a capsule or tableted to maintain stability of the nutraceutical compounds before oral administration.

A study undertaken by Maltais and coworkers (2010) detailed the development of cold-set soy protein hydrogel for the delivery of riboflavin in simulated gastrointestinal conditions. This study further highlighted the trend of using food biopolymers and proteins in the development of natural hydrogels. The proposed hydrogel was designed to be formulated without the bioactive being exposed to high temperatures, which will lead to structural degradation of the nutraceutical, rendering it ineffective to provide a functional health benefit, while still producing a product that would protect the bioactive against digestive enzymes and low pH and achieve zero-order release. Evaluation of the soy protein hydrogel in powder and tablet form showed little difference in riboflavin release in simulated intestinal fluid, with both systems reaching 60% drug release after 24 hours. Release of riboflavin in simulated gastric fluid, however, showed that the bioactive had influenced the release characteristics of the hydrogel matrix, with 30% of drug released within 24 hours, indicating a release mechanism other than swelling. The increased diffusion of riboflavin into dissolution media was therefore attributed to a lack of polymer–bioactive interaction as a result of the amphoteric properties of the bioactive, leading to a decreased net charge in addition to carboxyl groups being utilized in the crosslinking of matrix by Ca^{2+} to form the hydrogel (Figure 10.1). It was also noted that digestive enzymes had a significant effect on riboflavin release, a trend often seen in food biopolymeric matrices.

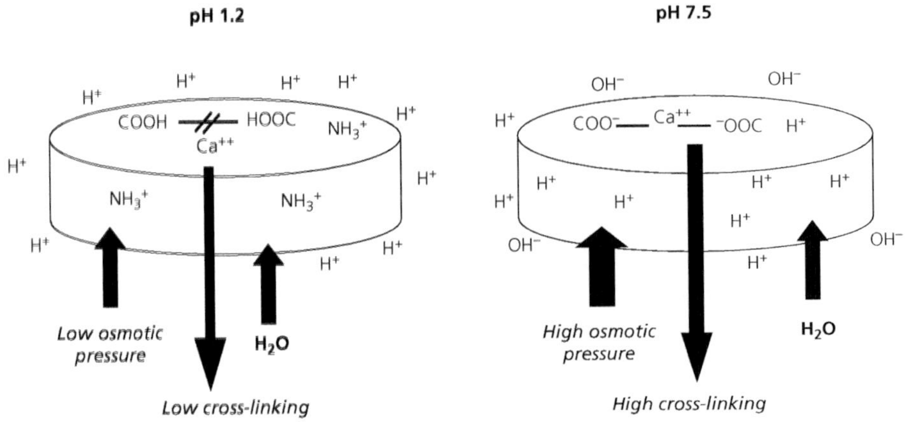

Figure 10.1 Schematic representation of the swelling of the hydrogel tablet in simulated gastric and intestinal fluid. Figure from Maltias *et al.*, 2010; reproduced with permission from Elsevier Ltd. © 2009.

Studies for the delivery of probiotics using hydrogel matrices have also been undertaken with xanthan gum and chitosan, an effective polymeric combination due to its high swelling capacity and ability to protect the probiotic bacteria against formulation and harsh physiological conditions (Argin *et al.*, 2014). Evaluation of the hydrogel formulation determined that release from the polymeric matrix was largely dependent on pH of the dissolution media and significantly less on digestive enzymes. Probiotic release analysis in simulated gastric conditions detailed negligible probiotic release in simulated gastric conditions at pH 2.0 after 2 hours attributed to decreased enzymatic degradation of the chitosan matrix as a result of conformational changes occurring with interaction with the enzymatically resistant xanthan gum. Complete release of the probiotic cells occurred in simulated intestinal conditions within 5 hours, leading to the hydrogel matrix being classified as enteric in nature and capable of delivering probiotic bacteria effectively to simulated human intestinal conditions. Release in this medium was attributed to chain relaxation in addition to swelling by a diffusion-controlled mechanism.

The production of emulsion-based nutraceutical hydrogels can also yield positive results when compared to other cross-linked hydrogel matrices (Carrillo-Navas *et al.*, 2012; Mun *et al.*, 2015). A study undertaken by Mun and coworkers (2015) prepared starch-based filled hydrogels incorporating lipophilic nutraceutical β-carotene. Two types of starch in the form of mung bean starch and rice starch were identified and evaluated to ascertain their effect on lipid digestion as well as the fraction of β-carotene solubilized within the mixed-micelle phase after lipid digestion had occurred. Further evaluated was the variation of surfactant whey protein isolate and polysorbate 20 (Tween-20) in the preparation of the oil-in-water emulsion and their effect on the two above-mentioned parameters. The method of formulating the hydrogels included incorporating the emulsions into the starch–hydrogel mixture and heating. This method, as previously stated, can have negative effects on the bioactives and might not be applicable to all nutraceuticals. Results of this evaluation showed the effectiveness of the emulsion formulation and the hydrogel system for the delivery of β-carotene. In comparison, the whey protein isolate emulsion had significantly lower bioaccessibility when compared to the polysorbate 20 formulation because the whey proteins were able to aggregate and precipitate micelles. It was, however, seen that upon incorporation into the hydrogel system, there was no significant difference between the two types of surfactants with regard to β-carotene bioaccessibility. It was also noted that the mung bean starch hydrogel showed a significant decrease in lipid digestion rate attributed to the high amylose and protein content of the starch when compared to the rice starch hydrogel.

It can therefore be noted that hydrogels are effective delivery systems for a broad range of nutraceutical bioactives. The type of hydrogel and the formulation process, however, are dependent largely on the chemical structure of the bioactive to ensure that the bio-effectiveness of the nutraceutical is maintained to provide health benefits.

10.2.3 Protein films

Nutraceutical films have become an innovative effective method to administer bioactives. Films are thin, orally administered, fast-dissolving polymeric strips that are instantly hydrated by saliva so that the film adheres to the intended site of delivery (Arya *et al.*, 2010). Plant protein films have been highlighted to effectively deliver bioactives because they are nontoxic, nonimmunogenic, and permeable to water vapor. The production of plant protein films is further advantageous because they are naturally abundant and because the production process is cost-effective and can be modified to have an increased structural integrity. Protein films, however, have naturally poor mechanical properties, which are decreased further due to the addition of glycerol, which has been found to promote elongation of films (Reddy *et al.*, 2012).

Production processes for formulating protein films include the nontreatment of proteins, such as gluten, whey protein, collagen, and gelatin, as well extraction of proteins, commonly castor bean cakes, from vegetable oil extractions (Makishi *et al.*, 2013). A study undertaken by Reddy and colleagues (2012) has provided the formulation and evaluation of solution-cast films derived from peanut proteins cross-linked with citric acid. The proteins that were extracted from protein meal were found to produce films with both good dry and wet tensile properties but poor biocompatibility when exposed to mouse fibroblast cells, indicated by poor spreading and cellular morphology (Figure 10.2). The study, however, showed that the protein films had an increased tensile strength, greater thermal resistance, and an increased meting

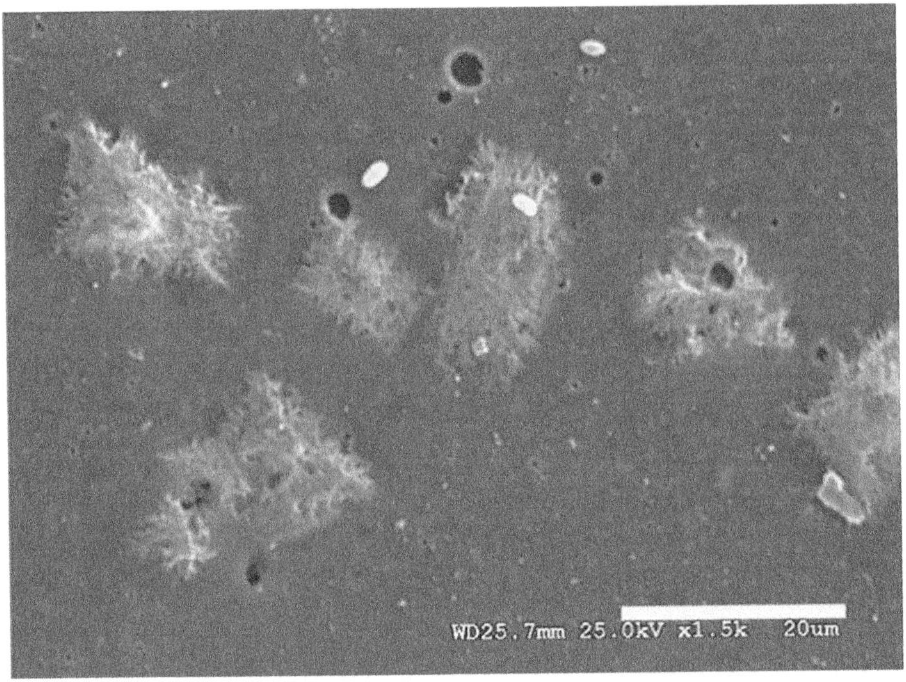

Figure 10.2 SEM image of fibroblast cells on peanut protein films after 5 days' exposure. Figure from Reddy *et al.*, 2012; reproduced with permission from Elsevier B.V © 2012.

point. This can be of significance in preparing nutraceutical products containing thermal labile bioactives.

Protein films derived from castor bean cake produced by Makishi and coworkers (2013) further highlighted the development of cross-linked plant protein films that can be used in the delivery of bioactives. In this study, different concentrations of proteins extracted from the castor bean cake were compared to various concentrations of two cross-linking agents, glutaraldehyde and glyoxal. An increase in protein concentration of the films was shown to positively influence the solubility and mechanical properties of the films with the crosslinked glyoxal showing the lowest minimum solubility value of 6% while still maintaining structural integrity when compared to the glutaraldehyde cross-linked films. This was due to the presence of arginine in the castor bean extract, which promoted glyoxal interaction, while the decreased concentration of cysteine, histidine, lysine, and tyrosine amino acids may have negatively affected glutaraldehyde interactions. The results of this study detailed another plant protein–based film with increased structural integrity and solubility. This is significant because it highlights that nutraceutical products can be incorporated and also included in product formulations to provide the delivery of bioactives through administration.

10.2.4 Formulation coatings

Coating of formulations provides a variety of functions including, among others, protection from gastric media, protection of moisture uptake, masking of bad tastes, improvement of formulation stability, and increased bioactive permeability (Castro *et al.*, 2015; Joshi and Petereit, 2013). Coatings used in pharmaceutical and nutraceutical development include enteric coats, film coats, compression coats, liquid melt, and powder coatings (Joshi and Petereit, 2013). With the large proportion of nutraceutical products using enteric coating, a shift has developed from natural products to semisynthetic and synthetic coatings (Czarnocka and Alhnan, 2015). Cellulose or acrylic-based polymers are examples of such coatings that have been used for their good film-forming and coating properties (Elzoghby *et al.*, 2011).

Compression coatings have also been documented to increase bioactive protection and delivery. A study undertaken by Chan and Zhang (2005) detailed the use of sodium alginate as the coating material for probiotic pellets. Results of the study indicated significant improvement in the survival of the encapsulated probiotic cells when exposed to acidic media, with the probiotic bacteria showing a 10^4- 10^5-fold increase in cell survival when compared to free unencapsulated bacterial cells under the test conditions. This was as a result of the formation of a hydrogel barrier, which retarded permeation of the acidic media into the pellets containing the probiotic cells. The mechanism of cellular release in conditions indicative of the intestinal ileum and early colon was due primarily to erosion of the alginate gel layer surface. This result detailed the effectiveness of dry powder compaction of enteric-coated nutraceutical products and its possible use in other gastric-labile bioactives.

An investigation conducted by Czarnocka and Alhnan (2015) on three generally regarded as safe (GRAS) coating systems was undertaken to determine if the available technologies effectively protected and delivered a model drug in tablet form. The three coatings evaluated included ethyl cellulose plus carboxymethyl cellulose, ethyl cellulose plus sodium alginate, and shellac plus sodium alginate. *In vitro* dissolution tests revealed an increased initial release in pH 6.8 (intestinal pH) for the ethyl cellulose–based coatings, and an extended drug release from the shellac plus sodium alginate coating was observed in both intestinal and colon pH (pH 7.4). When exposed to varying gastric pH conditions (pH 2, 3, and 4), the ethyl cellulose plus carboxymethyl cellulose and ethyl cellulose plus sodium alginate coatings were broken after 70 minutes and 30 minutes, respectively. The shellac plus sodium alginate–coated tablets demonstrated gastric resistance at all the gastric pH values analyzed. From this study, it was noted that the GRAS-grade coatings did not fully comply with the requirements for delayed drug release and that the use of these coating in nutraceutical products could lead to ineffective delivery of the bioactive.

10.3 Encapsulated systems

Encapsulation is a formulation technique that involves bioactives of interest being entrapped within a carrier matrix or wall material that may be macroscopic, microscopic, or nanoscopic in size. Such delivery mechanisms have been used to package nutraceuticals in defined configurations intended to improve their physicochemical properties to enhance the delivery and performance of the encapsulated bioactive. Biopolymers that are commonly used for encapsulation include proteins and polysaccharides. Because nature packages nutrients with other macromolecules in defined conformations, the use of polymeric biomolecules as an oral delivery vehicle for nutraceuticals is a logical methodology in formulation science.

The use of biopolymers in encapsulated systems has additional advantages, including improved biodegradability, reduced chemical manufacturing steps (ease of preparation), and reduced immunogenicity of organic compounds compared to their synthetic counterparts. Many studies have explicated the use of polysaccharides, protein-based polymers, and natural fibers to encapsulate nutraceutical agents for enhanced oral delivery. Nutraceuticals that have been packaged for oral release from encapsulated vehicles include lutein, lycopene, β-carotene, glucosamine, melatonin, chondroitin, vitamin D, green tea, coenzyme Q_{10}, melatonin, green tea extract, dehydroepiandrosterone (DHEA), lipoic acid, garlic, creatine, resveratrol, fat-soluble vitamins, water-soluble vitamins, herbal extracts, and polyphenols.

10.3.1 Bead-like conformations

Microbead structures using polyelectrolyte complexes of natural polysaccharides and cold-set internal gelation techniques are methods commonly used to encapsulate various nutraceuticals. Cocoa extract was encapsulated using sodium alginate, and this method to form microbeads with either smooth or rough surfaces was dependent upon the calcium source used during preparation (Lupo *et al.*, 2014). Such studies highlight that differences in calcium and emulsifier types influence morphology and size of the resultant beads, which in turn affects release rates of the encapsulated bioactive. Uniformity of structure, size, and stability of resultant microbeads dictates their applicability in food-based applications due to an effect on homogeneous distribution and thus sensory properties of the product.

Methodology is indeed critical also to reduce loss of bioactives from microbeads during synthesis – a limitation of this formulation technique that is well documented and necessitates strategies to negate this effect. Lupo and coworkers (2014) noted a pronounced premature loss of the polyphenol active from microbeads into the washing solution during their study. This type of procedure is an internal method of encapsulation involving the addition of a bioactive to the polymer solution prior to ionic induced gelation or addition of cross-linking agent to form beads. Leaching of bioactive during this stage is of more concern for lower-molecular-weight molecules than larger molecules due to an ability to pass through microbead pores and back into the cross-linker solution (Figure 10.3). Such formulation challenges result in beads with low bioactive encapsulation efficiency (EE) due to low nutraceutical retention. This limitation can render the internal process inefficient, unless methods are employed to rectify bioactive loss.

A second and alternative method of bead formation is an external addition process whereby the active is added after bead formation. During the external method, also termed *immobilization*, blank beads are submerged in a solution of the nutraceutical bioactive, which diffuses through bead pores, absorbing onto the bead matrices. Coating techniques have also been used to successfully hinder the leaching by coating surfaces of microbeads with biopolymers.

In certain cases, both internal and external microbead methodologies may be used to encapsulate nutraceuticals. O'Neill's group (2014) studied the encapsulation of riboflavin in whey hydrogel microbeads cross-linked with calcium chloride. These researchers found that whey microbeads were ideal biopolymers to absorb the B vitamin via a partition process that impeded B_{12} loss with an improved EE due to hydrophobic effects enhancing vitamin migration into the microbeads. Even when a maximum concentration of vitamin solution is added to microbead-forming solutions, there may be a significant diffusion out of the microbeads with no improvements in EE. This is not surprising because the high porosity of hydrogel structures used for bead formation allows fast leakage of bioactive. The internal method for encapsulation of smaller bioactives is therefore limited not only by the maximum solubility of the nutraceutical in the

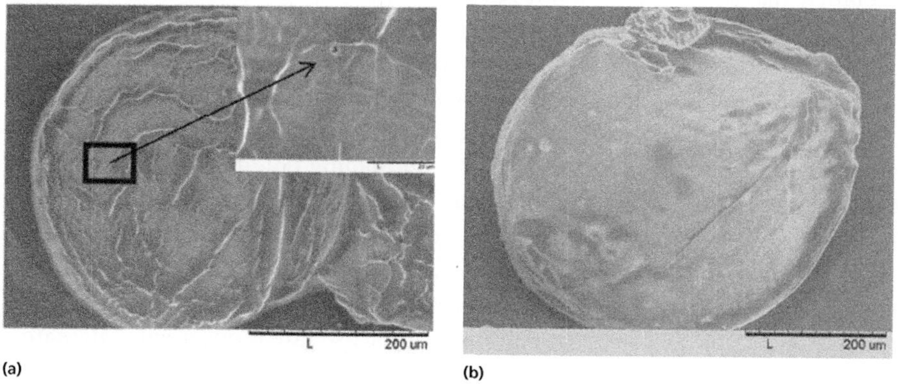

(a) (b)

Figure 10.3 SEM images of dry blank microspheres/microbeads at 0.05 M of calcium salts: **(a)** carbonate; **(b)** citrate. It is clear that alginate microspheres made using calcium carbonate had rough surfaces, whereas those made using calcium citrate had uniform surfaces and were smaller. The choice and concentration of emulsifier, cross-linker, and nutraceutical bioactive influence the morphology, size, and surface characteristics of the resultant biopolymeric microbeads. These characteristics affect the distribution, particle uniformity, and ultimately the release characteristics of nutraceuticals from microbeads. Figure from Lupo *et al.*, 2014; reproduced with permission from Elsevier B.V © 2014.

microbead-forming solution but also by the maximum loss through the gel pores during curing. In the study by O'Neill and coworkers (2014), it was postulated that the apolar ring of the riboflavin molecule interacted with high affinity with the hydrophobic portions of the whey protein beads during the external absorptive process. Thus the external method is more suitable for microbead encapsulation of smaller bioactives because preformed beads are able to successfully maintain a maximal ratio of vitamin solution to blank bead for optimal bead absorption.

The emulsion cross-linking technique for forming microbeads has been used by researchers who have used the biopolymer chitosan and the cross-linker glutaraldehyde to encapsulate the plant polyphenols in thyme (Trifkovic *et al.*, 2014). Encapsulation of thyme aqueous extract was achieved using an external method by immersing dry chitosan microbeads in an aqueous solution of thyme extract at acidic pH. The delivery of polyphenol from the microbead system saw a prolonged release in gastric medium. The study methods require optimization to incorporate an alternative less-noxious cross-linker and improve encapsulation efficiency. Such research reiterates the power of the cross-linker on bead morphology and also provides important information regarding the changes in surface morphology and porosity of resultant beads in the presence of nutraceuticals. The incomplete or complete release of nutraceuticals from microbeads is dependent upon interactions between the bioactive and the polymeric matrix, size and configuration of beads, and quantity and type of cross-linker, due to an effect on swelling behavior during hydration.

In certain scenarios, instead of a single cationic or anionic biopolymer, a combined approach may be employed by using two biopolymers to form nutraceutical microbeads. Some researchers have incorporated multiple herbal extracts (raspberry leaf, hawthorn, yarrow, olive leaf, ground ivy, and nettle extracts) in alginate–chitosan microbeads using an electrostatic extrusion method (Belscak-Cvitanovic *et al.*, 2011). Copolymer beads can provide improved encapsulation efficiency for higher loading potential when two polymers are combined or an alginate bead is reinforced with a chitosan layer. As demonstrated in many formulation studies , EE is influenced by microbead size, with the loading capacity being inversely proportional to bead size – a phenomenon that remains true in nutraceutical studies. The findings in copolymer studies include the fact that a prolonged release rate is observed if alginate–chitosan beads are synthesized instead of plain alginate beads, due to an electrostatic complexation between the two biopolymers, which hinders bioactive release. This is a mechanism that may be used for the controlled release of various vitamins and antioxidants for effective intake of substances over a chronic period for daily maintenance and health benefits. The aforementioned study illustrated versatility of microbeads to deliver multiple herbal extracts and also highlights the potential for nutraceuticals to interfere with the gelation process of biopolymers (Belscak-Cvitanovic *et al.*, 2011).

10.3.2 Microencapsulated systems

Microspheres composed of pectin, alginate, and chitosan or a combination thereof were used as a more effective mechanism to encapsulate and target delivery of both ascorbic acid and ketoprofen to the colon than waxy microspheres (Maestrelli *et al.*, 2015). The hydrophilic biopolymers were deemed more efficient vitamin-encapsulation materials than the synthetic waxy alternative and provided a higher colonic release rate. Many formulation techniques involve a pH-responsive coating being applied to microspheres, which prevents early release of bioactives, maintains particle integrity, prevents bioactive loss, and ensures targeted release. The study also tested enteric-coated microparticles for enhanced protection of the vitamin and to ensure release at the colon. A superior membrane permeability was also evident due to the presence of the cationic polysaccharide, chitosan. This finding reiterates the advantage that biopolymers offer over synthetic microsphere components due to their flexibility to allow double encapsulation of two bioactives with differing hydrophilic and lipophilic characteristics.

Table 10.1 shows how waxy microspheres were only able to encapsulate ketoprofen, whereas biopolymeric microspheres of pectin, alginate (coated with chitosan), and chitosan were adept at encapsulating both model agents, including the vitamin and the allopathic drug. Such comparative studies are interesting to note because they affirm the utility of biological macromolecules as encapsulation vehicles and may be preferable components to allow synergism when combining actives to treat specific pathologies.

Other research has shown the advantages of biopolymeric microparticles to improve efficacy through enhancements in cytotoxicity of herbal compounds. Microparticles composed of chitosan and casein cross-linked with glutaraldehyde were used to encapsulate plant extracts for improved anticancer effects *in vitro* (Amarnath *et al.*, 2014). When the study authors encapsulated the herbal extract *Acalypha indica* in chitosan–casein microparticles, it was found that an improved bioavailability and superior antiproliferative response was achieved for the delivery system as compared to the free extracts. Thus, biopolymeric

Table 10.1 Encapsulation efficiency (ee% s.D.) For each microsphere batch.

Batch	Description	Encapsulation Efficiency (EE%)	
		Ascorbic Acid	Ketoprofen
MS Pec	Calcium pectinate microspheres	50.8±1.5	96.2±2.3
MS AlgCs	Alginate microspheres covered in chitosan	19.5±0.7	94.4±3.5
MS CS	Chitosan microspheres	—	85.5±2.6
MS Pres	Precirol microspheres	—	62.6±3.1
MS Com	Compritol microspheres	—	91.7±6.5

Table from Maestrelli *et al.*, 2015; Reproduced with permission from Elsevier B.V © 2015.

encapsulation affects the pharmacodynamic effects of nutraceuticals in addition to improving kinetic delivery parameters.

Bioavailability and bioaccessibility enhancements were also seen with electrosprayed curcumin–gelatin microspheres (Gomez-Estaca *et al.*, 2015). Curcumin is a nutraceutical that boasts multiple health-related properties and is a natural food coloring but has low aqueous solubility. Physicochemical improvements in solubility were imparted to curcumin when encapsulated in gelatin microparticles in the aforementioned study. Gelatin is a mixture of proteins and peptides extracted from collagen and is therefore a gelling agent of natural origin that has high aqueous solubility intended to improve the solubility and functionality of many food industry compounds. In addition to solubility enhancements imparted by the gelatin–curcumin microparticles, microparticle curcumin demonstrated higher antioxidant activity than conventional commercial curcumin, again strengthening the argument for efficacy enhancements when using biopolymers as encapsulation vehicles.

Microcapsules have long since demonstrated an impact as superior delivery conformations. Microcapsules were prepared using varied concentrations of chitosan and poly(D,L-lactic-co-glycolic acid) (PLGA) and a water-oil-water double emulsion method for controlled release of resveratrol (Sanna *et al.*, 2015). The inclusion of chitosan improved loading of resveratrol due to microcapsules, slowed the release profile, and improved the stability of the nutraceutical compared to microcapsules containing PLGA only. This is not surprising because chitosan is a pH-responsive carbohydrate with various advantageous properties and with an ability to slow release in acid medium and to increase release in basic medium.

Not only can whey protein be used to form microbeads as discussed previously, but this protein polymer has also been successfully coformulated in combination with natural gums to form microcapsules to protect carotenoids from environmental degradation (Jain *et al.*, 2015). Microcapsules containing β-carotene demonstrated a sustained release of bioactive compared to the free vitamin and allowed efficient protection of the vitamin for sustained antioxidant activity due to protection within the microcarrier (Figure 10.4). This formulation was produced by a complex coacervation method; other researchers have used lyophilization or emulsification methods. Nanoemulsions can also be formed using whey protein isolate and gum arabic as biopolymer emulsifiers for the delivery of vitamin E in fortified food-based systems (Ozturk *et al.*, 2015). Proteins and carbohydrate polymers have varied uses relative to one another, with the main differences being the size of the resultant nanomolecules, rate of aggregation, and vulnerability to temperature. These considerations need to be evaluated when choosing biopolymers and are ultimately influenced by the fate of such systems in food-grade applications and commercial supplements.

Gallic acid may be microencapsulated using various biopolymer coating materials (chitosan or the polysaccharide xanthan) via a lyophilization technique

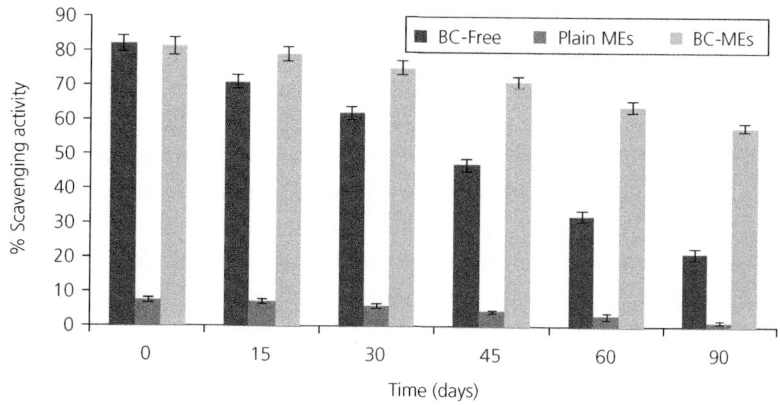

Figure 10.4 Antioxidant scavenging activity (%) of free β-carotene (BC-free), blank microencapsules (blank MEs), and β-carotene–loaded microencapsules (BC-MEs). Each data point represents mean ± SD ($n=6$). It is evident that over time, the functional stability of free β-carotene wanes, as observed by a rapid decline in % scavenging activity. The β-carotene–loaded microencapsules provided a prolonged antioxidant activity due to protective effects on the nutraceutical. Figure from Jain *et al.*, 2015; reproduced with permission from Elsevier B.V © 2015.

as an efficient means to produce microcapsules for improved bioactivity (Goncalves da Rosa *et al.*, 2013). The choice of coating material may vary but has a profound effect on the success of encapsulation. The aforementioned study noted that a chitosan matrix proved most superior in terms of higher EE, with no noticeable change in antioxidant activity compared to the pure compound.

10.3.3 Nanoencapsulated systems: Nanoparticles and nanocapsules

Chitosan has been used as a nanoparticle material because it has many attractive properties including hydrophilicity, bioadherence, biodegradability, and antimicrobial activity. However, a balance needs to be found between the protection of the entrapped nutraceutical from premature degradation and the ability of the system to liberate the bioactive for pharmacological benefit.

Researchers have reported significantly improved *in vitro* antioxidant effects and cytotoxicity when naringenin was encapsulated in chitosan nanoparticles when compared to free naringenin (Kumar *et al.*, 2015). The release of the flavonoid under simulated gastric conditions was low (15%), with the majority of the nutraceutical remaining entrapped within the nanoparticles at acid pH. However, entrapment of the bioactive with prolonged release and more-robust resistance to metabolic digestion provides limited benefit if the delivery mechanism does not liberate bioactive at the site of absorption in the intestine. Because release from chitosan-based systems preferentially occurs at alkaline conditions, it is vital to test release under intestinal conditions to ensure maximal bioavailability. A strong interaction between the incorporated nutraceutical and the nanoparticle may be noted, but quantifying the release at the site of absorption is required to ensure optimal solubilization, membrane transit, and systemic uptake to translate into *in vivo* efficacy of the of the nutraceutical. This is a critical step prior to inclusion of such systems in food-based applications.

Nanoliposomes also have appeal as delivery vehicles due to their ability to carry both hydrophilic and hydrophobic nutraceuticals and to improve penetration, stability, and solubility. Some researchers have used natural polymers as coatings of liposome surfaces to impart additional benefits (Xia *et al.*, 2013). Chitosan-coated nanoliposomes containing vitamin E demonstrated reduced aggregation and adverse morphological changes and improved shelf life compared to plain uncoated nanocomplexes. A cross-linked protonated layer of chitosan provides an electrostatic interaction between negative groups of liposomal surfaces and thus confers improved encapsulation efficiency and thermal protection and reduced capacity for deleterious aggregation and loss of included bioactives. Sodium tripolyphosphate (TPP) is a cross-linking and gelation agent commonly used to cross-link chitosan when forming beads, hydrogels, and scaffold-like structures. However, TPP, when used as a cooperative cross-linker within a chitosan layer, forms a more-rigid structure for successful synthesis of chitosan-decorated liposomes. The merging of technologies is therefore vital to achieving the most-evolved delivery mechanism: Natural polymers as coating agents thus provides important synergistic benefits to nanoparticulate systems.

Complex nanoencapsulation systems are also possible by combining polysaccharides with protein biomacromolecules. This is a strategy similar to the one already discussed when two or more polymers are combined to form beads with modified delivery properties. Chitosan may be used as a constituent of hybrid nanoparticles by combining the cationic polymer with proteins such as soy protein. Likewise, sodium alginate, also considered a common biopolymer, is an ideal anionic polysaccharide suitable for combining with proteins such as β-lactoglobulin. The formation of electrostatic complexes between a polysaccharide and a protein can in many cases result in biopolymers with different properties compared to the two individual polymers. In fact, the mixing of proteins and polysaccharide polymers often results in nanoparticles with synergistic characteristics for improved delivery of nutraceuticals.

Although chitosan has been extensively reported to be an ideal biopolymer to encapsulate vitamins and nutraceuticals, chitosan derivatives such as carboxymethyl chitosan (CMCS) are also conducive to nanoparticle formation. A study by Teng and coworkers (2013) prepared complex nanoparticles by ionic gelation using both CMCS and soy protein isolate (SPI) for encapsulation of vitamin D_3. The combined CMCS–SPI nanoparticles required less calcium for cross-linking integrity, demonstrated improved particle formation and EE, and conferred an increased release of vitamin D_3 under simulated intestinal conditions compared to nanoparticles consisting of the individual biopolymers. Work done using sodium alginate and β-lactoglobulin produced nanocomplexes that were able to encapsulate both hydrophobic and hydrophilic nutraceuticals (β-carotene, folic acid, vitamin D_2, and curcumin) (Hosseini *et al.*, 2015). This preliminary work highlighted the versatility of protein-polysaccharide–soluble nanocomplex systems to form stable vehicles for delivering nutraceuticals in liquid functional food products to enhance their health properties.

Modification of biopolymers can result in site-specific absorption of bioactives from the gastrointestinal tract and selective nutraceutical efficacy at the site of pathology while minimizing drug exposure to healthy tissues. For example, chitosan may be modified by grafting polycaprolactone side chains onto its backbone followed by galactosylation or lactsosylation to form nanoparticles with an ability to confer hepatocyte-targeted delivery of nutraceuticals (Zhou *et al.*, 2013). Curcumin was encapsulated with high efficiency in this novel chitosan-based nanoparticulate system, which resulted in a large increase (six-fold) in cytotoxic apoptosis and necrosis of cancerous liver cells compared to free nonencapsulated curcumin (Zhou *et al.*, 2013). These effects are not surprising because nanoparticles have long-since been shown to improve penetration into tumor cell sites due to their reduced size and passive diffusion effects. However, when biopolymers are further functionalized to actively target certain tumor cell receptors, then encapsulated natural chemotherapeutic agents show an improved efficacy with reduced nonselective toxicity. Such systems have potential for many useful applications in the oncology field, where the limitation of conventional formulations is due to a benefit-to-risk ratio that is negatively affected by nonselective distribution of drug.

Even within specific types of biopolymer there are various grades that differ in terms of molecular weight, viscosity, and structural conformation. Chitosan, for example, occurs in α and β forms that have different molecular weights and intermolecular bonds. These differences in polymer grades manifest in variations in mechanical properties, solubility, and reactivity of resultant encapsulation systems. One study used the less-available form of chitosan, namely β-chitosan, to form nanoparticles for the encapsulation of an herbal antioxidant, tea-polyphenol–zinc (TP–Z–) complex (Zhang *et al.*, 2015). Resultant microparticles achieved a high EE of TP-Zn, a sustained *in vitro* release profile, and high antioxidant activity, making this delivery system a useful mechanism to deliver gastrointestinal-insoluble antioxidants effectively from foodstuffs. These results are not surprising because different forms of chitosan result in nanoparticulate systems of different sizes, morphology, stability, and uniformity, which directly affects the success of the resultant systems at a microscopic level (Figure 10.5).

Proteins derived from food offer an additional advantage as biopolymers used for encapsulation, providing nutritional significance when consumed. Casein is one such protein that is the major milk protein and suitably structured to form nanoparticles with nutraceutical agents while offering a synergistic food-based value to the delivery mechanism. The water-soluble vitamin folic acid (vitamin B_9) was included in a casein nanoparticle, resulting in gastroresistant effects for

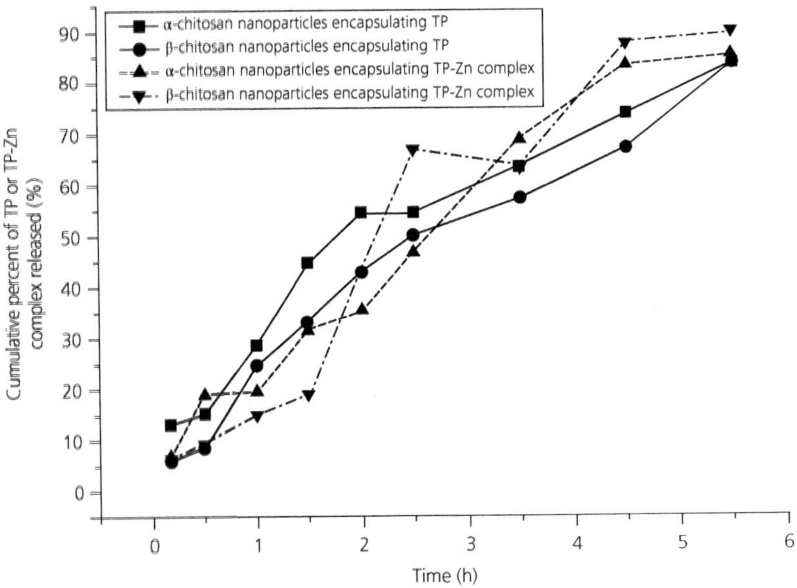

Figure 10.5 Releasing curves from various tea polyphenol (TP) and tea polyphenol–zinc complex (TP-Zn) loaded chitosan nanoparticles in phosphate buffer, pH 7.4. Chitosan nanoparticles succeeded in achieving sustained release of tea–polyphenol and the tea polyphenol–zinc complex over the course of 5.5 hours. These results are notable considering such herbal extracts have extremely low gastrointestinal oral bioavailability; however, when nanoencapsulated they can achieve a sustained *in vitro* release profile demonstrating up to 90% release. Figure from Zhang *et al.*, 2015; Reproduced with permission from Elsevier B.V © 2015].

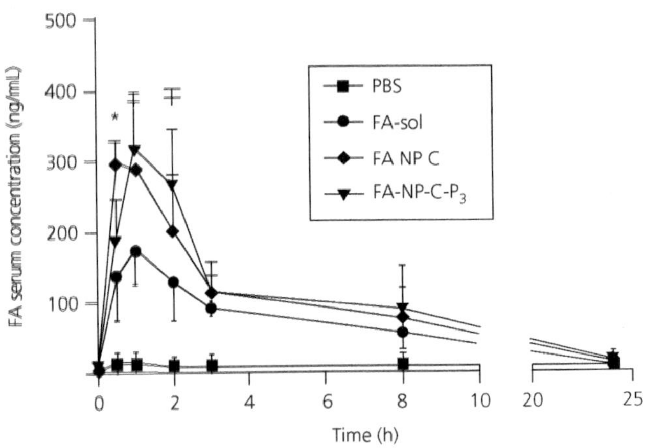

Figure 10.6 Folic acid serum concentration vs. time after oral administration of different formulations at a dosage of 1 mg/kg. Casein nanoparticles are gastro-resistant, evidenced by superior serum pK profiles following an *in vivo* animal study, resulting in significantly higher serum folic acid levels compared to an aqueous solution of the vitamin. The superior serum blood levels obtained in such a preclinical evaluation provide clear benefits for using biopolymeric nanoparticles over conventional formulations in oral delivery of nutraceuticals; FA NP C, Folic acid–loaded casein nanoparticles; FA-NP-C-P_3: folic acid–loaded casein nanoparticles treated by high hydrodynamic pressure. FA-Sol, folic acid solution; PBS, phosphate buffered saline. Figure from Penalva *et al.*, 2015; reproduced with permission from Elsevier B.V © 2015.

targeted release of folic acid in the intestine (Penalva *et al.*, 2015). *In vivo* release studies exemplified the bioavailability enhancement of the casein-encapsulated vitamin compared to a free folic acid solution. A 50% increase in bioavailability observed in preclinical studies make this encapsulation strategy a successful oral vehicle to improve folic acid serum levels while providing additive nutritional benefit from the casein encapsulation material (Figure 10.6).

10.4 Conclusion

The diverse nature of nutraceutical formulations allow increased effectiveness and treatment outcomes for patients. The use of monolithic matrix-based systems as well as nutraceutical-encapsulated archetypes has resulted in greater nutraceutical efficiency, with a large number of positive projects undertaken in this discipline. This has therefore allowed nutraceutical delivery to continuously improve, with a large number of innovative and novel techniques proposed annually, resulting in nutraceutical delivery being an exciting field of study going into the future.

Acknowledgments

This work was funded by the National Research Foundation (NRF) of South Africa.

References

Amarnath, K., Dhanabal, J., Agarwal, I., and Seshadry, S. (2014). Cytotoxicity induction by ethanolic extract of *Acalypha indica* loaded casein–chitosan microparticles in human prostate cancer cell line *in vitro*. *Biomedicine & Preventive Nutrition* 4: 445–450.

Argin, S., Kofinas, P., and Martin Lo, Y. (2014). The cell release kinetics and the swelling behavior of physically crosslinked xanthan–chitosan hydrogels in simulated gastrointestinal conditions. *Food Hydrocolloids* 40: 138–144.

Arya, A., Chandra, A., Sharma, V., and Pathak, K. (2010). Fast dissolving oral films: An innovative drug delivery system and dosage form. *International Journal of ChemTech Research* 2: 576–583.

Belscak-Cvitanovic, A., Stojanovic, R., Manojlovic, V., Komes, D., Cindric, I.J., *et al.*, (2011). Encapsulation of polyphenolic antioxidants from medicinal plant extracts in alginate–chitosan system enhanced with ascorbic acid with ascorbic acid by electrostatic extrusion. *Food Research International* 44: 1094–1101.

Bolhuis, G. K., Eissens, A. C., and Zoestbergen, E. (2001). DC calcium lactate, a new filler-binder for direct compaction of tablets. *International Journal of Pharmaceutics* 221: 77–86.

Carrillo-Navas, H., Cruz-Olivares, J., Varela-Guerrero, V., Alamilla-Beltrán, L., Vernon-Carter, E. J., and Pérez-Alonso, C. (2012). Rheological properties of a double emulsion nutraceutical system incorporating chia essential oil and ascorbic acid stabilized by carbohydrate polymer–protein blends. *Carbohydrate Polymers* 87: 1231–1235.

Castro, P. M., Fonte, P., Sousa, F., Madureira, A. R., Sarmento, B., and Pintado, M. E. (2015). Oral films as breakthrough tools for oral delivery of proteins/peptides. *Journal of Controlled Release* 211: 63–73.

Chan, E. S., and Zhang, Z., (2005). Bioencapsulation by compression coating of probiotic bacteria for their protection in an acidic medium. *Process Biochemistry* 40: 3346–3351.

Chen, L., Remondetto, G. E., and Subirade, M. 2006. Food protein–based materials as nutraceutical delivery systems. *Trends in Food Science & Technology* 17: 272–283.

Elzoghby, A. O., Abo El-Fotoh, W. S., and Elgindy, N. A. 2011. Casein-based formulations as promising controlled release drug delivery systems. *Journal of Controlled Release* 153: 206–216.

Gomez-Estaca, J., Gavara, R., and Hernandez-Munoz, P. (2015). Encapsulation of curcumin in electrosprayed gelatin microspheres enhances its bioaccessibility and widens its uses in food applications. *Innovative Food Science and Emerging Technologies* 29: 302–307.

Goncalves da Rosa, C., Borges, C. D., Zambiazi, R. C., Nunes, M. R., Benvenutti, E. V., *et al.*, 2013. Microencapsulation of gallic acid in chitosan, β-cyclodextrin and xanthan. *Industrial Crops and Products* 46: 138–146.

Govender, M., Choonara, Y. E., van Vuuren, S., Kumar, P., du Toit, L. C., and Pillay, V., 2015. A gastro-resistant ovalbumin bi-layered mini-tablet-in-tablet system for the delivery of *Lactobacillus acidophilus* probiotic to simulated human intestinal and colon conditions. *Journal of Pharmacy and Pharmacology* 67: 939–950.

Hosseini, S. M. H., Emam-Djomeh, Z., Sabatino, P., and van der Meeren, P. (2015). Nanocomplexes arising from protein–polysaccharide electrostatic interaction as a promising carrier for nutraceutical compounds. *Food Hydrocolloids* 50: 16–26.

Jain, A., Thakur, D., Ghoshal, G., Katare, O. P., and Shivhare, U. S. 2015. Microencapsulation by complex coacervation using whey protein isolates and gum acacia: An approach to preserve the functionality and controlled release of β-carotene. *Food and Bioprocess Technology* 8(8): 1635–1644.

Josef, E., Zilberman, M., and Bianco-Peled, H. (2010). Composite alginate hydrogels: An innovative approach for the controlled release of hydrophobic drugs. *Acta Biomaterialia* 6: 4642–4649.

Joshi, S., and Petereit, H-U. (2013). Film coatings for taste masking and moisture protection. *International Journal of Pharmaceutics* 457: 395–406.

Kumar, S.P., Birundha, K., Kaveri, K., and Ramya Devi, K.T. (2015). Antioxidant studies of chitosan nanoparticles containing naringenin and their cytotoxicity effects in lung cancer cells. *International Journal of Biological Macromolecules* 78: 87–95.

Lupo, B., Maestro, A., Porras, M., Gutierrez, J. M., and Gonzalez, C. (2014). Preparation of alginate microspheres by emulsification/internal gelation to encapsulate cocoa polyphenols. *Food Hydrocolloids* 38: 56–65.

Maestrelli, F., Zerrouk, N., Cirri, M., and Mura, P. (2015). Comparative evaluation of polymeric and waxy microspheres for combined colon delivery of ascorbic acid and ketoprofen. *International Journal of Pharmaceutics* 485: 365–373.

Makishi, G. L. A., Lacerda, R. S., Bittante, A. M. Q. B., Chambi, H. N. M., Costa, P. A., *et al.*, (2013). Films based on castor bean (*Ricinus communis* L.) proteins crosslinked with glutaraldehyde and glyoxal. *Industrial Crops and Products* 50: 375–382.

Maltais, A., Remondetto, G. E., and Subirade, M. (2010). Tabletted soy protein cold-set hydrogels as carriers of nutraceutical substances. *Food Hydrocolloids* 24: 518–524.

Mun, S., Kim, Y., Shin, M., and McClements, D.J. (2015). Control of lipid digestion and nutraceutical bioaccessibility using starch-based filled hydrogels: Influence of starch and surfactant type. *Food Hydrocolloids* 44: 380–389.

O'Neill, G. J., Egan, T., Jacquier, J. C., O'Sullivan, M., and O'Riordan E. D. (2014). Whey microbeads as a matrix for the encapsulation and immobilisation of riboflavin and peptides. *Food Chemistry* 160: 46–52.

Ozturk, B., Argin, S., Ozilgen, M., and McClements, D. J. (2015). Formation and stabilization of nanoemulsion-based vitamin E delivery systems using natural biopolymers: Whey protein isolate and gum arabic. *Food Chemistry* 188: 256–263.

Penalva, R., Esparza, I., Agueros, M., Gonzalez-Navarro, C. J., Gonzalez-Ferrero, C., and Irache, J. M. 2015. Casein nanoparticles as carriers for the oral delivery of folic acid. *Food Hydrocolloids* 44: 399–406.

Poulin, J. F., Caillard, R., and Subirade, M. 2011. β-Lactoglobulin tablets as a suitable vehicle for protection and intestinal delivery of probiotic bacteria. *International Journal of Pharmaceutics* 405: 47–54.

Reddy, N., Jiang, Q., and Yang, Y. (2012). Preparation and properties of peanut protein films crosslinked with citric acid. *Industrial Crops and Products* 39: 26–30.

Sanna, V., Roggio, A. M., Pala, N., Marceddu., S, Lubinu., G, *et al.* (2015). Effect of chitosan concentration on PLGA microcapsules for controlled release and stability of resveratrol. *International Journal of Biological Macromolecules* 72: 531–536.

Sultana, A., Hassan, F., Israr, F., Hasan, S. M. F., and Haque, N. (2014). Formulation and stability evaluation of immediate release antioxidant tablet. *Pakistan Journal of Pharmaceutical Sciences* 27: 1393–1400.

Teng, Z., Luo, Y., and Wang, Q. (2013). Carboxymethyl chitosan–soy protein complex nanoparticles for the encapsulation and controlled release of vitamin D_3. *Food Chemistry* 141: 524–532.

Trifkovic, K. T., Milasinovic, N. Z., Djordjevic, V. B., Krusic, M. T. K., Knezevic-Jugovic, Z. D., *et al.*, 2014. Chitosan microbeads for encapsulation of thyme (*Thymus serpyllum* L.) polyphenols. *Carbohydrate Polymers* 111: 901–907.

Villena, M. J. M., Lara-Villoslada, F., Martínez, M. A. R., and Hernández, M. E. M. (2015). Development of gastro-resistant tablets for the protection and intestinal delivery of *Lactobacillus fermentum* CECT 5716. *International Journal of Pharmaceutics* 487: 314–319.

Wankhade, V. P., Kale, N. S., and Tapar, K. K. (2014). Self microemulsifying nutraceutical and drug delivery systems. *International Journal of Pharmaceutical Sciences and Nanotechnology* 7(3): 2520–2528.

Xia, S., Tan, C., Xue, J., Lou, X., Zhang, X., and Feng, B. (2013). Chitosan/tripolyphosphate-nanoliposomes core–shell nanocomplexes as vitamin E carriers: Shelf-life and thermal properties. *International Journal of Food & Technology* 49(5): 1367–1374.

Zhang, H., and Zhao, Y. (2015). Preparation, characterization and evaluation of tea polyphenol–Zn complex loaded β-chitosan nanoparticles. *Food Hydrocolloids* 48: 260–273.

Zhou, N., Zan, X., Wang, Z., Wu, H., Yin, D., *et al.*, 2013. Galactosylated chitosan–polycaprolactone nanoparticles for hepatocyte-targeted delivery of curcumin. *Carbohydrate Polymers* 94: 420–429.

CHAPTER 11

Application of microencapsulated vitamins in functional food systems

Siew Young Quek and Cheng Peng
School of Chemical Sciences, University of Auckland, Private Bag 92019, Auckland 1142, New Zealand

11.1 Introduction

Vitamins are a group of micronutrients that play vital roles in maintaining human health and growth. Because most vitamins cannot be synthesized in the human body, the common way of satisfying the daily requirement is to get them from food or supplements. Nevertheless, daily consumption of food might not supply adequate vitamins. Some vitamins are not readily available in food, which makes it impossible for people who have special dietary or living habits to obtain adequate amounts. For instance, the daily intake of vitamin B_{12} is inadequate in some the strict vegans, because vitamin B_{12} exists in meat or other animal products. Moreover, for certain populations, the daily required amount of vitamins might be above normal requirements, which is difficult to fulfill through daily diet. For example, women in the first three months of pregnancy should consume 4.0 mg folic acid (vitamin B_9), which is four times higher than the requirement for nonpregnant adults (Food and Agriculture Organization, 2002). Additionally, low bioavailability of certain vitamins, inappropriate cooking methods, or antagonism between vitamins and the food matrix can all contribute to inadequate vitamin intake.

Vitamin deficiency can cause severe physiological malfunctions and has been manifested clinically. Table 11.1 shows the possible symptoms caused by vitamin deficiency.

There are three major solutions for overcoming vitamin deficiency (Li *et al.*, 2014): changing dietary habits, using vitamin supplements, and using functional foods (food fortification). Changing dietary habits is the best and most natural method but needs individual compliance and economic improvements, which cannot be controlled in the fast-paced lifestyle in certain countries. Using vitamin

New Polymers for Encapsulation of Nutraceutical Compounds, First Edition.
Edited by Jorge Carlos Ruiz Ruiz and Maira Rubi Segura Campos.

Table 11.1 Possible symptoms caused by deficiency of certain vitamins.

Vitamin	Possible Symptom of Deficiency	Major Sources
A	Blindness and visual impairment, susceptibility to infection	Liver, carrots, dark green leafy vegetables
B_2	Sore tongue, cracked lips, sore throat	Meat, mushrooms, spinach
B_3	High cholesterol, skin lesions, Diarrhea, insomnia	Red meat, white meat, fish, mushrooms
B_9	Megaloblastic anemia, stress-related disorders, infections	Beans, dark green leafy vegetables
B_{12}	Fatigue, depression, abnormal sensations	Fish, liver, red meat, eggs
C	Swollen gums, nosebleeds, scurvy	Dark green leafy vegetables, most berries, oranges
D	Rickets, muscle weakness	Fish, liver, eggs
E	Neuromuscular and neurological problems, anemia	Nuts, plant oil, seafood, spinach
K	Bruising, petechiae, hematomas	Green leafy vegetables, herbs, salad vegetables

supplements might rapidly alleviate vitamin deficiency; but it can cause side effects in the gastrointestinal (GI) tract and possibly a recurrence of the vitamin deficiency. Compared to changing the diet and using vitamin supplements, the functional food method (food fortification) stands as the most cost-effective and low-risk solution (Munin and Edwards-Lévy, 2011).

The water-soluble vitamins include the vitamin B family and vitamin C; the lipophilic (fat-soluble) vitamins include the vitamin A, D, E, and K families. The common difficulties of incorporating vitamins into food products include (Li *et al.*, 2014) poor solubility, reactions with existing ions, oxidation and degradation under ultraviolet (UV) light, heat degradation at processing, unstable chemical properties in alkaline and acidic environments, segregation from food carriers, undesirable sensory changes, off-flavors and off-colors noticeable to consumers, and low product stability. Several factors related to the degradation of each vitamin category are summarized in Table 11.2.

The four most successful applications of vitamins in food products are in bakery goods, bars, beverages, and breakfast cereals, known as the "4Bs" (Feder, 2006). Based on New Zealand and Australia food standard code and regulations, dairy products, cereal products, beverages, edible oils, juices, legume products, and formulated beverages are the major food types permitted to have added vitamins (Australian Government, 2014). Other than the traditional 4Bs, naturally derived substances like herbal extracts and animal- and marine-based derivatives could be the fastest-growing segment of the market. A more-pharmaceutical approach and less processing are also the current trend for designing novel functional foods. Personalized delivery systems, in which fortified foods are developed based on individual metabolic needs and genetics, rather than the common generic nanotechnology delivery systems, might be a future trend as well.

Table 11.2 Factors affecting instability in vitamins.

Vitamins	Metal Ion Reactions	Stability in Acidic Environment	Stability in Alkaline Environment	Heat	Light	Oxygen
A	U	U	S	U	S	U
B_6	U	S	U	S	U	S
B_9	U	U	U	U	U	U
B_{12}	S	S	S	S	U	S
C	U	U	U	U	U	U
D	U	U	S	U	U	U
E	U	S	S	S	U	U
K	U	S	U	S	U	U

S, stable; U, unstable
Data from Reference [4, 5]

The current existing method of incorporating vitamins into functional food includes (Patel and Bhandari, 2014) adding vitamins in solution form, adding vitamins in insoluble form without encapsulation, and adding microencapsulated vitamins into food. Adding vitamins in solution form has advantages and is convenient for incorporating vitamins into liquid-based food systems because the vitamins are ready for absorption and have better bioavailability; the inherent disadvantage of this method is that unpleasant color or taste might not be masked, and undesired chemical reactions could lead to instability of the final product. Adding insoluble vitamins without encapsulation might effectively protect vitamins from undesired chemical reactions and might be palatable, but the bioavailability might be reduced, the sensory properties could be negatively affected, and the stability of the product could be decreased as the greater mass of the dispersion could cause creaming and sedimentation (Patel and Bhandari, 2014).

The third solution, microencapsulating vitamins, has the special benefit of controlled targeted release (Champagne and Fustier, 2007; Gouin, 2004); stabilizing vitamins against damage from reactive and incompatible ingredients or degradation factors such as light, heat, and oxygen (Gunasekaran and Ko, 2014) and better palatability. The physical properties of the active ingredient's dispersion can be modified to prevent creaming and sedimentation, thus improving its stability Dubey *et al.*, 2009). Furthermore, the cost of microencapsulation techniques for fortifying food products has decreased due to the availability of more viable technology and raw materials (Global Industry Analysts, Inc., 2010). To sum up, microencapsulation has far more pros than cons and is superior to the other two methods.

This chapter gives an overview of the applications of various encapsulated vitamins incorporated in commonly used functional food systems including beverages, dairy products, and other fortified food systems. The common criteria of selecting wall materials, encapsulating technology, and incorporation methods for adding vitamins in various functional food systems is discussed with reference to case studies.

11.2 Common microencapsulation techniques for vitamins

The difficulties of formulating vitamins into microencapsulated forms includes finding the correct delivery dosage form and encapsulating technologies at formulating, and determining the appropriate wall materials and carriers, which vary in every case (Teleki *et al.*, 2014). When selecting the wall materials, there are several principles to follow: Wall materials should not react with the core, must be able to seal or to immobilize the inner structure, must provide maximum protection against adverse conditions, should not have an unpleasant taste, and should be economical. The commonly used wall materials are (Teleki *et al.*, 2014) carbohydrates (starch, modified starches, dextrin, sucrose, cellulose, and chitosan); gums (Arabic gum, alginate, and carrageenan); lipids (wax, paraffin, monoglycerides and diglycerides, hydrogenated oils and fats); inorganic materials (calcium sulfate and silicates), proteins (gluten, casein, gelatin, albumin).

Microencapsulation techniques can be divided into two types (Champagne and Fustier, 2007). The top-down method involves breaking large particles into smaller ones, for instance, forming a emulsion first (stabilizing with surfactants) and reducing the particle size by spray-drying or freeze-drying to form the final particles. The bottom-up approach involves assembling individual components into larger particles, for instance, precipitating crystals first and then extruding them. The advantages and disadvantages of some specific microencapsulation techniques are listed in Table 11.3.

Characterization studies of microencapsulated systems commonly include determination of particle size, size distribution, morphology, density, porosity, surface charge, shell thickness, mechanical strength, glass transition temperature, degree of crystallinity, flowability, and compressibility studies (Zhang *et al.*, 2010). The size of the microencapsulated particles can affect the interaction with other molecular species and can affect the stability, texture, appearance, and sensory quality of food products. It can also determine the formation technologies applied to testing the particle size of the microencapsulated particles, which is the most important practice among all the characterization studies (Liu *et al.*, 2013). Encapsulation efficiency testing is also used to evaluate the properties of the microencapsulation method and technology and the suitability of wall materials. Encapsulation efficiency (Liu *et al.*, 2013) is defined as the ratio between the weight of the encapsulated active compound and the whole of its total weight. *In vitro* studies using simulated gastric and intestinal fluid and the Caco-2

Table 11.3 Advantages and disadvantages of various microencapsulation techniques.

Microencapsulation Method	Advantages	Disadvantages
Spray-drying	Cheap and straightforward Stable Suitable for fine particles (10–100 nm) Mostly applicable for lipophilic vitamins	Unable to microencapsulate heat-sensitive products
Spray-cooling	Suitable for thermal-sensitive substances Can produce various particle sizes Easy to scale up	Low encapsulation capacity Expulsion of core materials
Lyophilization	Suitable for thermal-sensitive substances Widely used for flavorings	High cost Long process time
Coacervation	Suitable for high-value, active, and unstable substances	Limited range of PH, colloidal, electrolyte concentrations Nonspherical particles.
Extrusion	Longer shelf-life for flavor compounds because the barrier is almost impermeable	Limited wall materials Large particles affect mouth feel.
Emulsification	Simple, applied for all kinds of vitamins	Might use oftoxic organic solvents

Data from [10] [15] [14]

cell line test transport and uptake to evaluate the absorption rate and bioaccessibility of the core materials. *In vivo* studies can be used to provide direct data for evaluating the bioavailability of the microencapsulated system, despite the disadvantages of having ethical limitations, a lengthy approval process for clinical research, possible interactions with other elements in the diet, and uncertainty about the physiological state of the research subjects (Augustin, 2003).

11.3 Applications of incorporating encapsulated vitamins in dairy products

Fortifying dairy products with vitamins can enhance their quality and suitability and can reduce the loss of inherent nutrients during storage (Augustin, 2003). all dairy products lack vitamins E and K. Skim milk lacks VITAMIN A. Vitamin D levels in dairy products are affected by breed, diet, season, and exposure to sunlight (Augustin, 2003). In addition, vitamin C tends to be degraded during pasteurizing. In the United States, vitamin A and D fortification in pasteurized milk is mandated by the U.S. Food and Drug Administration (FDA) food regulations and guidance (U.S. Food and Drug Administration, 2005). In New Zealand, vitamins A and D may be added to dried milk, cheese products, yogurt, and dairy desserts based on Australia and New Zealand Food Standards Code 1.3.2 Vitamins and Minerals (Australian Government, 2014). Because vitamin D is the major regulator of calcium absorption, incorporating vitamin D in dairy products allows the body to optimally use the great amount of calcium in dairy products (Kwak *et al.*, 2014). Incorporating vitamin A in dairy products can prevent night blindness and visual impairment. Incorporating vitamin C with iron in dairy products can enhance the absorption of iron (Augustin, 2003).

11.3.1 Application in cheese

Cheese is derived from the curd of animal milk. It is manufactured by coagulating milk casein with enzyme or acid and further treating it by adding salt, placing the producting under pressure, and fermenting it (Vieira, 1996). Key factors determining the characteristics of a cheese are its moisture content (which determines its hardness), protein and lipid content, pH, species of fermentation bacteria, and the time taken for ripening (age). The procedures for manufacturing cheese includes adding acid and enzyme to form and solidify curds, cutting and cooking the curds (this step needs a high temperature), draining the whey, milling the curds and adding salt to get rid of the whey by osmosis and inhibit microorganisms, pressing the curds to get rid of the moisture, and ripening at a cool temperature.

Cheese is an ideal delivery system for most vitamins because it has higher pH and fat content, a stable semisolid form, and a strong buffering capacity that can protect the bioactive ingredients from the low pH environment in the stomach (Giroux *et al.*, 2013). In addition, the consumption of cheese has increased 100% since the end of the 20th century, which provides a greater marketing opportunity for functional cheese products (Upreti *et al.*, 2002). Vitamins, enzymes and antimicrobials commonly have already been used for making functional cheese (Mohammadi *et al.*, 2015). For pasteurization and sterilization purposes, most cheese has to go through a cooking step at which the temperature could reach above 50 °C over 20 minutes. The most common step of incorporating microencapsulated vitamins into cheese is at the initial step (step 1 before curd formation).

Delivering microencapsulated vitamin D and incorporating it into cheese could increase the retention of lipids and protein and enhance the quality of the cheese curd. Cheese contains a great amount of calcium, which has a synergistic effect on delivering vitamin D, as they enhance the absorption of each other in the human body. Milk fat can also enhance the stability of vitamin D.

Stratulat and colleagues (2012) studied the incorporation of vitamin D in flaxseed oil–based emulsion prepared by the micro-fluidization method. The emulsion was delivered into cheese as functional cream (before curd formation) in cheese manufacturing. A lipophilic substance, lecithin, was used as a surfactant to form an oil-in-water emulsion. Vitamin D delivered with lecithin shows greater stability than using other lipophilic surfactants whose hydrophilic–lipophilic balance (HLB) value is less than 6 (sorbitan monooleate, glyceryl monooleate, sugar esters). The reason might be that the lecithin and casein interactions strengthen the fat-droplet surface. Lecithin has a lower molecular weight, which allows it to compete against the other protein molecules absorbing on the droplets and repel them. Lecithin also limits the contact surface with the aqueous phase, which reduces the lipid oxidation and increases the yield of cheese (Stratulat *et al.*, 2012). Tippetts and coworkers (2012) found that more vitamin D could be retained in an emulsion-stabilized cheese compared to non-emulsifed oil vitamin D solution.

The quantification method for vitamin D is the saponification method, which is conducted as follows: Extract the vitamin D from the lipophilic layer, rotate to evaporate all the solvents, elute on a silica cartridge, and gather the elution and detect the vitamin D by high-performance liquid chromatography (HPLC) (Upreti *et al.*, 2002).

Banville's group (2000) compared the suitability of three different formulations (vitamin D emulsions, solutions, and liposomes) of microencapsulated vitamin D on the properties of cheese produced. The three forms of vitamin D were all incorporated into cheese before curd formation. Their findings showed that liposomes retain significantly greater amounts of vitamin D than the other microencapsulated dosage forms at the cheese-ripening stage (Banville *et al.*, 2000). Though using a liposome delivery system might have better vitamin retention and stability than emulsions do, the presence of liposomes increased the moisture of cheese and modified the microstructure of the product (Laloy *et al.*, 1998). As a result, the cheese was more elastic and brittle as its rheological properties changed (Laloy *et al.*, 1998).

There are a few potential challenges when incorporating hydrophilic vitamins into cheese. If the vitamins are directly delivered in aqueous solutions, they might be lost in the whey during the cheesemaking process. Hydrophilic substances might precipitate out in the salting and ripening process, and the non-retained vitamins might contaminate other products derived from the whey (Giroux *et al.*, 2013). A double-emulsion system developed by Giroux and colleagues (2013) solved these problems. They developed a water-in-oil-in-water double emulsion encapsulating vitamin B_{12} in the internal water phase of the double emulsion. The double emulsion was finely mixed with the skim milk delivered as functional cream at cheese making, which is similar to standard cheddar cheese making. The experiment results showed that the encapsulating efficiency of vitamin B_{12} reaches 96%, and the cheese has significantly lower fat content and higher protein content.

11.3.2 Application in yogurt

Yogurt is a liquid dairy product with a high nutritive value and rising consumption trends, especially among younger people (Kwak *et al.*, 2014). Yogurt is manufactured generally using the following steps: mixture of raw materials (texture modifiers, condensers, stabilizers, and milk), homogenization, pasteurization, fermentation, and cooling. The possible place to incorporate vitamins in yogurt manufacturing is at the fermentation or cooling stage to prevent the microencapsulates from degrading under high temperature and high pressure. Because the active ingredients are microencapsulated, they do not affect the pH of the fermentation environment (the key factor) and there is no significant influence on the viability of the probiotics during storage (Kim *et al.*, 2003). Microencapsulation also increases the product's overall antioxidant activity (Martins *et al.*, 2014) by decreasing and unifying the particle size and increasing stability and shelf-life (Wechtersbach *et al.*, 2012).

Two successful examples have been reported. Kim and colleagues (2003) used a spray-drying method of microencapsulating vitamin C with iron by using polyglycol monostearate (PGMS) as the wall material. The active ingredients were incorporated into yogurt at the fermentation step. The microencapsulated forms relatively improved the final product's sensory quality compared to the nonencapsulated forms. Wechtersbach and colleagues (2012) designed a dipomitoylphosphatidylcholine (DPPC)–cholesterol liposomal delivery system for microencapsulating vitamin C by the reverse-phase evaporation method and incorporated it into yogurt (fermented milk) after the cooling step. The oxidation rate of vitamin C was significantly decreased, and the half-life of microencapsulated vitamin C was increased three-fold in fermented milk. However, examples of successfully incorporating microencapsulated vitamins into yogurt is comparatively less.

Other studies of dairy products and other bioactive components (Chee *et al.*, 2005; McCowen *et al.*, 2010) reported the incorporation of microencapsulated lipophilic substances such as marine fish oils or omega-3 fatty acids into yogurt, which might provide motivation and inspiration for microencapsulating vitamins with similar physiochemical properties.

11.3.3 Application in ice cream

Ice cream is a frozen semisolid dairy product served as dessert, made by whipping air in a mixture of ingredients during the product's freezing process. The manufacturing process of ice cream generally has several steps: mixing liquid ingredients (including sweeteners, stabilizers, emulsifiers), homogenization, pasteurization, and cool down and hard freezing (during cool down and freezing, air is whipped into the ice cream). Ice cream's foamed colloidal structure and its low-temperature storage renders it an ideal carrier for beneficial microorganisms and nutraceuticals (Soukoulis *et al.*, 2014). The major principle of incorporating vitamins into ice cream must not adversely affect its colloidal air-whipped structure (Zhang *et al.*, 2010). It is crucial that the incorporating agents not impede sufficient air incorporation to prevent the agents from crystallizing and recrystallizing. Additionally, encapsulated particle size has to be controlled within a limited range to prevent the fat droplets from destabilizing.

Application of microencapsulated vitamins into ice cream is rarely found in the literature. Nevertheless, applications of other bioactive ingredients with similar physiochemical properties as vitamins could provide guidance for future formulation projects. Cam's group (Cam *et al.*, 2014) provided an application for polyphenols, which are hydrophilic bioactive ingredients similar to water-soluble vitamins. This group used maltodextrins as coating material and the spray-drying technique as the method for microencapsulating polyphenols. The microencapsulated polyphenol was incorporated into ice cream during the homogenization step. The final product enhanced antioxidant activity that almost equaled that of plant-based foods by simply adding phenolics. The sensory quality was improved, as the product showed no astringency. Mangolim and colleagues (Mangolim *et al.*, 2014) provided an application for similar hydrophobic ingredients to be incorporated into ice cream. They bound the colorant curcumin to chelating agents (β-CD) by co-precipitation, freeze-drying, and solvent-evaporation methods. The complexation was incorporated into ice cream during the homogenization step. The product was more obviously protected from UV light than its nonencapsulated form. In addition to these examples, other effective formulation strategies include liposomes, solid lipid nanoparticles (SLN), and coagulation (Jacobson *et al.*, 2002); other wall materials include pectin, cellulose, and carrageenan.

11.4 Application of microencapsulated vitamins in beverages

Based on their components, beverages can be classified into three groups (Potter and Hotchkiss, 1995): carbonated, noncarbonated mildly alcoholic, and noncarbonated mildly nonalcoholic. Beverages provide a convenience solution and can be used to meet consumer demands for container size and shape, appearance, and convenience of storage and refrigeration; in addition, it is easy to incorporate bioactive components into them. Therefore, beverages can be good candidates for designing as a functional food (Corbo *et al.*, 2014). Functional beverage market sales make up 59% of the total US functional food market (Corbo *et al.*, 2014). An international functional food consumption survey among German and Chinese consumers revealed that functional beverages are highly accepted by health-conscious consumers (Siegrist *et al.*, 2015).

Functional beverages can be divided into three groups: dairy-based beverages, vegetable and fruit beverages, and sports and energy drinks. Commonly used components in beverages include sweeteners, flavorings, colors, acid, preservatives, water, and carbon dioxide. Among all the ingredients, added acids and carbon dioxide can enhance beverage flavors, act as preservatives against microbial growth, and produce a tingling mouth feel, and it can decrease the pH of the beverage and affect the stability of bioactive ingredients incorporated into the beverage (Champagne and Fustier, 2007).

Microencapsulation as a protection for the naturally existing vitamins in fruit juice and concentrate has been found widely in the literature. The spray-drying process, which has the advantages of being economically viable and able to straightforwardly produce stable and uniform particles, is the first choice for directly encapsulating naturally existing vitamins in fruit juice (Murugesan and Orsat, 2012). In the spray-drying process, the fruit juice and wall materials are homogenized first to form a solution or emulsion, and then they go through the atomization process in which the liquid products are atomized in a hot gas, and water is evaporated.

Among the applications of encapsulating naturally existing vitamins by spray-drying, maltodextrin and gum arabic are the best choices for wall materials. Maltodextrin has film-forming capacity and plastic properties that are suitable for materials that are to dry hard. Gum arabic has mild taste and emulsifying properties, and its low viscosity gives it good flow properties, which aids the spray-drying process.

Rigetto's team (2006) microencapsulated West Indian cherry juice in a mixture of maltodextrin and gum arabic mixture (w/w = 3:1) by spray drying. They found that vitamin C degradation was less than in its nonencapsulated forms and in the synthetic vitamin C solution sample. Silva and colleagues (2013) used maltodextrin and gum arabic to encapsulate vitamin C and heat-sensitive phenolic compounds in camu-camu juice. In the process of direct microencapsulation in natural fruit juice or puree, the existing phenolics, carotenoids, or other antioxidants in the fruit puree could synergistically protect vitamins with wall materials from degradation. In another application (Sun-Waterhouse and Waterhouse, 2015) of microencapsulating vitamin C in kiwifruit puree, skim milk was added into the kiwifruit puree during the microencapsulation process; the whey protein in milk interacts with existing pectin and phenolics. This reaction induces complexation and strengthens microstructures, which has preservation effects for vitamin C.

Another method of formulating microencapsulated vitamins into beverages is to microencapsulate the bioactive ingredients in emulsions. In the current market, most of the functional emulsions are designed as low-calorie drinks, energy drinks, and beverage concentrates (Piorkowski and McClements, 2014). An emulsion is a mixture of two immiscible phases – a lipophilic phase and a hydrophilic phase – and surfactant. Among beverage emulsions, the lipophilic phase mainly contains fat-soluble vitamins, natural oils, edible hydrocarbons, or synthetic oil mixture of triglycerides with various chain lengths and degrees of saturation (McClements and Rao, 2011). The hydrophilic phase mainly contains water-soluble vitamins, water, and aqueous co-solvents. The emulsion is stabilized by the surfactant, a molecule composed of a hydrophilic group and hydrophobic group.

Based on the selected surfactant's physiochemical properties and its HLB value, emulsions can be designed into three types: oil–in-water, water-in-oil, and bicontinuous emulsions. Because water is the main component (around 92%) of the beverage formulation, oil-in-water emulsion is the most commonly applied form for functional beverages. Formulating the fat-soluble vitamins in the inner structure can protect the ingredients from oxidation.

The emulsion-manufacturing process includes the following steps (Piorkowski and McClements, 2014): preparing the water-phase and oil-phase solutions, homogenization, pasteurization, and dilution. The water-phase solution contains mostly water-soluble ingredients and a small amount of water; the oil-phase solution contains nutraceutical lipids and fat-soluble vitamins, vitamin E, pre-vitamin A. In the high-energy homogenization process, the water phase and oil phase are mixed together with surfactant. The dilution phase involves diluting the emulsion with a large amount of water; in this process, colorants and flavorings might be added.

Several studies (Chiu and Yang, 1992; Gonnet *et al.*, 2010; Guttoff *et al.*, 2015; Yang and McClements, 2013) describe the process of formulating fat-soluble vitamins and oil-in-water beverage emulsions. The studies' results show that emulsions could improve physiochemical stability and increase bioavailability, and they show potential for delivering other lipophilic ingredients. In addition to traditional coarse emulsions, microemulsions with particle size smaller than 100 nm (mainly between 10 nm and 100 nm) have been considered by the food industry. Compared to a coarse emulsion, a microemulsion is a thermodynamically and isotropic delivery system with the advantages of being transparent and palatable, prolonging shelf-life, and improving oral absorption of the delivered nutrients (Singh *et al.*, 2009). However, the smaller particle size has some risk of changing the absorption of certain bioactive components, causing side effects. For oil-in-water microemulsions, more-toxic surfactants with much higher HLB values might be used to stabilize the microemulsions (McClements and Rao, 2011).

For delivering vitamins in microencapsulated forms, nanoparticles and liposome systems are also applied. Liposomes can be described as closed and continuous bilayers enclosed by phospholipids (Mozafari *et al.*, 2008). Compared to emulsions and nanoparticles in functional beverages, liposomes have the advantage of being able to deliver nutrients with a wider range of oil–water partition coefficients (both lipophilic and hydrophilic vitamins) (Ma *et al.*, 2009). Liposomes can also prevent possible lipid oxidation in emulsions. Liposomes' polar lipids could enclose the nutrients within its inner compartments. While the inner phase of an emulsion is not immobilized as the liposome's inner structure, the reactive agents might penetrate through the phase boundaries in emulsions. Finally, the release pattern of the liposome can be predicted well, and entrapment efficiency is as good as that of nanoparticles.

The common method of preparing liposomes begins with evaporating an emulsion containing phospholipids and organic solvent to produce a thin film. After that, the compound is supplied with mechanical energy and hydrated. Finally, liposomes are formed by the separation of the film (Mozafari *et al.*, 2008). However, because of the lack of a continuous production process and the toxic ingredients (organic solvents are highly toxic, and phospholipids have a relatively high LD_{50} value) that have been used in the manufacturing process, scaling up of liposome manufacturing is limited in the food industry (Mozafari *et al.*, 2008). Using all-natural surfactants and less-toxic ingredients to replace synthetic ingredients might overcome these disadvantages.

Marsanasco's team (Marsanasco *et al.*, 2011) developed soy phosphatidylcholine–stearate–based liposomes to microencapsulate vitamin C and delivered it into Valencia orange juice. In this study, stearic acid partially replaced phosphatidylcholine in constructing the liposome's bilayer structure. Adding stearic acid increases the rigidity of the liposomes' bilayer, reduces the flow of water, and enhances the retention of vitamin C before and after pasteurization. The study results (Marsanasco *et al.*, 2011) show that the stearate-incorporated liposomes have greater encapsulation efficiency of vitamin C than the non–stearate-incorporated liposomes, and the organoleptic characteristics were not changed, which implied that stearic acid might be a good alternative for phosphatidylcholine in the food industry.

A nanoparticle delivery system is another possible way to delivery vitamins into beverages. A nanoparticle is defined as a small object that behaves as a whole unit and has dimensions between 1 and 2500 nm (Taylor *et al.*, 2013). Based on the particle size, thenanoparticles can be further classified as ultrafine, fine, or coarse (Taylor *et al.*, 2013). Spray-drying and freeze-drying techniques can be used to prepare smaller (1–500 nm) nanoparticles, and extrusion and coacervation techniques can be used to prepare larger (>500 nm) nanoparticles. Nanoparticle systems can be stabilized by electrostatic stabilization (as two charged particles approach each other, the electrostatic repulsion force increases), polymeric steric stabilization (as the particles approach each other, the polymer chains penetrate each other), electropolymeric steric stabilization (the combination of the two forces).

Chen and colleagues (Chen and Wagner, 2004) developed a nanoparticle delivery system containing vitamin E and incorporated the nanoparticles into apple juice. The system has a particle size of 100 nm. The powder was readily dispersed in juice by magnetic stirring, and turbidity was only slightly increased during storage. The beverage with vitamin E nanoparticles also has a clearer appearance than beverages with vitamin E emulsions. The nanoparticle delivery system could be a special candidate for beverage applications with decreased turbidity and greater physical stability, helping the industry to create new and innovative products.

Markman and colleagues (2012) used the Maillard reaction to form protein–polysaccharide nanoparticles. The particles of vitamin D conjugated in protein–polysaccharide are smaller than in the vitamin D solution, showing a clearer outer appearance. The conjugated nanoparticles offer better protection against oxidation, are more colloidally stable, and have an enteric delivery effect, with the interactions between the protein in the structure and loaded vitamin D causing its immobilization, reducing the oxidation and decomposition in reactions Markman and Livney, 2012).

11.5 Application of encapsulated vitamins in bakery products

Bakery products are one of the cheapest ready-to-eat products around the world, and consumption continues to increase (Nanditha and Prabhasankar, 2009). It is an ideal carrier for nutraceuticals because of its great popularity, ease of preparation, and ease of storage. Mandatory fortification of folic acid (vitamin B_9) in grain products was introduced in Canada and the United States in 1997 to prevent neural tube defects.

Bakery products are produced from dough or batters that typically contain flour, liquid, leaveners, fat, eggs, and sugar. Flour is normally all-purpose wheat flour, hard wheat flour for bread, or soft wheat flour for cake. Liquid is used to hydrate flour proteins and to dissolve other ingredients. Leaveners include baking soda, yeast, and baking powder. Fats and oils tenderize baked products by coating flour proteins. Eggs provide color and flavor, and they bind ingredients together. Sugar absorbs water. Other components such as milk or juice might be incorporated in the liquid (Vaclavik and Christian, 2003).

The gluten in flour contributes to the elastic properties of baked products (Vaclavik and Christian, 2003). The firmness of bakery products is mainly determined by the development of gluten in the dough-making process. A low liquid-to-flour ratio causes more gluten development, which produces larger holes in the crumb and increased firmness of the bakery product. The pH of the environment also has to be considered because many leavening agents need an acidic environment. Because the only way of incorporating vitamins into bakery products is at the dough-making stage, directly incorporating vitamins can affect the pH and liquid content of the dough, which indirectly affects gluten formation and the leavening process and changes the quality of the final product.

Encapsulating acidic ingredients such as vitamin C can prevent those acidic ingredients from inhibiting the growth of yeast, and it can protect the crumb texture from acid, because acid can prevent crumb extension (Ezhilarasi *et al.*, 2013). Additionally, adding lipophilic ingredients like fat-soluble vitamins and lipophilic-encapsulating wall materials into bakery products can modify the product's structure, increase the product's volume, and tenderize the final product, which might be due to lipid plasticization of gluten in the baking process (O'Brien *et al.*, 2000).

Fat content plays an important role in bakery products, including shortness, tenderness, richness, and stiffness of dough (Sudha *et al.*, 2014). The amount of the emulsification ingredients used in microencapsulation materials can affect the firmness of dough due to the binding of emulsifiers with fat-soluble ingredients, affecting the total free-fat content in the final product. Microencapsulating lipophilic ingredients can also allow good flowability during the kneading process and increase its oxidative stability (O'Brien *et al.*, 2000).

Proteins in the encapsulated wall materials can also affect the sensory qualities of the crust, which might become tougher as the concentration of protein increases. This might due to the Maillard reaction between the added amino acids and inherent reducing sugars (Costa de Conto *et al.*, 2012). The stability of the product could also improve by the binding effects between protein and the core materials.

Tomiuk and colleagues (O'Brien *et al.*, 2000) microencapsulated L-5-methyltetrahydrofolic acid (L-5-MTHF, the reduced form of vitamin B_9) by milk fat. Milk fat acts as coating as well as a bulking agent to improve the dispersion of L-5-MTHF. This process protects L-5-MTHF during the baking process (185 °C, 25 min) and increases the recovery of L-5-MTHF by 50%. Adding a co-encapsulated substance could also improve the tolerance of the vitamins for the baking process.

Liu's team (Liu *et al.*, 2013) fortified microencapsulated L-5-MTHF with microencapsulated vitamin C together into flour. They found the co-encapsulation sample had 39% higher microencapsulation efficiency than regular microencapsulation of L-5-MTHF. The experimental design could be used to optimize the best concentrations of the fat or proteins as wall materials added into the dough.

The common measurement of bread product quality includes the crumb - compression test, crumb texture profile analysis, firmness, volume yield, crust color, and baking loss. Several papers also provide the formulation process of incorporating microencapsulated vitamins or nutraceuticals into various bakery products, including bread (Costa de Conto *et al.*, 2012), biscuits (Umesha *et al.*, 2015), pasta (Liu *et al.*, 2015), and snacks (Caliskan *et al.*, 2015), and all these results in the studies have proved that the microencapsulation process could enhance the recovery of loaded nutrients.

11.6 Conclusions

The research in the area of incorporating microencapsulated vitamins into various functional food products has great potential to target vitamin-deficiency problems. At present, the developed food categories are dairy products, beverage products, and bakery products. The greatest difficulty with formulation is the use of high temperatures for pasteurization and baking.

Due to the flexibility of manufacturing techniques and delivery forms, beverages have the most abundant examples of successful application of microencapsulated vitamins that enhance product quality and stability. Because the mechanisms of bakery and dairy product manufacturing are well established, the space for research and development of novel products has been relatively narrowed. To study the method of incorporating microencapsulated vitamins into solid food products, semisolid products, and liquid products, it is reasonable to refer to the current existing examples in bakery products, dairy products, and beverages respectively. Microencapsulation of vitamins could also provide some insights into the encapsulation of other nutraceuticals with similar physiochemical properties, as well as their application in similar food matrices or systems.

References

Augustin, M. A. (2003). The role of microencapsulation in the development of functional dairy foods. *Australian Journal of Dairy Technology* 58(2): 156–160.

Australian Government. (2014). Australia New Zealand Food Standards Code – Standard 1.3.2 – Vitamins and Minerals. https://www.legislation.gov.au/Details/F2014C01184.

Banville, C., Vuillemard, J. C., and Lacroix, C. (2000). Comparison of different methods for fortifying Cheddar cheese with vitamin D. *International Dairy Journal* 10(5–6): 375–382.

Caliskan, G., Lim, A. S. L., and Roos, Y. H. (2015). Beta-carotene stability in extruded snacks produced using interface engineered emulsions. *International Journal of Food Properties* 18(10): 2256–2267.

Cam, M., Icyer, N.C., and Erdogan, F. (2014). Pomegranate peel phenolics: Microencapsulation, storage stability and potential ingredient for functional food development. *LWT – Food Science and Technology* 55(1): 117–123.

Champagne, C. P., and Fustier, P. (2007). Microencapsulation for the improved delivery of bioactive compounds into foods. *Current Opinion in Biotechnology* 18(2): 184–190.

Chee, C. P., Gallaher, J. J., Djordjevic, D., Faraji, H., McClements, D. J., *et al.* (2005). Chemical and sensory analysis of strawberry flavoured yogurt supplemented with an algae oil emulsion. *Journal of Dairy Research* 72(3): 311–316.

Chen, C. C., and Wagner, G. (2004). Vitamin E nanoparticle for beverage applications. *Chemical Engineering Research & Design* 82(A11): 1432–1437.

Chiu, Y.,C., and Yang, W. L. (1992). Preparation of vitamin E microemulsion possessing high resistance to oxidation in air. *Colloids and Surfaces* 63(3): 311–322.

Corbo, M. R., Bevilacqua, A., Petruzzi, L., Casanova, F. P., and Sinigaglia, M. (2014). Functional beverages: The emerging side of functional foods commercial trends, research, and health implications. *Comprehensive Reviews in Food Science and Food Safety* 13(6): 1192–1206.

Costa de Conto, L., Porto Oliveira, R. S., Pereira Martin, L. G., Chang, Y. K., and Steel, C. J. (2012). Effects of the addition of microencapsulated omega-3 and rosemary extract on the technological and sensory quality of white pan bread. *LWT – Food Science and Technology* 45(1): 103–109.

Dubey, R., Shami, T. C., and Rao, K. U. B. (2009). Microencapsulation technology and applications. *Defence Science Journal* 59(1): 82–95.

Ezhilarasi, P. N., Indrani, D., Jena, B. S., and Anandharamakrishnan, C. (2013). Freeze drying technique for microencapsulation of *Garcinia* fruit extract and its effect on bread quality. *Journal of Food Engineering* 117(4): 513–520.

Feder, D. (2006). Well noted: The four Bs of nutraceuticals. *Food Processing* http://www.foodprocessing.com/articles/2006/252.html.

Food and Agriculture Organization (FAO/WHO). (2002). *Human Vitamin and Mineral Requirements Folate and Folic Acid*. Bangkok: U.N. Food and Agriculture Organization/World Health Organization.

Giroux, H. J., Constantineau, S., Fustier, P., Champagne, C. P. St.-Gelais, D., *et al.* (2013). Cheese fortification using water-in-oil-in-water double emulsions as carrier for water soluble nutrients. *International Dairy Journal* 29(2): 107–114.

Global Industry Analysts, Inc. (2010). *Food Encapsulation: A Global Strategic Business Report.* San Jose, CA: Global Industry Analysts.

Gonnet, M., Lethuaut, L., and Boury, F. (2010). New trends in encapsulation of liposoluble vitamins. *Journal of Controlled Release* 146(3): 276–290.

Gouin, S. (2004). Microencapsulation: Industrial appraisal of existing technologies and trends. *Trends in Food Science & Technology* 15(7–8): 330–347.

Gunasekaran, S., and Ko, S. (2014). Rationales of Nano- and Microencapsulation for Food Ingredients. In: *Nano- and Microencapsulation for Foods,* pp. 43–64. H. S. Kwak, ed. Oxford: Blackwell Science.

Guttoff, M., Saberi, A. H., and McClements, D. J. (2015). Formation of vitamin D nanoemulsion-based delivery systems by spontaneous emulsification: Factors affecting particle size and stability. *Food Chemistry* 171: 117–122.

Jacobson, M. R., Reddy, S., Vadehra, D., Wedral, E. R., and Sher, A. (2002). Fortified foodstuff as e.g. dairy-based product, comprises complex of calcium, hydrolyzed polysaccharide, and acid. Vevey, Switzerland: Nestec SA (Nest-C).

Kim, S. J., Ahn, J., Seok, J. S., Kwak, H. S. (2003). Microencapsulated iron for drink yogurt fortification. *Asian–Australasian Journal of Animal Sciences* 16(4): 581–587.

Kwak, H. S., Al Mijan, M., and Ganesan, P. (2014). Application of Nanomaterials, Nano- and Microencapsulation to Milk and Dairy Products. In: *Nano- and Microencapsulation for Foods,* pp. 273–300. H. S. Kwak, ed. Oxford: Blackwell Science.

Laloy, E., Vuillemard, J. C., and Simard, R. (1998). Characterization of liposomes and their effect on the properties of Cheddar cheese during ripening. *Lait* 78(4): 401–412.

Li, Y. O., Gonzalez V. P. D., and Diosady L. L. (2014). Microencapsulation of Vitamins, Minerals, and Nutraceuticals for Food Applications. In: *Microencapsulation in the Food Industry: A Practical Implementation Guide,* pp. 501–522. A. G. Gaonkar, N. Vasisht, A. R. Khare, and R. Sobel, eds. London: Academic Press.

Liu, Y. Z., Green, T. J., and Kitts, D. D. (2015). Stability of microencapsulated L-5-methyltetrahydrofolate in fortified noodles. *Food Chemistry* 171: 206–211.

Liu, Y. Z., Green, T. J., Wong, P., and Kitts, D. D. (2013). Microencapsulation of L-5-methyltetrahydrofolic acid with ascorbate improves stability in baked bread products. *Journal of Agricultural and Food Chemistry* 61(1): 247–254.

Ma, Q. H., Kuang, Y., Z., Hao, X., Z., and Gu, N. (2009). Preparation and characterization of tea polyphenols and vitamin E loaded nanoscale complex liposome. *Journal of Nanoscience and Nanotechnology* 9(2): 1379–1383.

Mangolim, C. S., Moriwaki, C., Nogueira, A. C., Sato, F., Baesso, M. L., *et al.* (2014). Curcumin-β-cyclodextrin inclusion complex: Stability, solubility, characterisation by FT-IR, FT-Raman, X-ray diffraction and photoacoustic spectroscopy, and food application. *Food Chemistry* 153: 361–370.

Markman, G., and Livney, Y. D. (2012). Maillard-conjugate based core-shell co-assemblies for nanoencapsulation of hydrophobic nutraceuticals in clear beverages. *Food & Function* 3(3): 262–270.

Marsanasco, M., Marquez, A., Wagner, J. R., Alonso, S. del V., and Chiaramoni, N. S. (2011). Liposomes as vehicles for vitamins E and C: An alternative to fortify orange juice and offer vitamin C protection after heat treatment. *Food Research International* 44(9): 3039–3046.

Martins, A., Barros, L., Carvalho, A. M., Santos-Guelga, C., Fernandes, I. P., *et al.* (2014). Phenolic extracts of *Rubus ulmifolius* Schott flowers: Characterization, microencapsulation and incorporation into yogurts as nutraceutical sources. *Food & Function* 5(6): 1091–1100.

McClements, D. J., and Rao, J. (2011). Food-grade nanoemulsions: formulation, fabrication, properties, performance, biological fate, and potential toxicity. *Critical Reviews in Food Science and Nutrition* 51(4): 285–330.

McCowen, K. C., Ling, P. R., Decker, E., Djordjevic, D., Roberts, R. F., *et al.* (2010). A simple method of supplementation of omega-3 polyunsaturated fatty acids: Use of fortified yogurt in healthy volunteers. *Nutrition in Clinical Practice* 25(6): 641–645.

Mohammadi, R., Mahmoudzade, M., Atefi, M., Khosravi-Darani, D., and Mozafari, M. R. (2015). Applications of nanoliposomes in cheese technology. *International Journal of Dairy Technology* 68(1): 11–23.

Mozafari, M. R., Khosravi-Darani, K., Borazan, G. G., Cui, J., Pardakhty, A., and Yurdugul, S. (2008). Encapsulation of food ingredients using nanoliposome technology. *International Journal of Food Properties* 11(4): 833–844.

Munin, A., and Edwards-Lévy, F. (2011). Encapsulation of natural polyphenolic compounds: A review. *Pharmaceutics* 3(4): 793.

Murugesan, R., and Orsat, V. (2012). Spray drying for the production of nutraceutical ingredients – a review. *Food and Bioprocess Technology* 5(1): 3–14.

Nanditha, B., and Prabhasankar, P. (2009). Antioxidants in bakery products: A review. *Critical Reviews in Food Science and Nutrition* 49(1): 1–27.

O'Brien, C. M., Grau, H., Neville, D. P., Keogh, M. K., and Arendt, E. K. (2000). Functionality of microencapsulated high-fat powders in wheat bread. *European Food Research and Technology* 212(1): 64–69.

Patel, A. R., and Bhandari, B. (2014). Nano- and Microencapsulation of Vitamins. *Nano- and Microencapsulation for Foods*, pp. 223–248. H. S. Kwak, ed. Oxford: Blackwell Science.

Piorkowski, D. T., and McClements, D. J. (2014). Beverage emulsions: Recent developments in formulation, production, and applications. *Food Hydrocolloids* 42: 5–41.

Potter, N. N., and Hotchkiss, J. H. (1995). *Food Science*, 5th ed. New York: Springer.

Righetto, A. M., and Netto, F. M. (2006). Vitamin C stability in encapsulated green West Indian cherry juice and in encapsulated synthetic ascorbic acid. *Journal of the Science of Food and Agriculture* 86(8): 1202–1208.

Siegrist, M., Shi, J., Giusto, A., and Hartmann, C. (2015). Worlds apart. Consumer acceptance of functional foods and beverages in Germany and China. *Appetite* 92: 87–93.

Silva, N. K., Cornejo, F. E. P., Gomes, F. S., Pontes, S. M., Matta, V. M., and Freitas, S. P. (2013). Influence of shell material on vitamin C content, total phenolic compounds, sorption isotherms and particle size of spray-dried camu-camu juice. *Fruits* 68(3): 175–183.

Singh A. K., Chaurasiya A., Awasthi A., Mishra G., Asati D., *et al.* (2009). Oral bioavailability enhancement of exemestane from self-microemulsifying drug delivery system (SMEDDS). *AAPS PharmSciTech* 10(3): 906–916.

Soukoulis, C., Fisk, I. D., and Bohn, T. (2014). Ice cream as a vehicle for incorporating health-promoting ingredients: Conceptualization and overview of quality and storage stability. *Comprehensive Reviews in Food Science and Food Safety* 13(4): 627–655.

Stratulat, I., Britten, M., Salmieri, S., Fustier, P., St-Gelais, D., *et al.* (2012). Enrichment of cheese with vitamin D-3 and vegetable omega-3. *Journal of Functional Foods* 13: 300–307.

Sudha, M. L., Chetana, R., and Reddy, S. Y. (2014). Effect of microencapsulated fat powders on rheological characteristics of biscuit dough and quality of biscuits. *Journal of Food Science and Technology–Mysore* 51(12): 3984–3990.

Sun-Waterhouse, D., and Waterhouse, G. I. N. (2015). Spray-drying of green or gold kiwifruit juice-milk mixtures: Novel formulations and processes to retain natural fruit colour and antioxidants. *Food and Bioprocess Technology* 8(1): 191–207.

Taylor, R., Coulombe, S., Otanicar, T., Phelan, P., Gunaway, A., *et al.* (2013). Small particles, big impacts: A review of the diverse applications of nanofluids. *Journal of Applied Physics* 113(1): 011301.

Teleki, A., Hitzfeld, A., and Eggersdorfer, M. (2013). 100 Years of vitamins: The science of formulation is the key to functionality. *Kona Powder and Particle Journal* 30: 144–163.

Tippetts, M., Martini, S., Brothersen, C., and McMahon, D. J. (2012). Fortification of cheese with vitamin D_3 using dairy protein emulsions as delivery systems. *Journal of Dairy Science* 95(9): 4768–4774.

Umesha, S. S., Sai Manohar, R., Indiramma, A. R., Akshitha, S., and Akhilender Naidu, K. (2015). Enrichment of biscuits with microencapsulated omega-3 fatty acid (alpha-linolenic acid) rich garden cress *(Lepidium sativum)* seed oil: Physical, sensory and storage quality characteristics of biscuits. *LWT – Food Science and Technology* 62(1): 654–661.

U.S. Food and Drug Administration. (2005). Pasteurized Milk Ordinance 2005: Appendix O. Vitamin Fortification of Fluid Milk Products. Washington, DC: Food and Drug Administration.

Upreti, P., Mistry, V. V., and Warthesen, J. J. (2002). Estimation and fortification of vitamin D_3 in pasteurized process cheese. *Journal of Dairy Science* 85(12): 3173–3181.

Vaclavik, V., and Christian, E. W. (2003). *Essentials of Food Science*. New York: Springer.

Vieira, E. R. (1996). *Elementary Food Science*, 4th ed. Hathorne, MA Springer Science.

Wechtersbach, L., Poklar Ulrih, N., and Cigić, B. (2012). Liposomal stabilization of ascorbic acid in model systems and in food matrices. *LWT – Food Science and Technology* 45(1): 43–49.

Yang, Y., and McClements, D. J. (2013). Encapsulation of vitamin E in edible emulsions fabricated using a natural surfactant. *Food Hydrocolloids* 30(2): 712–720.

Zhang, Z., Law, D., and Lian, G. (2010). Characterization Methods of Encapsulates. In *Encapsulation Technologies for Active Food Ingredients and Food Processing*, pp. 101–125. N. J. Zuidam and V. Nedovic, eds. New York: Springer.

CHAPTER 12

Application of encapsulated compounds in functional food systems

M. K. Tripathi and S. K. Giri
APPD, Central Institute of Agricultural Engineering, Bhopal-462038, India

12.1 Introduction

Functional foods are food products, both naturally occurring and processed food, that contain bioactive compounds with a functionality beyond the essential daily nutritional requirements to improve human health. The industrial production of functional foods often requires the addition of different functional ingredients in the food matrix. Typically, these are used to control flavor, color, texture, and preservation properties, but increasingly ingredients with potential health benefits are also included.

Adding bioactive ingredients to functional foods presents many challenges (Champagne *et al.*, 2005), particularly with respect to the stability of the bioactive compounds during processing and storage and the need to prevent undesirable interactions with the carrier food matrix.

Encapsulation is an important process to entrap active compounds or agents within a carrier material and to improve the delivery of bioactive molecules and living cells into foods. Reactive, sensitive, or volatile additives can be turned into stable ingredients through microencapsulation. Microencapsulation has been defined as the process by which individual particles or droplets of solid or liquid material (the core) are surrounded or coated with a continuous film of polymeric material (the shell) to produce capsules in the micrometer to millimeter range, known as *microcapsules*. These capsules release their contents at controlled rates over prolonged periods of time. Such technologies are of significant interest to the pharmaceuticals sector (e.g., for drug and vaccine delivery), but they also have relevance for the food industry.

New Polymers for Encapsulation of Nutraceutical Compounds, First Edition.
Edited by Jorge Carlos Ruiz Ruiz and Maira Rubi Segura Campos.

Major advantages of microencapsulation process include

- Reducing the reactivity of the core with regard to the outside environment, for example oxygen and water
- Decreasing the evaporation or transfer rate of the core material with regard to the outside environment
- Controlling the release of the core material so as to achieve the proper delay until the right stimulus occurs
- Promoting the ease of handling of the core material
- Masking the taste of the core
- Diluting the core material when it is only used in very small amounts while achieving uniform dispersion in the host material

Microencapsulation can provide a physical barrier between the core compound and the other components of the product. More especially, in the food field, microencapsulation is a technique by which liquid droplets, solid particles, or gas compounds are entrapped into thin films of a food-grade microencapsulating agent. The core may be composed of just one or several ingredients, and the wall may be single or double layered. Microcapsule is a simplest form with a uniform wall around it. The material inside the microcapsule is referred to as the *core, internal phase,* or *fill,* whereas the wall is sometimes called *shell, coating, wall material,* or *membrane.* Practically, the core may be a crystalline material, a jagged adsorbent particle, an emulsion, a suspension of solids, or a suspension of smaller microcapsules.

The different types of microcapsules and microspheres are produced from a wide range of wall materials (monomers and/or polymers) and by a large number of different microencapsulation processes such as spray-drying, spray-cooling, spray-chilling, air suspension coating, extrusion, centrifugal extrusion, freeze-drying, coacervation, rotational suspension separation, co-crystallization, liposome entrapment, interfacial polymerization, and molecular inclusion, among others (Desi and Park, 2005).

12.2 Microencapsulation technologies and bioactive food ingredients

12.2.1 Nonmicrobial products

Spray-drying has been traditionally used to encapsulate oil-based vitamins and fatty acids (Augustin *et al.*, 2001). However, many emulsion, spray-chilling, and liposome techniques (Arnaud,1995) show potential for the controlled release of bioactive compounds such as retinol, omega-3 fatty acids, yeasts, vitamins, and enzymes.

Many emulsions can yield delivery systems with novel encapsulation and delivery properties. The functional component can be encapsulated within the inner phase (the oil phase) or the outer water phase after drying; thus, a single delivery system can contain multiple functional components. Lesser-used technologies for the microencapsulation of nonmicrobial bioactive ingredients include their incorporation into cyclodextrins and coacervation (Arneado, 1996). Nanoemulsions, with droplet sizes between 100 and 500 nm, are produced by microfluidization or micelle-formation techniques and are gaining popularity for both pharmaceutical and food applications (Weiss *et al.*, 2006). However, the lack of sufficient food-grade surfactants currently prevents the incorporation of many of these nanoemulsions into commercial food systems (Garti *et al.*, 2005).

12.2.2 Microbial products

Probiotic bacteria are defined as live microorganisms that, administered in adequate amounts, confer a beneficial physiological effect on the host. Probiotics present two sets of problems when considering microencapsulation: their size (typically between 1 and 5 µm diameter), which immediately excludes nanotechnologies, and the fact that they must be kept alive. This latter aspect has been crucial in selecting the appropriate microencapsulation technology. Because bioactive or encapsulating compounds can be in liquid form, many techniques are based on spraying. Methods such as spray-coating, spray-drying, extrusion, emulsion, and gel-particle technologies have been applied to microencapsulate probiotics.

In spray-coating, the core material needs to be in a solid form and is kept in motion in a specially designed vessel, either by injection of air at the bottom or by a rotary action. A liquid coating material is sprayed over the core material and solidifies to form a layer at the surface. The coating material can be injected from many angles, and this influences the properties of the coating.

In spray-chilling, a molten matrix with a low melting point (32–42 °C) containing the bioactive compound is atomized through a nozzle into a vessel. This process is similar to spray-drying with respect to the production of fine droplets; however, it is based on the injection of cold air into the vessel to enable solidification of the gel particle, rather than on hot air, which dries the droplet into a fine powder particle. The liquid droplet thus solidifies and entraps the bioactive product.

Of the various technologies mentioned, spray-coating and gel-particle technologies are most often used (Ubbink, 2003). The production of gel particles by spray-chilling is considered the least-expensive encapsulation technology (Gouin, 2004). Unfortunately, this approach has rarely been reported for probiotics, presumably because the current methods are much more easily carried out under laboratory conditions. Although most of the literature on the microencapsulation of probiotics relates to gel particles, most commercial products available are spray-coated products. However, spray-coating is a difficult technique to master, and most information on the technology is proprietary.

In addition to spray-coating and gel-particle technologies, methodologies that employ extrusion, emulsion, and spray-drying have also been explored for the microencapsulation of probiotics. Of these, spray-drying offers the most potential provided the cells can be stress-adapted to the high processing temperatures. Extrusion and emulsion technologies are not easily applied to probiotics because of their large particle size, but a very different picture emerges with respect to nonmicrobial bioactive compounds.

12.3 Delivery of bioactive ingredients into foods and to the gastrointestinal tract

12.3.1 Microbial-containing products

Yogurt and fermented milk products have spearheaded the development of probiotic functional foods. It is expected that cheese will be the next matrix opportunity for innovative dairy functional foods (Hayes *et al.*, 2006).

The microencapsulation of probiotics for their addition into foods and beverages offers many technological benefits (Box 12.1). It could be argued that

Box 12.1 Beneficial effects of probiotic microencapsulation in different products

Dried probiotic culture

Facilitates the production of oxygen-sensitive cultures
Facilitates the recovery of centrifugation-sensitive cultures and high exopolysaccharide-producing cultures
Fewer contamination problems
Cultures can be air-dried

Nutraceutical

Improved survival on exposure to gastric and bile solutions
Improved stability during storage in dried form

Dried sausages

Improved acidification rate

Biscuits, powder

Improved survival on heating

Ice cream, milk-based medium, cranberry juice

Improved survival on freezing

Cheese

Improved retention in the finished product

Fermented milks

Protection against bacteriophages and yeast contaminants

Yogurt, mayonnaise, milk

Improved survival during storage

microencapsulation serves to deliver viable cells into foods, even though they might not be released in the product. In addition to overcoming technological problems in the production of probiotics, cultures that are microencapsulated in alginate beads show improved resilience to acid in the gastric environment and to bile solutions (Chandramouli *et al.*, 2004). With gel particles, the cells are typically not released into the food products when added; *in vitro* and *ex vivo* studies showed that beads maintained their integrity in simulated stomach conditions, but they subsequently released their cargo in the GI tract (Iyer *et al.*, 2004). Therefore, microencapsulation can not only enhance the delivery of viable cells into the food during processing and storage, but it can also improve survival and facilitate controlled delivery in the GI tract. In some instances, microencapsulation might turn out to have multiple benefits in enhancing the viability of probiotics in functional foods.

It has been shown that the food matrix has a significant effect on the survival of the cells in the upper part of the GI tract (Saxelin *et al.*, 2003). Thus it must be stressed that a health effect noted with a nutraceutical probiotic product cannot be directly transposed to a food product. In some instances, functional foods might prove to be better than nutraceuticals. Data show that nonprotected cells consumed in a dried form have lower recovery levels in stools than those consumed in milk or cheese (Saxelin *et al.*, 2003). The high viability losses that occur when free cells in a powder hydrate enter the stomach explain why encapsulation is crucial for the functionality of probiotics in nutraceuticals. Microencapsulation offers the potential to extend this success to foods, reducing the effect of the food matrix on probiotic viability during processing and storage and following consumption.

Although the future use of microencapsulation in relation to probiotics seems bright, much research is still needed to validate its use. It was shown that the production and freeze-drying processes themselves had a greater effect than microencapsulation alone in promoting the survival of probiotics introduced into biscuits, frozen cranberry juice, and vegetable juices (Reid *et al.*, 2007). Therefore, microencapsulation can also serve to co-entrap prebiotics (i.e., nondigestible food ingredients that can beneficially affect the host by selectively stimulating the growth and/or the activity of bacteria in the gut), raising the possibility of using microencapsulation to deliver multiple bioactive ingredients. However, co-encapsulation with prebiotics has so far not proven better than with glucose in enhancing the resilience of lactobacilli to GI conditions. Moreover, data suggest that at least 3 g of prebiotics in a sample (which is rarely attained in microencapsulation products) are required to significantly affect the probiotic population in the GI tract. Therefore, the benefits of co-entrapment with prebiotics do not seem high. Nevertheless, this approach could be extended to antioxidants, peptides, or immune-enhancing polymers, which are active at lower concentrations than prebiotics.

Co-encapsulation with antioxidants would be a logical combination, because such compounds would help protect the viability of the probiotic cells, particularly bifidobacteria, which are sensitive to exposure to oxygen during storage and in the stomach. Thus, such a combination would provide two sets of bioactive ingredients that would also interact to enhance the functionality of the probiotic culture itself. Bioactive peptides, such as bacteriocins, are also candidates for co-encapsulation; they could enhance or complement the antimicrobial activities of the probiotic bacteria, especially if the health target is protection against diarrhea. In summary, co-encapsulation not only offers the possibility of introducing multiple bioactive ingredients, but it also enables the creative selection of ingredients that will interact to enhance their mutual biological value.

Once the bioactive components responsible for the health-beneficial effects of probiotics are known, it might be found that cell viability is not in fact a prerequisite for the health-promoting effect (Stanton *et al.*, 2005). In such instances, dead bacterial cells could serve as the microencapsulation delivery vehicle for the probiotic-derived bioactive components. This would be particularly appropriate for intracellular ingredients, such as enzymes, which would be inactivated by the acid of the stomach. The use of highly autolytic cells, like those used to accelerate ripening in cheese making, could subsequently promote the release of the intracellular ingredients in the GI tract.

12.3.2 Nonmicrobial products

Microencapsulation promotes the delivery of vitamins and minerals to foods mainly by preventing their interaction with other food components; for example, iron bioavailability is severely affected by interactions with food ingredients (e.g., tannins, phytates, and polyphenols). Additionally, iron catalyzes the oxidative degradation of fatty acids and vitamins. Liposome technology is often used to deliver fluid food products, because it reduces the ability of iron to react with food components. By encapsulating calcium lactate in lecithin liposomes, it was possible to fortify soymilk with levels of calcium equivalent to those found in cow's milk (Hirotsuka *et al.*, 1984) while preventing undesirable calcium–protein reactions.

As with probiotics, the co-encapsulation of vitamins and minerals could be beneficial. Thus, the presence of calcium in a hydrophilic phase and vitamins A or D in a hydrophobic phase could promote calcium absorption in the GI tract. In one such example, encapsulation of ascorbic acid in a liposome together with vitamin E produced a synergistic antioxidant effect. In this case, the vitamin E is incorporated into the liposome wall, and the ascorbic acid is entrapped in the aqueous interior.

Omega-3 and omega-6 fatty acids used for food fortification having considerable health benefits; however, major issues have been encountered with regard to the taste and smell of these oils and their propensity to oxidize rapidly (Augustin and Sanguansri, 2003). It was demonstrated that the consumption of food enriched with microencapsulated fish oil obtained by emulsion spray-drying was as effective as the daily intake of fish oil gelatin capsules in meeting the dietary requirements of this omega-3 long-chain fatty acid (Wallace *et al.*, 2000).

Spray-chilling and fluidized-bed coating are the most popular methods for encapsulating water-soluble vitamins (e.g., ascorbic acid), whereas spray-drying of emulsions is generally recommended for the encapsulation of lipid-soluble vitamins (e.g., β-carotene, vitamins A, D, and E). The glass transition (T_g) properties of various polymers (polysaccharides, proteins, and their mixtures) used as encapsulating matrices is important while selecting it, because these are crucial to the stability of the spray-dried products. Amorphous glassy matrices are generally recommended, because they are more stable due to the low water mobility of the matrices, thereby slowing down the oxygen diffusion that alters the stability of the bioactive compounds.

12.4 Techniques of microencapsulation

The various microencapsulation processes can be broadly divided into chemical, physicochemical, and physicomechanical processes, though the method of preparation and the techniques employed overlap considerably. Chemical processes include the interfacial and *in situ* polymerization methods. Physicochemical processes include the coacervation phase separation, complex emulsion, meltable dispersion, and powder bed methods. Mechanical processes include the air-suspension method, pan coating, and spray-drying, spray-congealing, micro-orifice system, and rotary fluidization bed granulator method. The spheronization is sometimes included under the mechanical process of microencapsulation. Sustained-release polymer microcapsules containing drugs with various solubility characteristics were prepared with colloidal polymer dispersion in a completely aqueous environment as an alternative to the conventional microencapsulation technique.

A number of techniques are available for encapsulating food compounds. The choice of microencapsulation method depends on the nature of the polymeric or monomeric material used. Appropriate combination of starting materials and synthesis methods can be chosen to produce microencapsulated products with a wide variety of compositional and morphological characteristics. For example, poly(alkylcyanoacrylate) nanocapsules are obtained by emulsion polymerization (Damge *et al.*, 1997), whereas reservoir-type nylon microcapsules are usually prepared by interfacial polymerization (Persico *et al.*, 2005). Some of the important and most common microencapsulation techniques used nowadays is discussed below.

12.4.1 Emulsion polymerization

In emulsion polymerization technique, the monomer (alkyl acrylates) is added dropwise to the stirred aqueous polymerization medium containing the material to be encapsulated (core material) and a suitable emulsifier. The polymerization begins, and the initially produced polymer molecules precipitate in the aqueous medium to form primary nuclei. As the polymerization proceeds, these nuclei grow gradually and simultaneously entrap the core material to form the final microcapsules. Generally, lipophilic materials are found to be more suitable for encapsulation using this technique.

12.4.2 Interfacial polycondensation

The interfacial polycondensation technique involves the polycondensation of two complementary monomers at the interface of a two-phase system (Janssen and Nijenhuis, 1992). For the preparation of microcapsules, this two-phase system is mixed under carefully controlled conditions to form small droplets of one phase (dispersed phase) in the other one (continuous phase/suspension medium). The material to be encapsulated must be chosen in such a way as to be present in the droplets. It is also necessary to use a small amount of a suitable stabilizer to prevent droplet coalescence or particle coagulation during the polycondensation process and capsule formation. Thus if the polymer is soluble in the droplets, matrix-type microcapsules are formed. On the other hand, if the polymer is not soluble, it precipitates around the droplets and leads to the formation of monocore-type microcapsules. Preparation of microcapsules by interfacial polycondensation is applicable to a large number of polymers, including polyamides (Argillier *et al.*, 2004), polyureas (Chao, 1993), polyurethanes (Ramanathan, 1998), and polyesters (Wang *et al.*, 1991).

12.4.3 Suspension cross-linking

Suspension cross-linking is the method of choice for the preparation of protein and polysaccharide microcapsules (Katti and Krishnamurti, 1999). Microcapsule formation by this technique involves dispersion of an aqueous solution of the polymer-containing core material in an immiscible organic solvent in the form of small droplets. The suspension medium contains a suitable stabilizer to maintain the individuality of the droplet. The droplets are subsequently hardened by covalent cross-linking and are directly converted to the corresponding microcapsules. The cross-linking process is accomplished either thermally (at >500 °C) or by the use of a cross-linking agent. Suspension cross-linking is a versatile method and can be adopted for microencapsulation of soluble, insoluble, liquid, or solid materials and for the production of microcapsules and nanocapsules.

12.4.4 Solvent extraction

Microcapsule formation by solvent extraction is very similar to suspension cross-linking, but in this case the polymer is usually hydrophobic polyester (Bodmerier and Mcginity, 1987). The polymer is dissolved in a water-immiscible volatile organic solvent like dichloromethane or chloroform, into which the core material is also dissolved or dispersed. The resulting solution is added dropwise to a stirring aqueous solution having a suitable stabilizer, like poly or polyvinyl pyrrolidone, to form small polymer droplets containing encapsulated material. With time, the droplets are hardened to produce the corresponding polymer microcapsules. This hardening process is accomplished by the removal of the solvent from the polymer droplets either by solvent evaporation or by solvent extraction. Solvent extraction produces microcapsules with higher porosities than those obtained by solvent evaporation. Solvent extraction processes are suitable for the preparation of drug-loaded microcapsules based on the biodegradable polyesters such as polylactide, poly(lactidecoglycolide), and polyhydroxybutyrate (Gursel and Hasirci, 1995).

12.4.5 Phase separation

The phase-separation method is widely employed for the preparation of gelatin microcapsules, as well as for a large number of products based on cellulose derivatives and synthetic polymers (Nimmannit and Suwanpatra,1996). Phase-separation processes are divided into simple and complex phase separation. Simple phase separation involves the use of a single polymer such as gelatin or ethyl cellulose, in aqueous or organic media, respectively. Complex phase separation involves two oppositely charged polymeric materials such as gelatin and acacia, both of which are soluble in aqueous media. In both cases, phase separation is brought about by gradual dissolvation of the fully solvated polymer molecules. Microencapsulation by phase separation is carried out by preparing an aqueous polymer solution (1%–10%) at 40 to 50 °C into which the core material is also dispersed.

A suitable stabilizer may also be added to the mixture to maintain the individuality of the final microcapsules. A suitable phase-separation agent is gradually introduced to the mixture, which leads to the formation of partially dissolved polymer molecules and hence their precipitation on the surface of the core particles. The phase-separation mixture is cooled to about 5 to 20 °C, followed by the addition of a cross-linking agent to harden the microcapsule wall formed around the core particles. Gelatin microcapsules loaded with carboquone as well as gelatin acacia microcapsules loaded with sulfamethoxazole have been produced by phase separation (Takenaka *et al.*, 1980).

12.4.6 Emulsification

Emulsification is defined as a process of dispersing one liquid in a second immiscible liquid. By including the core material in the first liquid, we can encapsulate the bioactive component. In most cases, the encapsulating agent is a molecule already present in the food (Augustin & Hemar, 2009). The addition of a surfactant that induces encapsulation by forming micelles, vesicles, bilayers, and reverse micelles around the bioactive molecules is commonly proposed as a solution (Augustin & Hemar, 2009). Usually it protects the bioactive molecules in products and facilitates their release in the duodenum as soon as lipase is being released. The type and digestibility of the applied biopolymer determines its exact release in the gut (Champagne and Fustier, 2007).

12.4.7 Coacervation

Coacervation is a modified emulsification technology that has a relatively simple principle. When a solution of bioactive components is mixed with a matrix molecule of an opposite charge, a complex is formed. The size of the capsule and its characteristics can be varied by changing the pH, the ion concentration, the ratio of matrix molecule and the bioactive component, and the type of matrix. The technique is mainly driven by electrostatic interaction, but hydrophobic interactions are also involved (Augustin and Hemar, 2009). This is an immobilization rather than an encapsulation technology and is therefore mostly used for bioactive food molecules rather than for bioactive living cells. The technique is applied mainly for flavors, oils, and some water-soluble bioactive molecules.

12.4.8 Spray-drying

Spray-drying is one of the oldest and the most widely used encapsulation techniques in the food industrial sector. It is a flexible, continuous, and most importantly an economical operation. This feature is desired from the standpoint of sensory and textural characteristics of final products. Although spray-dryers are widespread in the food industry, there are several disadvantages of this technique: the equipment is complex, the conditions in the drying chamber are not uniform, and it is not always easy to control particle size.

Spray-drying is used for both bioactive food molecules and living probiotics. It is a fast and relatively cheap procedure with high reproducibility. The principle of spray drying is dissolving the core in a dispersion of a chosen matrix material. The dispersion is subsequently atomized in heated air. The powdered particles are separated from the drying air at the outlet at a lower temperature. Spray-drying has many advantages over other technologies for other bioactive food components such as vitamins, minerals, flavors, unsaturated oils, and enzymes. It is a relatively gentle methodology in terms of application of solvents and matrix molecules. Only water-based dispersions are applied in spray-drying. Usually the product is very stable and has a long shelf life (Augustin and Hemar, 2009).

12.4.9 Spray-cooling

Spray cooling is a technology in which an opposite principle of spray-drying is applied. In this technology, a dispersion of a matrix and the bioactive product is made. In this process, instead of evaporating, the dispersion is cooled in order to allow immobilization. Usually fats with a high melting point are used in this technology. Also this is an immobilization rather than an encapsulation technique. At present it is only used for dry products to conserve enzymes, flavors, minerals, and proteins.

12.4.10 Fluid-bed coating

Fluid bed coating methodology is modified spray-dry methodology that enlarges the field of application. In this technology, the bioactive food components are suspended in air and the matrix molecules are sprayed onto the bioactive components (Champagne and Fustier, 2007). The choice of matrix molecules is broader than for traditional spray drying. It may be fats, proteins, carbohydrates, or emulsifiers. It may even be used to produce spray-dried products or a sensitive core for example oils as a second coating. Also it is useful for applying an additional layer of molecules for targeted release in the gut.

12.4.11 Extrusion technologies

Extrusion is nothing more than producing a small droplet of an encapsulation material by forcing the solution through nozzles or small openings in droplet-generating devices. The smaller the inner diameter of the nozzle or openings, the smaller the capsules. Industry-oriented groups quite often have the incorrect assumption that this procedure does not allow large-scale production and is only suitable for laboratory-scale processes. However, enormous advances have been made in the up-scaling of encapsulation processes using extrusion technology. Large-scale droplet production can be achieved by multiple-nozzle systems, spinning disc atomizers, or jet-cutter techniques (Kailasapathy, 2002). An advantage of the extrusion technology is that it is in most cases a true encapsulation procedure instead of an immobilization technology. An alternative extrusion technology is co-extrusion. It might be used to prepare spherical microbeads with a hydrophobic core and a hydrophilic or hydrophobic shell (Zuidam and Shimoni, 2009).

12.5 Materials used for encapsulation

A numbers of substances are known that can be used to entrap, coat, or encapsulate solids, liquids, or gases of different types, origins, and properties. However, only a limited number of substances have been certified for food applications as generally recognized as safe (GRAS). Some compounds that are widely accepted for drug encapsulation have not been approved for use in the food industry. The majority of materials used for microencapsulation in the food sector are biomolecules. Carbohydrate polymers and polysaccharides are the most abundant in comparison to other sources. Proteins and lipids are also biomolecules reported to be suitable for microencapsulation in the food sector. Table 12.1 lists groups of biomolecules, arranged according to their origin, that are found to be most suitable either when used alone or when used in combination with others for microencapsulation in the food industry.

12.6 Selection and safety evaluation of encapsulation materials

The creation of novel functionalities of active ingredients in complex food matrices is of increasing importance for the food industry. Some important traditional active ingredients are flavors, vitamins, and minerals. Relatively novel ones are

Table 12.1 Materials suited for microencapsulation in the food industry.

Origin	Protein	Carbohydrate Polymer	Lipid
Plant	Gluten (corn) Isolates (pea, soy)	Starch derivatives Cellulose derivatives Plant exudates: gum arabic, gum karaya, mesquite gum Plant extracts: galactomannans, soluble soybean Polysaccharide	Fatty acids/alcohols Glycerides Waxes Phospholipids
Animal, microbe	Caseins Whey proteins Gelatin	Xanthan Gellan Dextran Chitosan	Fatty acids/alcohols Glycerides Waxes Phospholipids (Shellac)

probiotic microorganisms and various classes of bioactive compounds (Ubbink and Krüger, 2006). The application of microencapsulation in the food industry can have various goals such as the creation of a totally new product, improvement of an existing product, protection of a known ingredient, improvement of an existing process, or replacement of an existing technology. All of these aspects also affect the strategies for selecting a matrix and wall material. The fundamental knowledge of the chemistry and physicochemical properties of the materials remain the prerequisite for successful product development. A number of well-established industrial technologies for the microencapsulation of food ingredients have been reported (Table 12.2). Some important recommendations for the selection of materials are mentioned in Table 12.3.

12.7 Nutritional and nutraceutical compounds and microencapsulation

The use of microencapsulation to protect, isolate, or control the release of a given substance is of growing interest in the food industry. The many available technologies for microencapsulation can be divided into two categories: one that uses liquid as a suspending medium (complex coacervation, interfacial and *in situ* polymerization, or solvent evaporation from emulsions), and one that uses a gas as a suspending medium into which a liquid phase is sprayed (spray-drying or spray-cooling, fluidized-bed coating, or coextrusion).

12.7.1 Bioactive food components

The commonly applied bioactive food molecules that are encapsulated in industrial applications are carbohydrates, lipids, and proteins (Burey *et al.*, 2008). These ingredients are encapsulated mainly to resist the high acidity and enzyme activity of the stomach and duodenum.

Table 12.2 Application of materials reported recently.

Active Material	Material for Encapsulation	Technology	Reference
Oil			
Vegetable oil	Maltodextrin/GA, 3/2, w/w	Spray-drying + agglomeration in an air fluidized-bed	Fuchs *et al.* (2006)
Fish oil	Modified cellulose, skim milk powder, mixture of fish gelatin/corn starch	Spray-drying	Kolanowski *et al.* (2007)
	MC, HPMC, maltodextrin		Kolanowski *et al.* (2004)
Lipids			
Conjugated linoleic acid (CLA)	WPC, GA, blend WPC/ maltodextrin 10DE (1:1, w/w)	Spray-drying	Jimenez *et al.* (2006)
Linoleic acid	GA	Spray-drying	Fang *et al.* (2005)
Lipids: oleic acid, linoleic acid, stearic acid	Potato starch, waxy maize starch, tapioca starch	Microwave heating	Kapusniak and Tomasik (2006)
Vitamins			
Vitamin C, acerola, synthetic ascorbic acid	Maltodextrin DE20, mixture DE20/GA Maltodextrin DE25, GA, or mix of both	Spray-drying	Righetto and Netto (2005, 2006)
Vitamin C	Tripolyphosphate/chitosan	Spray-drying	Desai and Park (2006)
Vitamin E	Starch	High-pressure homogenization	Chen and Wagner (2004)
Vitamin A acetate dissolved in coconut oil	hi-CAP 100 (starch octenylsuccinate, OSA- starch)	Effect of humidity	Xie *et al.* (2007)
Folic acid	Alginate-pectin	Coacervation	Madziva *et al.* (2006)
Aroma and Flavor			
Oregano, citronella, and marjoram flavors	Milk-protein–based matrices: WPC, skim milk powder	Spray-drying	Baranauskiene *et al.* (2006)
Limonene	Gum arabic–sucrose–gelatin	Freeze-drying	Kaushik and Roos (2007)
Cardamom oil	Mesquite gum	Spray-drying	Beristain *et al.* (2001)
Probiotics			
Bifidobacterium lactis	Hydrated gellan, xanthan gums	Extrusion	McMaster *et al.* (2005)
Bifidobacterium PL1	Starch	Spray-coating, spray-drying	O'Riordan *et al.* (2001)
Lactobacillus acidophilus Bifidobacterium lactis	Alginate/Hi-Maize starch	Emulsion	Kailasapathy (2006)

(Continued)

Table 12.2 (Continued)

Active Material	Material for Encapsulation	Technology	Reference
Lactobacillus acidophilus 547B, *Bifidum* ATCC 1994, *Lactobacillus casei* 01	Alginate/$CaCl_2$/chitosan		Krasaekoopt *et al.* (2006)
Lactobacillus spp.	GA, gellan gum, mesquite gum, and binary mixtures thereof	Interfacial polymerization	Yáñez-Fernández *et al.* (2008)
Others			
Isoflavone, β-galactosidase	Medium-chain triacylglycerol (MCT), polyglycerol monostearat (PGMS)		Kim *et al.* (2006)
Anthocyanin pigments of black carrot	Maltodextrins: DE 10, DE 20–23, DE 28–31	Spray-drying	Ersus and Yurdagel (2007)
Immunoglobulin Y	Whey protein concentrates (WPC-34, 50 and 80); whey protein isolate (WPI)	Emulsification, heat gelation	Lee *et al.* (2004)

GA, gum arabic; HPMC, hydroxypropyl methylcellulose; MC, methylcellulose; WPC, whey protein concentrate

Table 12.3 Recommendations for the selection of materials.

Material	Technological aspects	Application	Reference
Hybrid polymer coated with inorganic oxide layer (SiOx, AlOx)	Sol–gel technology	Barrier against oxygen, water vapor, flavor permeation	Amberg Schwab *et al.* (2006)
Starch–linear amylose	Complexation	Inclusion complexes with a wide variety of flavor compounds; controlled favor release	Heinemann *et al.* (2005)
Whey protein concentrate	Spray-drying	Soy oil	Hogan *et al.* (2001a)
Beeswax, carnauba wax	Emulsion, solid or liquid preparation	Water-soluble compounds	Mellema *et al.* (2006)

The carbohydrates that are considered bioactive components are mainly dietary fibers (Redgwell and Fischer, 2005). The fiber components that would benefit most from encapsulation are the soluble nondigestible polysaccharides. These fibers have been included for reduction of cholesterol and of glycemic fluctuations, for prevention of constipation, for their prebiotic effects, and for the prevention of cancer (McClements *et al.*, 2009a,b).

Lipids are a broad family of food components that are insoluble inorganic solvents. These are mainly fatty acids, phospholipids, carotenoids, and oil-soluble vitamins (McClements, *et al.*, 2009a). Bioactive proteins are the second family of bioactive molecules that might require encapsulation. Many food-derived peptides act as growth factors, antihypertensive agents, antioxidants, and immune regulatory factors (McClements *et al.*, 2009b).

Proteins are considered the most susceptible bioactive molecules for biodegradation in the GI tract. Most peptides even require hydrolysis in the stomach and small intestine in order to release specific bioactive peptides or amino acids. Thus, encapsulation for proteins depends on the type of protein, its envisioned health effect, and the product that serves as a vehicle for the bioactive protein.

12.7.2 Antioxidants

Ascorbic acid is often used as an antioxidant in foods. By putting it in a liposome together with vitamin E, with which ascorbic acid can have a synergistic antioxidant effect, it can be used for protection of emulsion-type foods (Reineccius, 1995). Vitamin E is incorporated into the liposome wall (Berrocal and Abeger, 1999), whereas the ascorbate is entrapped in the aqueous interior. This system is then used as an emulsifier in an emulsion, and it adsorbs at the water–oil interface. In this way, the antioxidants are targeted at the site where oxidative reactions generally occur (Pothakamury and Barbosa-Cánovas, 1995).

12.7.3 Minerals

12.7.3.1 Iron

From a nutritional point of view, iron is one of the most important elements, and its deficiency affects about one third of the world's population. The best way to prevent iron deficiency is through the iron fortification of food. However, the bioavailability of iron is negatively influenced by interactions with food ingredients such as tannins, phytates, and polyphenols. Moreover, iron catalyzes oxidative processes in fatty acids, vitamins, and amino acids, and consequently it alters sensory characteristics and decreases the nutritional value of the food.

Microencapsulation can be used to prevent these reactions, although bioavailability should be checked carefully. The bioavailability of readily water-soluble iron salts such as $FeSO_4$ or ferrous lactate is higher than that of poorly water soluble (e.g., ferrous fumarate) or water-insoluble iron (e.g., $FePO_4$). Suitable encapsulation techniques depend on the water solubility of the compound. Liposome technology is the method of choice for iron fortification of fluid food products. An iron bioavailability study on milk enriched with $FeSO_4$ encapsulated in a lecithin liposome has been conducted (Uicich *et al.*, 1999). Heat treatment and storage for 6 months did not result in decreased iron bioavailability of the iron-fortified milk. Bioavailability was similar to absorption of iron from high-bioavailable $FeSO_4$.

12.7.3.2 Calcium fortification

Soymilk contains much less calcium (12 mg/100 g soymilk) than does cow's milk (120 mg/100 g cow's milk), which is undesirable from a nutritional point of view. Attempts to fortify soy milk with calcium salts have been unsuccessful because this process causes the soybean proteins to coagulate and precipitate (Weingartner *et al.*, 1983). By encapsulating the calcium salt (calcium lactate) in a lecithin liposome, it was possible to fortify 100 g soy milk with up to 110 mg calcium, thereby reaching levels equivalent to those in normal cow's milk (Hirotsuka *et al.*, 1984). The soy milk remained stable at 4 °C for at least 1 week. It would be desirable to know how stable fortified long-shelf-life soy milk would be and how the calcium bioavailability of soy milk compares with that of cow's milk.

12.7.3.3 Vitamins

Both lipid-soluble (e.g., vitamin A, β-carotene, vitamins D, E, and K) and water-soluble (e.g., ascorbic acid) vitamins can be encapsulated using various technologies. The most common reason for encapsulating these ingredients is to extend the shelf life, either by protecting them against oxidation or by preventing reactions with components in the food system in which they are present.

A good example is ascorbic acid (vitamin C), which is added extensively to a variety of food products as either an antioxidant or a vitamin supplement (Kirby *et al.*, 1991). Its application as a vitamin supplement is impaired by its high reactivity and, hence, poor stability in solution. Oxidation of ascorbic acid is a free radical–mediated process, which results in a series of reactive intermediates. It is catalyzed by transition metal ions and is accelerated at neutral to alkaline pH. Furthermore, losses due to enzymic or anaerobic destruction of vitamin C can occur.

It is a true challenge to encapsulate water-soluble food ingredients to protect them against deterioration during the shelf-life of the food product in which they are used. The most obvious way to encapsulate these compounds is by spray-cooling and spray-chilling. Another technique that can be used to encapsulate water-soluble ingredients is fluidized-bed coating. Here, the dry water-soluble ingredient is suspended in an upward moving stream of air, which is temperature and humidity controlled. For vitamin C encapsulation, both spray-cooling or spray-chilling and fluidized-bed coating can be used when the vitamins are added to solid foods, such as cereal bars, biscuits, or bread. For application in liquid food systems, the best way to protect water-soluble ingredients is by encapsulation. Lipid-soluble vitamins such as vitamin A, β-carotene and vitamins D, E, or K are much easier to encapsulate than water-soluble ingredients.

12.7.3.4 Polyunsaturated fatty acids

n-3 polyunsaturated fatty acids (PUFAs) have been identified as essential to human. A high intake of PUFAs is associated with a low incidence of coronary heart disease and a reduced risk of cancers (Wallace *et al.*, 2000). Thus, enrichment of food with fish oil has been studied intensively as an acceptable and effective means of increasing the levels of *n*-3 PUFAs in the general population.

However, *n*-3 PUFAs are prone to oxidation because of the high number of unsaturated double bonds in the fatty acyl chains. Encapsulation by emulsion spray-drying has been used successfully to increase the shelf-life of this type of ingredient, and it allows PUFAs to be used in a large variety of foods such as infant formulas and bread mixes (Andersen, 1995).

It was demonstrated in two studies that consuming food enriched with microencapsulated fish oil obtained by emulsion spray-drying was as effective as the daily intake of fish oil gelatin capsules in increasing dietary levels of *n*-3 long-chain PUFAs (Wallace *et al.*, 2000). This finding indicates that the bioavailability of *n*-3 PUFAs added to the food matrix is maintained by microencapsulation. It was also found that the shelf life of the fatty acids could be increased to more than 2 years by microencapsulation.

12.7.4 Polyphenols and carotenoids

An important role for consumer health, disease prevention, and even treatment is being played by phytochemicals (Howells, *et al.*, 2007). Polyphenols and carotenoids as bioactive ingredients are readily available for a wide range of products. In determining a suitable encapsulation method for carotenoids, the specific food system determines the initial basis on which to decide. The specific food production process has to be taken into account, as well as the food characteristics, sensory aspects, production costs, and bioavailability of the carotenoids after storage and consumption.

Several encapsulation methods have demonstrated their suitability to encapsulate carotenoids (including β-carotene, lycopene, astaxanthin, zeaxanthin, and lutein, which are common ingredients used for food coloration and added nutritional value due to their antioxidant behavior). These methods include various emulsification processes, high-pressure homogenization, liposome entrapment, microbead production, spray-drying, and freeze-drying (Ribeiro *et al.*, 2010) (Table 12.4). Studies have shown that the encapsulation of polyphenols does protect their functionality and stability, and it can induce a health benefit by tailoring the encapsulation mechanism for increased bioavailability (de Vos *et al.*, 2010). For example, lycopene has been encapsulated using emulsion technology to enhance the solubility and bioavailability.

Most of encapsulation methods available have been adapted successfully to polyphenols (Fang and Bhandari, 2010). Polyphenols, carotenoids, and other food components with the potential to constitute further upcoming nutraceuticals in relation to the growing knowledge on their functional properties and health benefits will play an important role in the development of novel food products with several health benefits.

Table 12.4 Microencapsulated food ingredients and food applications.

Ingredient Category	Food Ingredient	Preferred Encapsulation Method	Food Applications and Benefits
Flavoring agents	Citrus oil, mint oils, onion oil, garlic oil	Extrusion, spray drying	To transfer liquid flavorings into easy-to-handle and stable free-flowing powders
Colorants	Annatto, β-carotene, turmeric	Extrusion, emulsion	Easier handling and improved solubility Protection from oxidation and improved application in dry mixing
Sweeteners	Sugars, artificial sweeteners (e.g., aspartame)	Co-crystallization, fluidized-bed coating	To reduce hygroscopicity, resulting in an improved flowability Prolonged sweetness perception
Acidulants	Lactic acid, glucono-δ-lactone, vitamin C, acetic acid, potassium sorbate, sorbic acid, calcium propionate, sodium chloride	Fluidized-bed coating, extrusion	Applied to assist in the development of color and flavor in meat emulsions, dry sausage products, uncooked processed meats, and other meat containing products Acids and baking soda is used in wet and dry mixes to control release of carbon dioxide during processing in the bakery industry
Enzymes and microorganisms	Lipase, invertase, *Brevibacterium linens, Penicillium roqueforti*	Coacervation, spray methods, liposomes	To improve stability and control time and point of release
Vitamins and minerals	Vitamins A, D, E, K (fat soluble) Vitamins C, B_1, B_2, B_6, B_{12}, niacin, folic acid (water soluble)	Coacervation, inclusion complexation, spray-drying, liposomes	Reduction of off-flavors To control release time To enhance stability To protect from interaction with other ingredients

Adapted from Desai and Park, 2005.

12.7.5 Living bioactive food components

Probiotic bacteria at present are playing a major role in designing functional foods, especially in dairy products, and maintaining their functional effects for supporting human health. The application of encapsulation approaches with living probiotics is very limited. The size of probiotic colonies (1–5 mm) excludes many of the nanotechnological approaches of encapsulation. The microencapsulation of many types of probiotics may be important steps for achieving the promised health benefits.

The survival of probiotics is influenced by many factors such as variations in pH, and oxygen toxicity during processing and packaging (Tripathi and Giri,

2014; Kailasapathy, 2002). An important critical issue that limits survival of probiotics in many dairy products is incompatibility with the bacteria involved in the starting culture and lack of a nitrogen source due to the absence of functional proteases in the product (Shah, 2000) and other issues that are associated with the processing that interfere with the survival rate. Several studies indicate low viability count of probiotics in products and less recovery of viable cells in products (Kailasapathy, 2002).

During recent years it has become clearer that probiotic effects are determined by the presence of specific bioactive molecules or effector molecules in the cell envelope of probiotic bacteria (Kleerebezem and Vaughan, 2009). These effector molecules are proteins and their functional effects can be preserved (Konstantinov *et al.*, 2008). The survival of these effector molecules in the product is more important than the survival of numbers of probiotics. Preserving and protecting these effector molecules is major challenge in probiotic development (Ledeboer *et al.*, 2006). Therefore, encapsulation promotes not only viability but also more functional properties of probiotics.

12.8 Spray-drying in microencapsulation of food ingredients

Although many techniques have been developed to microencapsulate food ingredients, spray-drying is the most common technology used in the food industry due to low cost and available equipment. Microencapsulation by spray-drying has been successfully used in the food industry (Gouin, 2004), and this process has been used since the 1930s to prepare the first encapsulated flavors using gum acacia as wall material.

The spray-drying process involves three basic steps in microencapsulation: preparation of the dispersion or emulsion to be processed, homogenization of the dispersion, and atomization of the mass into the drying chamber.

The first stage is the formation of a fine and stable emulsion of the core material in the wall solution. The mixture to be atomized is prepared by dispersing the core material, which is usually hydrophobic, into a solution of the coating agent with which it is immiscible. In the spray-drying process, the initial emulsion droplets are on the order of diameter 1 to 100 μm. Before the spray-drying step, the formed emulsion must be stable over a certain period of time, oil droplets should be rather small, and viscosity should be low enough to prevent air inclusion in the particle (Drusch, 2006).

Emulsion viscosity and particle size distribution have significant effects on microencapsulation by spray-drying. High viscosities interfere with the atomization process and lead to the formation of elongated and large droplets that adversely affect the drying rate. The core material retention during microencapsulation by spray-drying is affected by the composition and the properties of the emulsion and by the drying conditions. As the sprayed particles fall through the gaseous medium, they assume a spherical shape with the oil encased in the aqueous phase (Dziezak, 1988). The short time exposure and the rapid evaporation of water keep the core temperature below 40 °C, in spite of the high temperatures generally used in the process. The main factors in spray-drying that must be optimized are feed temperature, air inlet temperature, and air outlet temperature (Liu *et al.*, 2004).

When the feed temperature is increased, viscosity of feed materials is decreased. High temperatures can cause volatilization or degradation of some heat-sensitive ingredients. The rate of feed delivered to the atomizer is adjusted to ensure that each sprayed droplet reaches the desired drying level before it comes in contact with the surface of the drying chamber. Air inlet temperature is directly proportional to the microcapsule drying rate and the final water content. When the air inlet temperature is low, the low evaporation rate causes the formation of microcapsules with high-density membranes, high water content, poor fluidity, and easiness of agglomeration. Table 12.5 summarizes the optimized conditions for the encapsulation of different food ingredients by spray-drying.

12.8.1 Food ingredients microencapsulated by spray-drying

12.8.1.1 Lipids and oleoresins

In general, lipids are difficult to disperse in food products, in addition and especially polyunsaturated fatty acids are susceptible to auto-oxidation, which results in off-flavors and toxic compounds. Lipids can be used as solvents in which one can solubilize hydrophobic substances such as volatile aromatic compounds. There are several advantages of lipid encapsulation: retarding auto-oxidation, enhancing stability, controlling lipid-soluble flavor release, masking the bitter taste of lipid-soluble substances, and protecting dissolved substances against enzyme hydrolysis.

Spray-drying is quite suitable for encapsulating oils and oleoresins. Stability of black pepper oleoresin encapsulated in gum arabic and emulsifying modified starches by spray-drying has been reported (Shaikh *et al.*, 2006). Sodium caseinate–carbohydrate blends were used to encapsulate soy oil by spray-drying, and the obtained results showed that microencapsulation efficiency can be improved by increasing the dextrose equivalence of the carbohydrates (Hogan *et al.*, 2001b). Study of spray-dried powders with 50% butter oil encapsulated in sucrose and double encapsulated in a matrix of vegetable waxes shows that the double encapsulation method could improve capsule resistance to moisture sorption, but it also decreases powder flow properties (Onwulata *et al.*, 1998). The oxidative and thermal stabilities of crude squid oil have been effectively enhanced by spray-drying microencapsulation (Lin *et al.*, 1995). Fat properties, such as crystal forms and habit in spray-dried microcapsules, were also investigated as a function of storage time.

Table 12.5 Experimental conditions for encapsulating different food ingredients by spray-drying.

Encapsulated Ingredient	Wall Material	Feed Temperature (°C)	Air Inlet Temperature (°C)	Air Outlet Temperature (°C)	References
Ethyl butyrate Ethyl caprylate	Whey proteins, lactose	5	160	80	Rosenberg and Sheu (1996)
Anhydrous milk fat	Whey proteins, lactose	50	160	80	Young *et al.* (1993)
Soy oil	Sodium caseinate, carbohydrates	NR	180	95	Hogan *et al.*, 2001b Hogan *et al.*, 2001c
Calcium citrate Calcium lactate	Cellulose derivatives, polymethacrylic acid	NR	120–170	91–95	Oneda and Ré (2003)
Lycopene	Gelatine, sucrose	55	190	52	Shu *et al.* (2006)
Cardamom essential oil	Mesquite gum	Room temperature	195–205	105–115	Beristain *et al.* (2001)
Fish oil	Starch derivatives, glucose syrup	NR	170	70	Drusch *et al.* (2006)
Arachidonyl L-ascorbate	Maltodextrin, gum arabic, soybean polysaccharides	NR	200	100–110	Watanabe *et al.* (2004)
D-Limonene	Gum arabic, maltodextrin, modified starch	NR	200	100–120	Soottitantawat *et al.* (2005a)
L-Menthol	Gum arabic, modified starch	NR	180	95–105	Soottitantawat *et al.* (2005b)
Black pepper oleoresin	Gum arabic, modified starch	NR	176–180	105–115	Shaikh *et al.* (2006)
Short-chain fatty acid	Maltodextrin, gum arabic	NR	180	90	Teixeira *et al.* (2004)
Cumin oleoresin	Gum arabic, maltodextrin, modified starch	NR	158–162	115–125	Kanakdande *et al.* (2007)
Fish oil	Sugar beet pectin, glucose syrup	NR	170	70	Drusch (2006)

NR, not relevant

12.8.1.2 Flavoring compounds

Most of the flavoring compounds are highly volatile with respect to water. Several methods have been reported for microencapsulation of flavors, but the most common technique employed is spray-drying. Spray-drying is generally used to for production of flavor powders in a short time. Many studies have been carried out on the influence of wall material compositions and the operating conditions on the retention and controlled release of encapsulated flavors (Madene *et al.*, 2006). Flavors of oregano, citronella, and marjoram were successfully encapsulated by spray-drying in wall systems of skim milk powder and whey protein concentrate (Baranauskiene *et al.*, 2006). Sumac flavor has been successfully encapsulated by spray-drying in sodium chloride as wall material (Bayram *et al.*, 2005), but the salty property of this carrier and the acidic property of sumac limit the applications of the obtained particles to salted cookies, salads, and crackers.

12.8.1.3 Other food ingredients

Lycopene was successfully microencapsulated by spray-drying using a wall system consisting of gelatin and sucrose. Spray-drying is also considered the most effective technique for encapsulating iodine, and the best results were obtained with dextrin as an encapsulating agent (Diosady, 2002). Light stability of spray-dried bixin encapsulated with gum arabic and maltodextrin was studied, and results prove that bixin microencapsulated in gum arabic was more stable to photo-degradation than that in maltodextrin with polysorbate-80 (Tween 80) (Barbosa *et al.*, 2005). Spray-drying has been considered an excellent means of preserving nutritive value of vitamins, and this technique has been found to be suitable to encapsulate most vitamins (Hartman, 1967).

12.9 Nanoencapsulation of food ingredients using lipid-based delivery systems

A delivery system is defined as one in which a bioactive material is entrapped in a carrier to control the rate of bioactive release. Nanocarriers can protect a bioactive component from unfavorable environmental conditions such as oxidation and pH and enzyme degradation (Ghosh *et al.*, 2009). Nanocarriers provide more surface area and have the potential to enhance solubility and to improve bioavailability and controlled release and targeting of the encapsulated food ingredients. Typically, food-applicable nanocarrier systems can be carbohydrate, protein, or lipid based. Despite different advantages of carbohydrate- and protein-based nanocapsules, they do not have the potential to fully scale up due to the requirement of applying different complicated chemical or heat treatments that cannot be completely controlled. Lipid-based nanocarriers could be used in industrial production and have the advantage of more encapsulation efficiency and low toxicity.

12.9.1 Nanoemulsions

Nanoemulsions are nano-scale droplets of multiphase colloidal dispersions formed by dispersing one liquid in another immiscible liquid by physical share-induced rupturing (Mason *et al.*, 2006). Nanoemulsions have some interesting physical properties that can be applied to distinguish them from microemulsions. For instance, microemulsions typically show multiple scattering of visible light, and therefore have a white opaque appearance. The droplet sizes in nanoemulsions are much smaller than visible wavelengths; hence, most nanoemulsions are optically transparent. Nanoemulsions are good candidates for delivery of poorly water-soluble food ingredients, such as fish oil and lipophilic vitamins, because of their ability to improve bioactive solubilization and potential for enhancing absorption in the GI tract caused by surfactant-induced permeability changes. Soybean oil–based nanoemulsion has been shown to have bactericidal properties against gram-positive bacteria (Hamouda and Baker, 2000). The location of a drug or any other bioactive compound within the capsule or carrier influences the stability, release, and thus the bioavailability of the nanocarrier formulation.

12.9.2 Liposomes

The liposome method has many benefits, such as the possibility of large-scale production using natural ingredients and entrapment and release of water-soluble, lipid-soluble, and amphiphilic materials (Huwiler *et al.*, 2000). The mechanism of liposome formation is based on the interactions between amphiphilic compounds (mainly phospholipids) and water molecules, where the polar head groups of phospholipids are subjected to the aqueous phases of the inner and outer media, and the hydrophobic hydrocarbon tails are associated into the bilayer (Goyal *et al.*, 2005).

Liposomes are classified based on their number of bilayers and size. According to their bilayer structure, vesicles can be classified as unilamellar vesicles (ULV) or as multilamellar vesicles (MLV) that consist of one or more concentric lipid bilayer(s) (Nagle *et al.*, 2000). Liposomes can generally provide greater chemical stability compared to other encapsulation technologies and protection to sensitive bioactives such as ascorbic acid and glutathione at high water-activity conditions (Kirby 1993). Liposome-based delivery has significant potential in the food industry, for example for the release of antimicrobials upon pH changes as a result of increased microbial activity. Many methods for the stabilization of liposomes have been investigated: lyophilization, freezing, spray-drying, and supercritical fluid technology (Mishima, 2008).

12.9.3 Solid lipid nanoparticles

Solid lipid nanoparticles have some distinct advantages, which include having high encapsulation efficiency, avoiding use of organic solvents in their preparation, the possibility of large-scale production and sterilization, providing high flexibility in controlling the release profile due to solid matrix. The slower degradation rate allows bioactive release for prolonged times, and the solid matrix can protect the incorporated bioactive ingredients against chemical degradation (Saupe and Rades, 2006).

Several methods have been reported for solid lipid nanoparticle production in pharmaceuticals, but only two basic production techniques are likely to be used for large-scale production of solid lipid nanoparticles in food processing: hot homogenization and cold homogenization (Muller *et al.*, 1993). There are mainly three models for incorporating bioactive components into solid lipid nanoparticles: the homogeneous matrix model, the bioactive enriched shell model, and the bioactive enriched core model.

12.9.4 Nanostructure lipid carrier

The nanostructure lipid carrier, a novel lipid carrier for overcoming the limitations of solid lipid nanoparticles, was developed by Radtke and Muller (2001). A pharmaceutical study for the investigation of chemical stability enhancement of ascorbyl palmitate after incorporation into nanostructure lipid carriers showed that addition of antioxidants as well as selection of suitable surfactants and solid lipids improved the chemical stability of ascorbyl palmitate.

12.10 New techniques and ingredients that improve effectiveness of encapsulation

Dry packaged foods are often formulated with added flavors to enhance their quality. However, many flavor components are volatile liquids that are lost by evaporation, oxidation, or ingredient interactions. The extent of these effects can be sufficient to dramatically alter the quality of a food product, especially when packages are repeatedly opened over an extended period of time. As a result, it is beneficial to encapsulate volatile flavors prior to use in foods. Encapsulation can be defined as any method employed to entrap flavors in a carrier to convert it to a more useful form or to impart some degree of protection against evaporation, reaction, or migration in a food.

The ability of carbohydrates to bind flavors is complemented by their diversity, low cost, and widespread use in foods. Sugars, maltodextrins, modified starches, and gums are all used as encapsulation substrates (Godshall, 1988). Although a variety of methods are used to manufacture encapsulated flavors, spray-drying and extrusion are the most common techniques (Reineccius, 1991). The goal in spray-drying is to trap flavors within the solid walls of hollow spheres, and the goal in extrusion is to trap flavors in an impermeable glass.

Many factors are responsible for the efficiency of these encapsulation techniques. During spray-drying, highly volatile flavor components are less effectively encapsulated and more quickly lost than less-volatile ones (King, 1990).

Table 12.6 Different encapsulation methods and carriers.

Method	Carbohydrate Substrate
Spray-drying	Wall of hollow sphere
Extrusion	Solid glassy melt
Co-crystallization	Crystal agglomerate
Absorption	Macroporous carrier
Adsorption	Microporous carrier
Molecular inclusion	Cyclodextrin

Diffusion of flavors out of extruded carbohydrates is enhanced by structural defects such as cracks, thin walls, or pores formed during or after processing (Wampler, 1992). Structural imperfections in both spray-dried and extruded substrates limit shelf life due to slow diffusion and oxidation of encapsulated flavors. Improvements in formulation of substrates continue to be made to reduce defects, increase encapsulation capacity, and lengthen shelf life (Inglett *et al.*,1988).

Crystalline sucrose is a poor flavor carrier, but co-crystallization with flavors forms aggregates of very small crystals that incorporate the flavors either by inclusion within the crystals or, more commonly, by entrapment between the crystals; entrapment still serves to enhance flavor stability (Chen *et al.*, 1988). Crystals of lactose and glucose have been moistened and heated to form porous crystalline granules that can later be used to absorb liquid flavors. Low-density spherical granules of sucrose, corn sugars, and maltitol having a highly porous crystalline structure and reportedly large surface area for absorbing liquid flavors have been prepared using specialized melt-solidification or spray-drying techniques (Kawashima *et al.*, 1994). An emerging encapsulation technique to reduce oxidation and volatility involves the inclusion of flavors as guest molecules in the interior cavity of cyclodextrins (Szejtli, J. 1984). A simplified overview of these encapsulation techniques is provided in Table 12.6.

Perhaps the least-developed encapsulation method involves the physical adsorption of flavors onto the surfaces of high-surface-area substrates. Physical adsorption can be defined as the reversible condensation of a gas onto the surface of a solid due to weak attractive forces and accompanied by release of heat. Only highly microporous substrates, also known as molecular sieves, possess sufficient surface area to efficiently adsorb volatile flavors. The effectiveness of these materials is demonstrated by the extensive reduction of equilibrium vapor pressure that accompanies physical adsorption of volatile flavors. This technique is rarely a viable encapsulation option because the use of conventional microporous substrates such as activated carbon and silica is severely regulated in foods. Desorption of adsorbed flavors can maintain a nearly constant level of package aroma throughout product use by replenishing the equilibrium vapor levels in the headspace after the package is opened and resealed.

References

Amberg-Schwab S., Weber U., Burger A., Nique S., and Xalter R. (2006). Development of passive and active barrier coatings on the basis of inorganic–organic polymers. *Monatshefte für Chemie* 137: 657–666.

Anonymous. (1984). Flavors and Oils Carried on Maltodextrin Buds. *Food Engineering* 56: 78.

Argillier, J. F., Soto-Portas, M. L., Zydowicz, N., Mechin, F., and Chomard A; Institut Francais du Petrole. (2004). Process for manufacturing microcapsules by interfacial polycondensation with polyoxyalkyleneamine and acid chlorides. U.S. Patent 6,706,397. 16 March 2004. 6 pp.

Arneado, C. J. F. (1996). Microencapsulation by complex coacervation at ambient temperature. Patent no. FR 2732240 A1; 1996.

Augustin M. A., and Sanguansri L. (2003). Polyunsaturated fatty acids: Delivery, innovation and incorporation in foods. *Food Australia* 55: 294–296.

Augustin M. A., Sanguansri L., Margetts C., and Young B. (2001). Microencapsulation of food ingredients. *Food Australia* 53: 220–223.

Augustin, M. A., and Hemar, Y. (2009). Nano- and micro-structured assemblies for encapsulation of food ingredients. *Chemical Society Reviews* 38: 902–912.

Baranauskiené, R., Venskutonis, P. R., Dewettinck, K., and Verhé, R. (2006). Properties of oregano (*Origanum vulgare* L.), citronella (*Cymbopogon nardus* G.) and marjoram (*Majorana hortensis* L.) flavors encapsulated into milk protein–based matrices. *Food Research International* 39: 413–425.

Barbosa, M. I. M. J., Borsarelli, C. D., and Mercadante, A. Z. (2005). Light stability of spray-dried bixin encapsulated with different edible polysaccharide preparations. *Food Research International* 38: 989–994.

Bayram, O. A., Bayram, M., and Tekin, A. R. (2005). Spray drying of sumac flavour using sodium chloride, sucrose, glucose and starch as carriers. *Journal of Food Engineering* 69: 253–269.

Beristain C. I., Garcia H. S., and Vernon-Carter E. J. (2001). Spray dried encapsulation of cardamom (*Elettaria cardamomum*) essential oil with mesquite (*Prosopis juliflora*) gum. *Food Science Technology* 34: 398–401.

Beristain, C. I., García, H. S., and Vernon-Carter, E. J. (2001). Spray-dried encapsulation of cardamom (*Elettaria cardamomum*) essential oil with mesquite (*Prosopis juliflora*) gum. *Lebensmittel-Wissenschaft und- Technologie* 34: 398–401.

Bodmerier, R., and Mcginity, J. W. (1987). Polylactic acid microspheres containing quinidine base and quinidine sulphate prepared by the solvent evaporation techniques. *Journal of Microencapsulation* 4: 279–286.

Burey, P., Bhandari, B. R., Howes, T., and Gidley, M. J. (2008). Hydrocolloid gel particles: Formation, characterization, and application. *Critical Reviews in Food Science and Nutrition* 48: 361–377.

Champagne C. P., Roy D., and Gardner N. (2005). Challenges in the addition of probiotic cultures to foods. *Critical Review of Food Science and Nutrition* 45: 61–84.

Champagne, C. P., and Fustier, P. (2007). Microencapsulation for the improved delivery of bioactive compounds into foods. *Current Opinion in Biotechnology* 18: 184–190.

Champagne, C. P., and Fustier, P. (2007). Microencapsulation for the improved delivery of bioactive compounds into foods. *Current Opinion in Biotechnology* 18: 184–190.

Chandramouli V., Kailasapathy K., Peiris P., and Jones M. (2004). An improved method of microencapsulation and its evaluation to protect *Lactobacillus* sp. in simulated gastric environments. *Journal of Microbiological Methods* 56: 27–35.

Chao, D. Y. (1993). The role of surfactants in synthesizing polyurea microcapsules. *Journal of Applied Polymer Science* 47: 645–651.

Chen C. C., and Wagner G. (2004) Vitamine E nanoparticles for beverage applications. *Chemical Engineering Research and Design* 82: 1432–1437.

Chen, A. C., Veigra, M. F., and Anthony, B. R. (1988) Cocrystallization: An encapsulation process. *Food Technology* 42: 87–90.

Damge, C., Vranckx, H., Balschmidt, P., and Couvreur, P. (1997). Poly(alkylcyanoacrylate) nanospheres for oral administration of insulin. *Journal of Pharmaceutical Sciences* 86(12): 1403–1409.

de Vos, P., Faas, M. M., Spasojevic, M., and Sikkema, J. (2010). Encapsulation for preservation of functionality and targeted delivery of bioactive food components. *International Dairy Journal* 20: 292–302.

Desai K. G. H., and Park H. J. (2006). Effect of manufacturing parameters on the characteristics of vitamin C encapsulated tripolyphosphate–chitosan microspheres prepared by spray-drying. *Journal of Microencapsulation* 23(1): 91–103.

Desai, K. G. H., and Park, H. J. (2005). Recent developments in microencapsulation of food ingredients. *Drying Technology* 23: 1361–1394.

Desobry, S. A., Netto, F. M., and Labuza, T. B. (1997). Comparison of spray-drying, drum drying and freeze-drying for (1–3,1–4)-β-carotene encapsulation and preservation. *Journal of Food Science* 62: 1158–1162.

Dewettinck K., and Huyghebaert A. (1999). Fluidized bed coating in food technology. *Trends in Food Science Technology* 10: 163–168.

Diosady, L. L., Alberti, J. O., and Venkatesh Mannar, M. G. (2002).Microencapsulation for iodine stability in salt fortified with ferrous fumarate and potassium iodide. *Food Research International* 35: 635–642.

Doleyres Y., and Lacroix C. (2005). Technologies with free and immobilised cells for probiotic bifidobacteria production and protection. *International Dairy Journal* 15:973–988.

Drusch, S. (2006a). Sugar beet pectin: A novel emulsifying wall component for microencapsulation of lipophilic food ingredients by spray-drying. *Food Hydrocolloids* doi:10.1016/j. foodhyd.2006.08.007.

Drusch, S. (2006b). Sugar beet pectin: A novel emulsifying wall component for microencapsulation of lipophilic food ingredients by spray-drying. *Food Hydrocolloids* doi:10.1016/j. foodhyd.2006.08.007.

Drusch, S., Serfert, Y., Van Den Heuvel, A., and Schwarz, K. (2006). Physicochemical characterization and oxidative stability of fish oil encapsulated in an amorphous matrix containing trehalose. *Food Research International* 39: 807–815.

Dziezak, J. D. (1988). Microencapsulation and encapsulated ingredients. *Food Technology* 42(4): 136–151.

Ersus S., and Yurdagel U. (2007) Microencapsulation of anthocyanin pigments of black carrot (*Daucuscarota* L.) by spray drier. *Journal of Food Engineering* 80(3): 805–812.

Fang X., Shima M., Adachi S. (2005). Effects of drying conditions on the oxidation of linoleic acid encapsulated with gum arabic by spray-drying. *Food Science and Technology Research* 11(4): 380–384.

Fang, Z., and Bhandari, B. (2010). Encapsulation of polyphenols: a review. *Trends in Food Science and Technology* 21(10): 510–523.

Fuchs M., Turchiuli C., Bohin M., Cuvelier M. E., Ordonnaud C., *et al.* (2006) Encapsulation of oil in powder using spray drying and fluidised bed agglomeration. *Journal of Food Engineering* 75(1): 27–35.

Garti N., Spernath A., Aserin A., and Lutz R. (2004). Nano-sized self assemblies of non-ionic surfactants as solubilization reservoirs and microreactors for food systems. *Soft Matter* 1: 206–218.

Ghosh, A., Mandal, A. K., Sarkar, S., Panda, S., and Das, N. (2009). Nanoencapsulation of quercetin enhances its dietary efficacy in combating arsenic-induced oxidative damage in liver and brain of rats. *Life Sciences* 84: 75–80.

Gibbs B. F., Kermasha S., Alli I., and Mulligan C. N. (1999a). Encapsulation in the food industry: A review. *International Journal of Food Science and Nutrition* 50: 213–224.

Gibbs B. F., Kermasha S., Alli, I., and Mulligan, C. N. (1999b). Encapsulation in the food industry: A review. *International Journal of Food Science and Nutrition* 50: 213–224.

Godshall, M. A. (1988). The role of carbohydrates in flavor development. *Food Technology* 42: 71–78.

Gouin S. (2004). Microencapulation: Industrial appraisal of existing technologies and trends. *Trends in Food Science and Technology* 15: 330–347.

Goyal, P., Goyal, K., Kumar, S. G. Y., Singh, A., Ktare, O. P., and Mishra, D. N. (2005). Liposomal drug delivery systems – clinical applications. *Acta Pharmaceutica* 55: 1–25.

Gursel, I., and Hasirci, V. (1995). Properties and drug release behavior of poly(3-hydroxybutyric acid) and various poly(3-hydroxybutyrate-hydroxyvalerate) copolymer microcapsules. *Journal of Microencapsulation* 12: 185–193.

Hamouda, T., and Baker J. R. Jr. (2000). Antimicrobial mechanism of action of surfactant lipid preparations in enteric gram-negative bacilli. *Journal of Applied Microbiology* 89: 397–403.

Hartman, G. H., Akeson, J. W. R., and Stahmann, M. A. (1967). Leaf protein concentrate prepared by spray-drying. *Journal of Agricultural and Food Chemistry* 15: 74–79.

Hayes M., Coakley M., O'Sullivan L., Stanton C., Hill C., *et al.* (2006). Cheese as a delivery vehicle for probiotics and biogenic substances. *Australia Journal of Dairy Technology* 61: 132–141.

Heinemann C., Zinsli M., Renggli A., Escher F., and Conde-Petit W. (2005). Influence of amylose-flavor complexation on build-up and breakdown of starch structures in aqueous food model systems. *Food Science Technology* 38: 885–894.

Hirotsuka M., Taniguchi H., Narita H., and Kito M. (1984). Calcium fortification of soy milk with calcium–lecithin liposome system. *Journal of Food Science* 49: 1111–1112, 1127.

Hogan S. A., McNamee B. F., O'Riordan E. D., O'Sullivan M. (2001a) Microencapsulating properties of whey protein concentrate 75. *Journal of Food Science* 66: 675–680.

Hogan, S. A., McNamee, N. F., O'Riordan, E. D., and O'Sullivan, M. (2001b). Emulsification and microencapsulation properties of sodium caseinate/carbohydrate blends. *International Dairy Journal* 11, 137–144.

Hogan, S. A., McNamee, B. F., O'Riordan, E. D., and O'Sullivan, M. (2001c). Microencapsulation properties of sodium caseinate. *Journal of Agricultural and Food Chemistry* 49: 1934–1938.

Howells, L. M., Moiseeva, E. P., Neal, C. P., Foreman, B. E., Andreadi, C. K., *et al.* (2007). Predicting the physiological relevance of *in vitro* cancer preventive activities of phytochemicals. *Acta Pharmacologica Sinica* 28(9): 1274–1304.

Huwiler, A., Kolter, T., Pfeilschifter, J., and Sandhoff, K. (2000). Physiology and pathophysiology of sphingolipid metabolism and signaling. *Biochimica et Biophysica Acta* 1485: 63–99.

Inglett, G. E., Gelbman, P., and Reineccius, G. A. (1988) Encapsulation of orange oil. In *Flavor Encapsulation*, pp. 29–36. S. J. Risch and G. A. Reineccius, eds. Washington, D.C.: American Chemical Society.

Iyer C., Kailasapathy K., Peiris P. (2004). Evaluation of survival and release of encapsulated bacteria in *ex vivo* porcine gastrointestinal contents using a green fluorescent protein gene–labelled *E. coli*. *Lebensmittel Wissensschaft & Technologie* 37: 639–642.

Janssen, J. M., and Nijenhuis, K. (1992). Encapsulation by interfacial polycondensation II. The membrane wall structure and the rate of the wall growth. *Journal of Membrane Science* 65: 69–75.

Jimenez M., Garcia H. S., Beristain C. I. (2006). Spray-dried encapsulation of conjugated linoleic acid (CLA) with polymeric matrices. *Journal of the Science of Food and Agriculture* 86: 2431–2437.

Kailasapathy K. (2006). Survival of free and encapsulated probiotic bacteria and their effect on the sensory properties of yoghurt. *LWT – Food Science and Technology* 39: 1221–1227.

Kailasapathy, K. (2002a). Microencapsulation of probiotic bacteria: Technology and potential applications. *Current Issues in Intestinal Microbiology* 3: 39–48.

Kailasapathy, K. (2002b). Microencapsulation of probiotic bacteria: Technology and potential applications. *Current Issues in Intestinal Microbiology* 3: 39–48.

Kanakdande, D., Bhosale, R., and Singhal, R. S. (2007). Stability of cumin oleoresin microencapsulated in different combination of gum arabic, maltodextrin and modified starch. *Carbohydrate Polymers* 67: 536–541.

Kapusniak J., Tomasik P. (2006). Lipid microencapsulation in starch. *Journal of Microencapsulation* 23: 341–348.

Katti, D., and Krishnamurti, N. (1999). Preparation of albumin microspheres by an improved process. *Journal of Microencapsulation* 16(2): 231–242.

Kawashima, S., Magara, M., Ishii, Y., and Kato, S. (1994). Crystalline Mixture Solid Containing Maltitol and a Process for Preparing It. U. S. patent 5,354,856.

Kim N. C., Jeon B. J., Ahn J., Kwak H. S. (2006). *In vitro* study of microencapsulated isoflavone and beta-galactosidase. *Journal of Agricultural and Food Chemistry* 54(7): 2582–2586.

King, C. J. (1990). Spray drying food liquids and the retention of volatiles. *Chemical Engineering Progress* 86: 33–39.

Kirby, C. J. (1993). Controlled delivery of functional food ingredients: Opportunities for liposomes in the food industry. In: *Liposome Technology*. G. Gregoriadis, ed. London: CRC Press.

Kleerebezem, M., and Vaughan, E. E. (2009). Probiotic and gut lactobacilli and bifidobacteria: molecular approaches to study diversity and activity. *Annual Reviews of Microbiology* 63: 269–290.

Kolanowski W., Jaworska D., Weissbrodt J., Kunz B. (2007). Sensory assessment of microencapsulated fish oil powder. *Journal of the Americal Oil Chemists' Society* 84(1): 37–45.

Kolanowski W., Laufenberg G., Kunz B. (2004). Fish oil stabilisation by microencapsulation with modified cellulose. *International Journal of Food Science and Nutrition* 55(4): 333–343.

Konstantinov, S. R., Smidt, H., de Vos, W. M., Bruijns, S. C., Singh, S. K., *et al.* (2008). S layer protein A of *Lactobacillus acidophilus* NCFM regulates immature dendritic cell and T cell functions. *Proceedings of the National Academy of Sciences of the United States of America* 105: 19474–19479.

Krasaekoopt W., Bhandari B., Deeth H. C. (2006). Survival of probiotics encapsulated in chitosancoated alginate beads in yoghurt from UHT- and conventionally treated milk during storage. *LWT – Food Science and Technology* 39(2): 177–183.

Ledeboer, A. M., Nauta, A., Sikkema, J., Laulund, E., Niederberger, P., and Sijbesma, W. (2006). Survival of probiotics. *European Dairy Magazine* 31–32

Lee J. J., Park I. B., Cho Y. H., Huh C. S., Baek Y. J., Park J. (2004). Whey protein–based IgY microcapsules prepared by multiple emulsification and heat gelation. *Food Science and Biotechnology* 13(4): 494–497.

Lin, C. C., Lin, S. Y., and Hwang, L. S. (1995). Microencapsulation of squid oil with hydrophilic macromolecules for oxidative and thermal stabilization. *Journal of Food Science* 60: 36–39.

Liu, Z., Zhou, J., Zeng, Y., and Ouyang, X. (2004). The enhancement and encapsulation of *Agaricus bisporus* flavor. *Journal of Food Engineering* 65: 391–396.

Madene, A., Jacquot, M., Scher, J., and Desobry, S. (2006). Flavour encapsulation and controlled release – A review. *International Journal of Food Science and Technology* 41: 1–21.

Madziva H., Kailasapathy K., Phillips M. (2006). Evaluation of alginate–pectin capsules in Cheddar cheese as a food carrier for the delivery of folic acid. *LWT – Food Science and Technology* 39: 146–151.

Mason, T. G., Wilking, J. N., Meleson, K., Chang, C. B., and Graves, S. M. (2006). Nanoemulsions: Formation, structure, and physical properties. *Journal of Physics: Condensed Matter* 18: R635–R666.

Masters, K. (1968). Spray drying: The unit operation today. *Industry Engineering and Engineering Chemistry* 60: 53–63.
McClements, D. J., Decker, E. A., and Park, Y. (2009a). Controlling lipid bioavailability through physicochemical and structural approaches. *Critical Reviews in Food Science and Nutrition* 49: 48–67.
McClements, D. J., Decker, E. A., Park, Y., and Weiss, J. (2009b). Structural design principles for delivery of bioactive components in nutraceuticals and functional foods. *Critical Reviews in Food Science and Nutrition* 49: 577–606.
McMaster L. D., Kokott S. A., Slatter P. (2005). Micro-encapsulation of *Bifidobacterium lactis* for incorporation into soft foods. *World Journal of Microbiology and Biotechnology* 21: 723–728.
Mellema M., Van Benthum W. A. J., Boer B., Von Harras J., Visser A. (2006). Wax encapsulation of water-soluble compounds in food. *Journal of Microencapsulation* 23: 729–740.
Mishima, K. (2008). Biodegradable particle formation for drug and gene delivery using supercritical fluid and dense gas. *Advances in Drug Delivery Reviews* 60: 411–432.
Morris, C. E. (1981) New form of maltodextrin has unique properties. *Food Engineering* 53: 94–95.
Mullers, R. H., Schwarz, C., Mehnert, W., and Lucks, J. S. (1993). Production of solid lipid nanoparticles (SLN) for controlled drug delivery. *Proceedings of International Symposium on Controlled Release Bioactive Materials* 20: 480–481.
Nagle, J. F., and Tristram-Nagle, S. (2000). Structure of lipid bilayers. *Biochimica et Biophysica Acta (BBA) - Reviews on Biomembranes* 1469: 159–195.
Nimmannit, U., and Suwanpatra, N. (1996). Microencapsulation of drugs by the coacervation technique using ethyl cellulose and acrylate methacrylate copolymer as wall materials. *Journal of Microencapsulation* 13(6): 643–649.
O'Riordan K., Andrews D., Buckle K., Conway P. (2001). Evaluation of microencapsulation of a *Bifidobacterium* strain with starch as an approach to prolonging viability during storage. *Journal of Applied Microbiology* 91: 1059–1066.
Oneda, F., and Ré, M. I. (2003). The effect of formulation variables on the dissolution and physical properties of spray-dried microspheres containing organic salts. *Powder Technology* 130: 377–384.
Onwulata, C. I., Konstance, R. P., and Holsinger, V. H. (1998). Properties of single- and double-encapsulated butteroil powders. *Journal of Food Science* 63: 100–103.
Persico, P., Carfagna, C., Danicher, L., and Frere, Y. (2005). Polyamide microcapsules containing jojoba oil prepared by interfacial polymerization. *Journal of Microencapsulation* 22(5): 471–486.
Porzio M. A. (2007). Flavor delivery and product development. *Food Technology* 61(1): 22–29.
Radtke, M., and Müller, R. H. (2001). NLSTM nanostructured lipid carriers: The new generation of lipid drug carriers. *New Drugs* 2: 48–52
Ramanathan, L. S., Shukla, P. G., and Sivaram, S. (1998). Synthesis and characterization of polyurethane microspheres. *Pure and Applied Chemistry* 70(6): 1295–1299.
Redgwell, R. J., and Fischer, M. (2005). Dietary fiber as a versatile food component: An industrial perspective. *Molecular Nutrition and Food Research* 49: 521–535.
Reid A. A., Champagne C. P., Gardner N., Fustier P., Vuillemard J. C. (2007). Survival in food systems of *Lactobacillus rhamnosus* R011 microentrapped in whey protein gel particles. *Journal of Food Science* 72: M31–M37.
Reineccius, G. A. (1991). Carbohydrates for flavor encapsulation. *Food Technology* 45: 144.
Ribeiro, H. S., Schuchmann, H. P., Engel, R., Walz, E., and Briviba, K. (2010). Encapsulation of Carotenoids. In: *Encapsulation Technologies for Active Food Ingredients and Food Processing*, pp. 211-252. N. J. Zuidam and V. A. Nedović, eds. New York: Springer Science Business Media.
Righetto A. M., Netto F. M. (2005). Effect of encapsulating materials on water sorption, glass transition and stability of juice from immature acerola. *International Journal of Food Properties* 8(2): 337–346.

Righetto A. M., Netto F. M. (2006). Vitamin C stability in encapsulated green West Indian cherry juice and in encapsulated synthetic ascorbic acid. *Journal of the Science of Food and Agriculture* 86: 1202–1208.

Rosenberg, M., and Sheu, T-Y. (1996). Microencapsulation of volatiles by spray-drying in whey protein–based wall systems. *International Dairy Journal* 6: 273–284.

Saltmarsh M. (ed). (2000). *Essential Guide to Food Additives*. Leatherhead, UK: Leatherhead Food RA Publishing, Surrey.

Saupe, A., and Rades, T. (2006). Solid lipid nanoparticles. In: *Nanocarrier Technologies: Frontiers of Nanotherapy*, pp. 41–50. M. R. Mozafari, ed. Dordrecht: Springer.

Saxelin M., Korpela R., Mayra-Makinen A. (2003). Introduction: Classifying Functional Dairy Products. In: *Functional Dairy Products*, pp. 1–15. S.Mattila-Sandholm, ed. Boca Raton, FL: CRC Press/Woodhead Publishing Ltd.

Shah, N. P. (2000). Probiotic bacteria: Selective enumeration and survival in dairy foods. *Journal of Dairy Science* 83: 894–907.

Shaikh, J., Bhosale, R., and Singhal, R. (2006). Microencapsulation of black pepper oleoresin. *Food Chemistry* 94: 105–110.

Shu, B., Yu, W., Zhao, Y., and Liu, X. (2006). Study on microencapsulation of lycopene by spray-drying. *Journal of Food Engineering* 76: 664–669.

Soottitantawat, A., Bigeard, F., Yoshii, H., Furuta, T., Ohkawara, M., and Linko, P. (2005a). Influence of emulsion and powder size on the stability of encapsulated D-limonene by spray drying. *Innovative Food Science and Emerging Technologies* 6: 107–114.

Soottitantawat, A., Takayama, K., Okamura, K., Muranaka, D., Yoshii, H., and Furuta, T. (2005b). Microencapsulation of L-menthol by spray drying and its release characteristics. *Innovative Food Science and Emerging Technologies* 6: 163–170.

Stanton C., Ross R. P., Fitzgerald G. F., Sinderen D. V. (2005). Fermented functional foods based on probiotics and their biogenic metabolites. *Current Opinion in Biotechnology* 16: 198–203.

Szejtli, J. (1984). Industrial Applications of Cyclodextrins. In: *Inclusion Compounds*, pp. 337–346. Vol. 3, Physical Properties and Applications. J. L. Atwood, J. E. D. Davies, and D. D. MacNicol, eds. London: Academic Press.

Takenaka, H., Kamashima, Y., and Lin, S. Y. (1980). Micromeritic properties of sulfamethoxazole microcapsules prepared by gelatin–acacia coacervation. *Journal of Pharmaceutical Sciences* 69(5): 513–516.

Teixeira, M. I., Andrade, L. R., Farina, M., and Rocha-Leao, M. H. M. (2004). Characterization of short chain fatty acid microcapsules produced by spray drying. *Materials Science and Engineering* 24: 653–658.

Ubbink J. B., Schaer-Zmmaretti P., Cavadini C. (2003). Probiotic delivery system. European Patent # EP 1 244 458 A1.

Ubbink J., Krüger J. (2006). Physical approaches for the delivery of active ingredients in foods. *Trends in Food Science and Technology* 17: 244–254.

Wallace J. M. W., McCabe A. J., Robson P. J., Keogh M. K., Murray C. A., *et al.* (2000). Bioavailability of *n*-3 polyunsaturated fatty acids in foods enriched with microencapsulated oils fish oil. *Annals of Nutrition and Metabolism* 44: 157–162.

Wampler, D. J. (1992). Flavor encapsulation: A method for providing maximum stability for dry flavor systems. *Cereal Foods World* 37: 817–820.

Wang, H. T., Schmitt, E., Flanagan, D. R., and Linhardt, R. L. (1991). Influence of formulation methods on the *in vitro* controlled release of protein from poly(ester) microspheres. *Journal of Controlled Release* 17: 23–32.

Watanabe, Y., Fang, X., Adachi, S., Fukami, H., and Matsuno, R. (2004). Oxidation of 6-*O*-arachidonoyl–ascorbate microencapsulated with a polysaccharide by spray-drying. *Lebensmittel-Wissenschaft und Technologie* 37: 395–400.

Weiss J., Takhistov P., McClements J. (2006). Functional materials in food nanotechnology. *Journal of Food Science* 71: 107–116.

Xie Y. L., Zhou H. M., Zhang Z. R. (2007). Effect of relative humidity on retention and stability of vitamin A microencapsulated by spray drying. *Journal of Food Biochemistry* 31: 68–80.

Yáñez-Fernández J., Ramos-Ramirez E. G., Salazar-Montoya J. A. (2008). Rheological characterization of dispersions and emulsions used in the preparation of microcapsules obtained by interfacial polymerization containing *Lactobacillus* sp. *European Food Research and Technology* 226(5): 957–966.

Young, S. L., Sarda, X., and Rosenberg, M. (1993). Microencapsulation properties of whey proteins. 1. Microencapsulation of anhydrous milk fat. *Journal of Dairy Science* 76: 2868–2877.

Zuidam, N. J., and Shimoni E. (2009). Overview of Microencapsulates for Use in Food Products or Processes and Methods to Make Them. In: *Encapsulation Technologies for Food Active Ingredients and Food Processing*, pp. 3–31. N. J. Zuidam and V. A. Nedovic, eds. Dordrecht: Springer.

CHAPTER 13

Encapsulation of polyunsaturated omega-3 fatty acids for enriched functional foods

Jorge Carlos Ruiz Ruiz[1] and Maira Rubi Segura Campos[2]

[1] *Departamento de Ingeniería Química-Bioquímica, Instituto Tecnológico de Mérida, Av. Tecnológico Km 4.5 S/N, C.P. 97118, Mérida, Yucatán, México*

[2] *Facultad de Ingeniería Química, Universidad Autónoma de Yucatán, Periférico Norte. Km. 33.5, Tablaje catastral 13615, Col. Chuburná de Hidalgo Inn, Mérida, Yucatán, México, CP. 97203*

13.1 Introduction

The incorporation of functional ingredients in a given food system and the processing and handling of such foods are associated with nutritional challenges for their healthy delivery. Encapsulation is one example of technology that has the potential to meet the challenge of successfully incorporating and delivering functional ingredients into a range of food types.

Polyunsaturated omega-3 fatty acids are a group of naturally occurring lipids that are present in high concentrations in certain fishes and plants (Cunnane *et al.*, 1995). The term *omega-3* signifies that the first double bond exists at the third carbon–carbon bond from the terminal methyl end of the carbon chain. The three most common omega-3 fatty acids are alpha linolenic acid, eicosapentaenoic acid, and docosahexaenoic acid. Alpha linolenic is present in vegetable oils, whereas eicosapentaenoic and docosahexaenoic acids are present in fish and in more-concentrated amounts in fish oil (Mantzioris *et al.*, 2000). The origin of the omega-3 fatty acids found in these species of fishes is the chloroplasts of marine phytoplankton and algae (Stamey, 2010; Cohen, 1995).

Fish consumption and omega-3 supplementation have attracted considerable interest in the past few decades in relation to their health benefits. Fish oils provide a source of eicosapentaenoic and docosahexaenoic acids, two fatty acids now recognized as an important part of the human diet (Calder, 2006). Eicosapentaenoic and docosahexaenoic acids are highly unsaturated fatty acids

New Polymers for Encapsulation of Nutraceutical Compounds, First Edition.
Edited by Jorge Carlos Ruiz Ruiz and Maira Rubi Segura Campos.

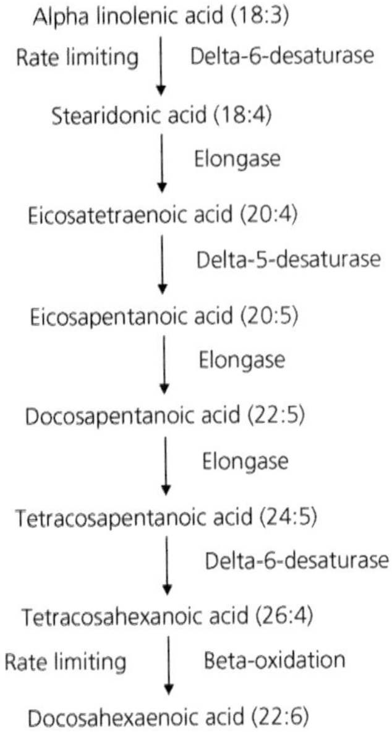

Figure 13.1 A series of elongation and desaturation reactions allows conversion of short-chain omega-3 fatty acids into the longer-chain polyunsaturated fatty acids such as eicosapentaenoic acid and docosahexaenoic acid. The delta-6-desaturase catalyzes the rate-limiting enzymatic reaction, leading to inefficient conversion to stearidonic acid in humans.

synthesized from alpha linolenic and other fatty acids in the omega-3 pathway (Figure 13.1).

Over thousands of years of an agriculture-based existence, the dietary ratio of omega-3 to omega-6 remained stable at about l:1. However, in the past 100 years changes in the food supply and dietary habits have caused this ratio to fall dramatically to less than 0.1. Within a range of total caloric intake of 2000 to 2500 Kcal, a proper safety ratio of oleic to linoleic to alpha-linolenic could be expressed as 11–16:4–6:1. Recent data show that a diet including about 13% of oleic acid in the total caloric intake could provide protection against the occurrence of new cardiovascular events, but an increase of oleic acid intake to more than 20% could limit this beneficial intake by inducing an increase of low-density lipoprotein in blood (Stuchlík and Žák, 2002). Today this consumption ratio is about 10–20:1, indicating a deficiency in n-3 polyunsaturated fatty acids (PUFAs) compared with the diet on which humans evolved and their genetic patterns were established. The omega-3 and omega-6 fatty acids are not interconvertible in the human body, and therefore appropriate amounts of both acids need to be considered in making dietary recommendations. The food industry is already taking steps to return polyunsaturated omega-3 fatty acids to the food supply by enriching various products with safety sources of omega-3 fatty acids (Simopoulos *et al.*, 1999).

13.2 Functional effects of omega-3 fatty acids

More-recent studies suggested that omega-3 PUFA supplementation could be helpful against many inflammatory diseases. The key link between PUFAs and inflammation is that eicosanoids, which are among the mediators and regulators of inflammation, are generated from 20-carbon PUFAs. Because inflammatory cells typically contain a high proportion of arachidonic acid (20:4 omega-6) and low proportions of other 20-carbon PUFAs, arachidonic acid is usually the major substrate for eicosanoid synthesis. Eicosanoids, which include prostaglandins, thromboxanes, leukotrienes, and other oxidized derivatives, are generated from arachidonic acid (Calder, 2006). The metabolic processes is summarized in Figure 13.2.

Although their action in antagonizing arachidonic acid metabolism is a key antiinflammatory effect of omega-3 PUFAs, these fatty acids have several other

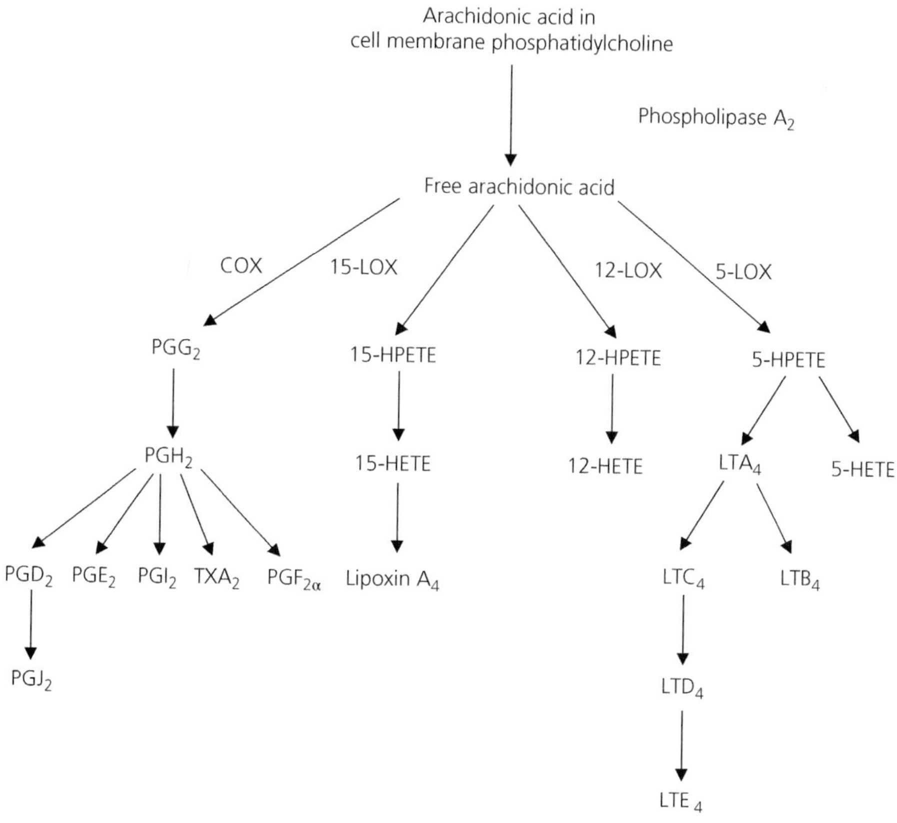

Figure 13.2 Generalized pathway for the conversion of arachidonic acid to eicosanoids. COX, cyclooxygenase; HETE, hydroxyeicosatetraenoic acid; HPETE, hydroperoxyeicosatetraenoic acid; LOX, lipoxygenase; LT, leukotriene; PG, prostaglandin; TX, thromboxane (Calder, 2006).

antiinflammatory effects that might result from altered eicosanoid production or might be independent of this. For example, studies have shown that when it is consumed in sufficient quantities, dietary fish oil results in decreased leukocyte chemotaxis, decreased production of reactive oxygen species and proinflammatory cytokines, and decreased expression of adhesion molecules (Calder, 2001).

13.3 Susceptibility to oxidation

The polyunsaturated nature of omega-3 and omega-6 fatty acids is critical to their functioning in terms of health benefits, but this same property also renders them highly susceptible to oxidative deterioration. Oxidation is a free-radical process and can be initiated by a variety of factors including heat, light, metals, and enzymes. Oxidation reduces the nutritive quality of the lipid and produces off-flavor and -aroma compounds through the breakdown of lipid hydroperoxides.

The structure of the fatty acid greatly affects its susceptibility to oxidation. Polyunsaturated lipids are much more susceptible to oxidation than saturated lipids due to their high content of bis-allylic methylene groups (Kulas *et al.*, 2006). Oleic acid, with a single double bond, reacts approximately 10 times faster than its saturated counterpart, stearic acid, whereas linoleic (two double bonds) reacts more than 100 times faster, and linolenic (three double bonds) reacts almost 200 times faster (Pokorny *et al.*, 2001). Eicosapentanoic (five double bonds) and docosahexaenoic (six double bonds) are extremely susceptible to oxidation.

The highly unsaturated nature of long-chain omega-3 fatty acids not only effects the rate at which oxidation occurs but also results in a highly complicated outcome in terms of the products generated. Each double bond is a site for hydrogen abstraction, ultimately enabling formation of greater than 16 hydroperoxide isomers for eicosapentanoic and 20 hydroperoxide isomers for docosahexaenoic acid (Kulas *et al.*, 2006). The extreme sensitivity of oils to oxidation can easily lead to the development of off-flavors and cause significant loss of product quality, stability, nutritional value and bioavailability, and the overall acceptability of the food product. Consequently, encapsulation has been successfully used to encapsulate oils in order to prevent oxidation and to improve stability and bioavailability (Wakil *et al.*, 2010).

13.4 Methods for encapsulating oil

One way of protecting or delivering oils is by encapsulating them in a matrix that acts as a barrier (Ye *et al.*, 2009). Commonly, oils are encapsulated for controlled release, masking off-flavors or colors, increasing shelf-life stability, evaporation and incompatibilities with reactive substances, easy handling by converting sticky oils to free-flowing particles, and easy storage of dry particles compared to frozen oils (Abang *et al.*, 2012). Encapsulation of omega-3 oils minimizes oxidative deterioration and allows their use in stable and easy-to-handle forms (Kaushik *et al.*, 2014).

Oils can be encapsulated in two structures: beads or capsules. A capsule consists of a well-defined core and an envelope, whereas a bead is made of a continuous phase of one or more miscible polymers in which encapsulants are dispersed (Mathiowitz *et al.*, 1999). Oils have been entrapped in capsules using spray-drying and freeze-drying (Dzondo-Gaget *et al.*, 2005; Jafari *et al.*, 2008), emulsification/internal gelation (Ribeiro *et al.*, 1999), cocrystallization (Beristain *et al.*, 1996), emulsion extrusion (Yilmaz *et al.*, 2001), solvent evaporation (Aliabadi *et al.*, 2007), emulsification (Miyazawa *et al.*, 2000), and ionic gelation (Chan, 2011). Oils can be encapsulated in capsules using a coacervation method (Katona *et al.*, 2010), extrusion through concentric nozzles (Wyss *et al.*, 2004), condensation and interfacial polymerization (Bouchemal *et al.*, 2006), and microfluidic devices (Ren *et al.*, 2010). The key parameter in any of these processes is the selection of wall material (Kaushik et al., 2014).

13.5 Nonconventional wall materials for encapsulating oil

13.5.1 Chitosan

Chitosan is a naturally occurring polysaccharide of D-glucosamine and *N*-acetyl-D-glucosamine joined through a $\beta(1\rightarrow4)$ linkage. The main sources of chitin and chitosan are crustacean exoskeletons, but these polysaccharides are also structural components in fungal cell walls (Agullo *et al.*, 2003). Chitosan is classified by the quantity of amine groups present on the chain. This property is referred to as either the degree of acetylation (DA) or the degree of deacetylation (DD). Generally, a material is considered chitosan rather than chitin if the degree of deacetylation is greater than 60% (Muzzarelli and Muzzarelli 2005).

The amine groups along the chitosan backbone contribute to unique and beneficial properties including antimicrobial properties, the ability to chelate metal ions, bioadhesion, and immunostimulatory activity (Agnihotri *et al.*, 2004). The amine groups have a pKa in the range of 6.2 to 6.8 such that the material acts as a cationic polyelectrolyte under acidic conditions (Agullo *et al.*, 2003). Chitosan is nontoxic, is biocompatible, is biodegradable, and can be recovered from waste materials.

The use of chitosan in food applications is growing, and food preservation is a primary interest. Chitosan has been evaluated as an antimicrobial agent (Shahidi *et al.*, 1999). When applied as a coating to fruits and vegetables, chitosan not only reduces microbial growth but also extends product shelf life by delaying ripening, controlling moisture transfer, limiting oxygen transmission, and preventing browning reactions (Shahidi *et al.*, 1999; Agullo *et al.*, 2003). Chitosan has been used as an encapsulant for food ingredients, but it has been explored much more widely as a pharmaceutical encapsulant (Uragami and Tokura, 2006). Food applications evaluated include pigments, antioxidants, and polyunsaturated omega-3 fatty acids.

Klaypradit and Huang (2008) developed an encapsulation technique using an ultrasonic atomizer and three processing steps: emulsification, ultrasonic atomization, and freeze-drying. The size and stability of the emulsion droplet and the properties of the encapsulated powders after freeze-drying were characterized by these authors. At 20 g per 100 g tuna oil, the optimum ratio of chitosan to maltodextrin was 1:10. The combination of chitosan and maltodextrin gave the smallest particle size and the highest emulsion stability. The eicosapentaenoic and docosahexaenoic content (240 mg/g) of the encapsulated powder were slightly higher than commercial specification (100 mg/g) and they had low moisture content and water activity, and they had acceptable appearance and encapsulation efficiency. The use of chitosan together with other conventional polymers could lead to its application in the food industry improving the stability of oils.

13.5.2 Pullulan

Pullulan is a water-soluble linear polysaccharide formed from $\alpha(1\rightarrow6)$ linked maltotriose units. Extensive research has shown that pullulan is an excellent film former (Kshirsagar *et al.*, 2009). Furthermore, pullulan films have been shown to exhibit substantial oxygen barrier properties (Leathers, 2005). Pullulan has also been shown to act as a dietary fiber and prebiotic (Knapp *et al.*, 2008).

Kshirsagar and colleagues (2009) found that pullulan had a stabilizing effect on turmeric oleoresin emulsions prepared with gum arabic. These researchers found that incorporating pullulan at a level of 1% (w/w) resulted in an emulsion index (ESI) of 1, indicating no oil separation after 24 hours of storage in a cylinder. The emulsion contained 30% (w/w) gum arabic and turmeric oleoresin at 5% (w/w) based on gum arabic content. ESI of the emulsion without pullulan was 0.4. The enhanced stability was attributed to increased viscosity and polymer–polymer interactions.

Kshirasagar and colleagues (2009) incorporated pullulan in gum arabic and turmeric oleoresin emulsions to generate turmeric oleoresin microcapsules. The microcapsules were prepared by spray-drying at an inlet temperature of 140 °C and an outlet temperature of 88 °C. The authors found that spherical microcapsules formed when pullulan was incorporated at 1% (w/w) for emulsions containing 30% (w/w) gum arabic and 5% oleoresin (w/w, based on gum arabic weight) but that at higher levels, fiber-like structures started to form, with cobweb structures resulting for pullulan concentrations of 3% to 5% (w/w). The authors evaluated blends of gum arabic and maltodextrin, all of which contained

1% pullulan, and found that gum arabic and pullulan alone produced microcapsules with the highest encapsulation efficiency (72%). This was also the most stable emulsion of those evaluated.

Hannah (2009) encapsulated fish oil as source of omega-3 PUFAs using chitosan–pullulan and chitosan–high amylose starch–pullulan systems. According to this author, pullulan incorporation resulted in fiber-like structures that wrapped around and between the microcapsules. Blending different polymers may provide more favorable capsule properties and easier-to-process emulsions than if a polymer is used alone. This author reported favorable properties for chitosan blends compared to chitosan alone (oxidation-induction time, oil droplet size), but some properties did not improve (encapsulation efficiency). Pullulan can produce fibrous materials and if it is used as a wall material it should be kept at a concentration lower than 20% of the total wall composition to avoid production of fibers, or used at levels higher than 20% if fibers are desirable.

13.5.3 *Salvia hispanica* mucilage

Salvia hispanica seeds soaked in water release a viscous material called mucilage, which is of interest from the nutritional point of view and is important as a thickening agent in the food industry. In 1996, the Food and Agriculture Organization of the United Nations (FAO) described *S. hispanica* seeds as a potential source of polysaccharide gum because of its exceptional mucilaginous properties at low concentration in aqueous solutions (Hulse, 1996). A tentative structure of the basic unit of the polysaccharide was proposed by Lin and colleagues (1994) as a tetrasaccharide with 4-*O*-metil-α-D-glucoronopyranosyl residues occurring as branches of β-D-xylopyranosyl on the main chain (Figure 13.3).

The monosaccharides β-D-xylose, α-D-glucose, and 4-*O*-metil-α-D-glucoronic acids were obtained by acid hydrolysis in the proportion 2:1:1, respectively. The monosaccharide composition was 16.8% D-xylose + D-mannose, 2.1% D-arabinose, 6.8% D-glucose, 3.9% galacturonic acid, and 12.1% glucuronic acid, with 41.66% of total sugars. The mucilage contains functional groups: hydroxyl and

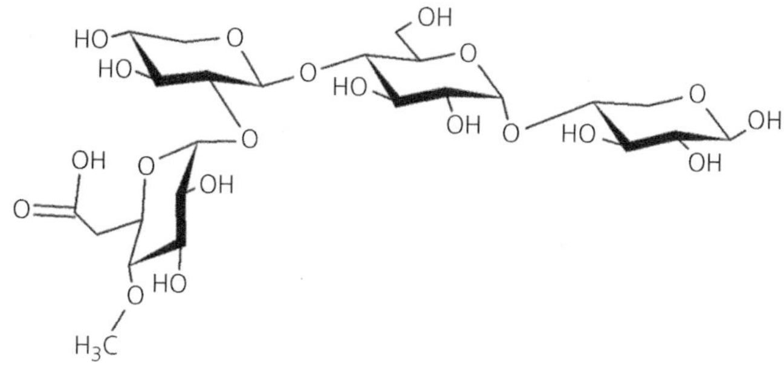

Figure 13.3 Tentative structure of the basic unit of the *Salvia hispanica* mucilage proposed by Lin *et al.* (1994).

carbonyl groups of carboxylates and carboxylic acid similar to those found in xanthan gum. In general, hydrocolloids are widely used in different applications in the food industry, due to their ability to retain water. They are also notable for their thickening and gelling properties, syneresis control, and emulsion stabilization, among other features (Phillips and Williams, 2000). *S. hispanica* seeds contain 5% to 6% mucilage.

Us-Medina (2015) obtained capsules of *Salvia hispanica* oil by the external ionic gelation method using alginate–*S. hispanica* mucilage systems at a concentration of polymers (50/50, w/w) of 2% (w/v), a calcium chloride concentration of 2% (w/v) and a crosslinking time of 20 minutes (Figure 13.4). Capsules were spherical, averaging 2.16 mm in diameter. Encapsulation efficiency was 82.92% and method yield was 92.17%. Encapsulated oil exhibited low total oxidation (TOTOX) values during storage at different relative humidities. Thermograms of capsules indicates three consecutive glass transitions. The first onset is close to 49.4 °C and corresponds to the *S. hispanica* oil. The second glass transition temperature of 86.2 °C is attributable to *S. hispanica* mucilage. And the third onset is close to 119 °C, corresponding to alginate. These results indicate that *S. hispanica*

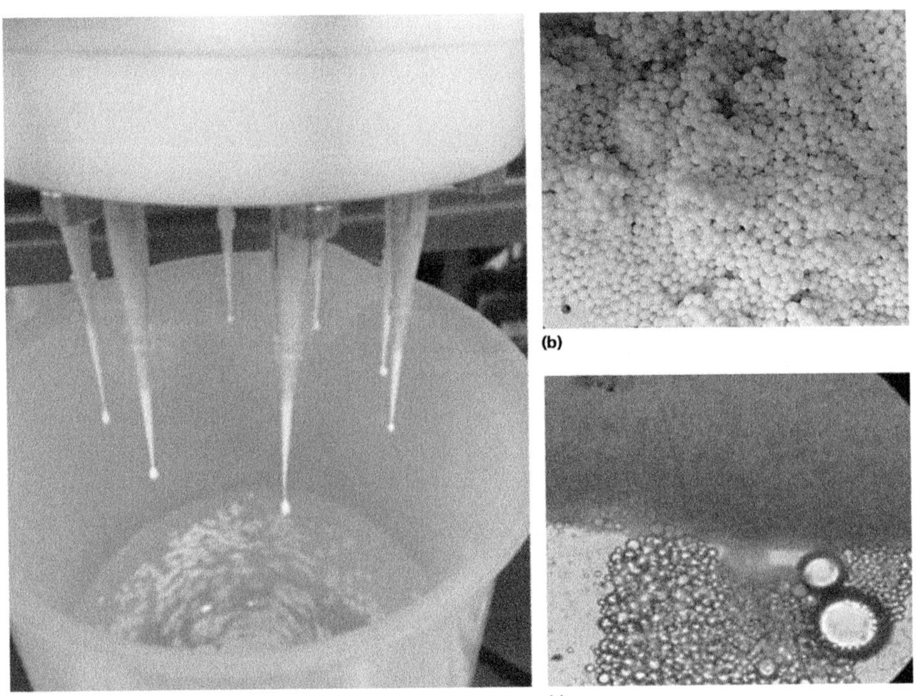

(a) (b) (c)

Figure 13.4 (a) Multinozzle extruder used for dripping emulsions of alginate–*Salvia hispanica* mucilage–*S. hispanica* oil. **(b)** Wet capsules of alginate–*S. hispanica* mucilage containing *S. hispanica* oil. **(c)** Micrograph of a capsule of alginate–*S. hispanica* mucilage containing *S. hispanica* oil.

mucilage could be used in polymeric systems as wall material for capsules containing high oil content to improve their stability and incorporation into functional food systems.

13.5.4 *Opuntia ficus-indica*

Opuntia ficus-indica is a cactaceae from arid and semi-arid regions, in the form of shrub or tree up to 5 m tall, forming a sturdy trunk when aging. This species is native to Mexico (Torres *et al.*, 2012). The mucilage from *O. ficus-indica* is an interesting and promising alternative due to its emulsifying properties (Medina Torres *et al.*, 2000). It is used as an additive in the food industry, specifically as an edible coating to extend the shelf life of food products (Del Valle *et al.*, 2005). Previous studies have shown that chemical composition of *O. ficus-indica* mucilage is a complex mixture of polysaccharides such as L-arabinose, D-galactose, D-xylose and L-rhamnose, and D-galacturonic acid, which represent up to 10 g/100 g of total sugars (Medina Torres *et al.*, 2006).

Multiple applications have been developed for this material, ranging from a thickener of foods to a turbidity remover in contaminated water. The usefulness of this heteropolysaccharide of high molecular weight (2.31×10^4 g/mol) relies on its physicochemical properties, which have been described by many research groups, emphasizing its electrolyte-thickener capacity and its flow characteristics (Cárdenas *et al.*, 1997). High moisture content in the mucilage limits its applications, generating the need for previous treatments such as spray-drying to increase its potential uses (Medina Torres *et al.*, 2013). Medina-Torres and colleagues (2013) produced microcapsules of gallic acid by spray-drying with an aqueous extract of *O. ficus-indica* mucilage, which acted as an encapsulating agent. The mechanical spectra showed that the sample with gallic acid was stable long term (>2 days) and presented a bimodal particle size distribution. This study demonstrated the effectiveness of nopal mucilage when used as wall biomaterial in microencapsulation of gallic acid by the spray-drying process.

13.6 Properties of oil as omega-3 polyunsaturated fatty acids capsules

Spray-drying and coacervation are the two most commonly reported methods for the encapsulation of vegetable oils. The first method is widely used for drying heat-sensitive foods, pharmaceuticals, and other substances because of the rapid evaporation of the applied solvent from the droplets. The second method was the first reported process to be adapted for the industrial production of microcapsules. Sometimes both methods are used consecutively to obtain oil microcapsules.

Yu and colleagues (2012) obtained olive oil capsules by complex coacervation using gelatin and acacia gum as wall materials and glutaric dialdehyde as the cross-linking agent. The authors evaluated process parameters, such as the dosage of the cross-linking agent, concentration of the wall materials, pH value, and the ratio between core and wall materials. The optimum process parameters were as follows: The dosage of the cross-linking agent was 3 mL, the concentration of wall materials was 3%, the pH value of coacervation was 4.0, and the ratio of core to wall material was 1:1. To obtain microcapsules with good mobility and dispersal, a spray-drying process was used to dry the product. The capsules had a mean particle size of 6 μm and a loading oil rate of 60%. At 80 °C, the microcapsules had a fast-release stage in the first 5 hours and then remained almost steady. The higher decomposition temperature (180 °C) of the microcapsules was obtained under higher concentration of wall materials. This is because the wall materials play an important role in the heat-resistant microcapsule. According to Yu and colleagues (2012), using the method of complex coacervation, the first elastic layer of the microcapsule was obtained, and then the second glass layer was obtained through spray-drying. The two double-wall constructures resulted in a good heat-resistant property of the microcapsules.

In another study, Devi's group (2012) encapsulated olive oil by complex coacervation using gelatin, sodium alginate, and glutaraldehyde as cross-linking agents. For these authors, the optimum ratio between gelatin A–sodium alginate and pH to form the maximum coacervate complex was found to be 3.5:1 and 3.5:8, respectively. In these conditions the oil load, the oil content, and the encapsulation efficiency were 188%, 58%, and 89%, respectively. Through scanning electron microscopy analysis, the formation of free-flowing spherical microcapsules of different sizes was confirmed. With the increase of the amount of polymer concentration, the size of the microcapsules increased. According to Devi and Maji (2010), this might be due to the increase of the thickness of the wall of the microcapsules. The Fourier transform infrared and thermogravimetric analysis carried out by the authors did not exhibit any remarkable interaction between olive oil and the gelatin–sodium alginate complex. This indicates that the encapsulated material retains all its properties.

A major property of encapsulated powders manufactured for consumer use is their ease of reconstitution. The reconstitution process in water can be divided into four steps: wetting, submersion, dispersion, and dissolving (Schubert *et al.*, 2003). Wettability is understood as the ability of a bulk powder to imbibe a liquid under the influence of capillary forces. Generally, it depends on powder particle size, density, porosity, surface charge, surface area, and the presence of amphipathic substances. Fast wetting is also favored by large particles of high porosity (Domian, 2005).

Domian and Wąsak (2008) encapsulated rapeseed oil by spray-drying using maltodextrin and acacia gum. The emulsions were dried at a constant temperature of inlet and outlet air – 200 °C and 100 °C, respectively – and at a spray disk speed reaching 34,000 rpm. The capsules were characterized by a regular and spherical shape, a smooth surface with visible cavities, and constituted powder particles with sizes ranging from 10 to 90 μm. The encapsulation yield ranged between 71% and 94% and the encapsulation efficiency ranged between 83% and 95%. According to the authors, directly after drying, the powders demonstrated low water activity (a_w) of 0.04 to 0.15 at a moisture content w of 2.5% to 4.8%. Loose and tapped bulk density as well as a porosity of loosely poured and packed bed reached ρL 430–489 kg/m^3 and ρT 695–765 kg/m^3 as well as εL 0.60–0.65 and εT 0.35–0.45, respectively. Particles of microencapsulated oil powder were characterized by density ρ ranging from 1184 to 1288 kg/m^3. The authors concluded that spray-drying microencapsulation of rapeseed oil onto a maltodextrin carrier with the addition of acacia gum enabled the obtaining of a powdered product with complete water reconstitution and very poor wettability and flowability.

13.7 Oxidation stability and fatty acid composition of encapsulated vegetable oils

Lipid oxidation in microencapsulated lipids is of paramount importance because it can result in a loss of nutritional value and the development of flavors unacceptable to consumers in a significant number of products such as infant formulas, bakery products, milk powders, dried eggs, and dehydrated soups and sauces (Velasco *et al.*, 2003). In this sense, Dzondo-Gaget and coworkers (2005) encapsulated oil extracted from the safou fruit by using spray-drying and freeze-drying. These authors evaluated the storage stability by determining parameters such as iodine value, peroxide value, and the content of thiobarbituric reactive species in the oil for a period of 2 months at four storage temperatures from 4 to 50 °C. According to the authors, the freeze-dried particles were more efficient against oil oxidation than spray-dried particles.

In another study, Beristain and colleagues (1996) encapsulated orange peel oil by cocrystallization using sucrose syrups. According to these authors, at proportions of 100 to 250 grams of oil per kilogram of sugar it was possible to obtain encapsulation capacities greater than 90%. When oil was encapsulated without antioxidants, a sensory evaluation detected oxidized flavors in oils after storage at 35 °C for one day. When BHA was added to the oil prior to cocrystallization, no signs of oxidized flavors were detected after 2 months of storage at ambient temperature. This suggests that encapsulation with the addition of antioxidant additives could prolong the storage time of the encapsulated oils.

Calvo's team (2010) encapsulated extra virgin olive oils by spray-drying using sodium caseinate and lactose as wall materials. The spray-drying conditions were as follows: The pressure of compressed air for the flow of the spray was 5 bars. The inlet and outlet air temperatures were maintained at 165 and 80 °C, respectively, with a feed rate of 540 mL/h. With these conditions, the oil encapsulation yield was 53%. For the extra virgin olive oil that had highest amounts of total phenolic contents (459.64 mg caffeic acid/kg oil), oxidative stability index (83.89 h), and a ratio between C18:1 and C18:2 (12.82), the fatty acid profile was unaltered after the microencapsulation process.

Fatty acid profile and vitamin E contents could be used as parameters to evaluate the nutritional value and to regulate the marketing of oil-encapsulated base products. In this sense, Hirashima and colleagues (2013) evaluated the identity (fatty acid profile) and the compliance with nutritional labeling (fatty acid and vitamin E contents) of 21 commercial encapsulated oils. Samples included flaxseed (6), evening primrose (5), safflower (8), borage (1) and blackcurrant (1) oils. Nine samples were adulterated (five samples of safflower oil, three of flaxseed oil, and one of evening primrose). Among them, three flaxseed and two safflower oil samples were probably adulterated by the addition of soybean oil. Only two samples presented all values in compliance with nutritional labeling (one safflower oil sample and one borage oil sample). The results show that a continuous monitoring of commercialized encapsulated oils is necessary.

It is difficult to foresee the rate of oxidation in heterogeneous systems due to the high number of variables involved. In particular, the evolution of oxidation in the noncontinuous or dispersed lipid phase may become very complex due to the heterogeneity in the lipid droplets isolated one from another in the matrix. Consequently, different oxidation rates can occur in different droplets. However, after extraction of the encapsulated fraction, a continuous oily phase is analyzed and substantial information on the oxidation in the different droplets is lost (Velasco *et al.*, 2003). Some authors have reported that oxidation proceeded more rapidly in freeze-dried samples than in spray-dried samples, attributing such results to the greater surface area of the former (Fioriti *et al.*, 1975; Taguchi *et al.*, 1992). Other researchers have found the opposite (Desobry *et al.*, 1999; Stapelfeldt *et al.*, 1999), even starting from samples with similar microencapsulation efficiency (Desobry *et al.*, 1999), then attributing the lower oxidative stability of spray-dried samples to the high temperatures used during the atomization process.

Minemoto's group (2001) compared freeze-drying with hot-air drying at 50 °C, finding freeze-dried samples more resistant to oxidation, even though they showed lower microencapsulation efficiency. This research group suggested that the effect of the drying method might be closely related to the type of encapsulating agent and oxidative conditions. According to De Barros-Fernandes and coworkers (2013), the use of higher temperatures and low feed flow rate contributed to the decrease of particle moisture content and, in general, it was related to the variation of the hygroscopicity and wettability of the resulting powders. A higher moisture content can lead to oxidation of the encapsulated material.

Torres-Giner and colleagues (2012) studied the stabilization by encapsulation of docosahexaenoic acid (DHA) in zein ultrathin capsules produced by electrospraying. The zein ultrathin DHA encapsulation was observed by ATR-FTIR spectroscopy to be more efficient against degradation under both ambient conditions and in a confined space. In the latter case, which more closely simulates a sealed food packaging situation, the bioactive DHA was considerably more stable. By fitting the degradation data to a specific autodecomposition food lipids kinetic model, it was seen that the encapsulated omega-3 fatty acid showed a 2.5-fold reduction in the degradation rate constant and also had much higher degradation induction time. Moreover, the ultrathin zein–DHA capsules were more stable across relative humidity and temperature. Finally, headspace analysis by gas chromatography coupled with mass spectrometry showed that the presence of three main flavor-influencing aldehydes in the headspace was much lower in the zein-encapsulated DHA, suggesting that the encapsulated bioactive also releases much less off-flavor. Electrosprayed ultrathin capsules of zein are shown to exhibit potential in the design of novel functional foods or bioactive packaging strategies to enhance the stability of polyunsaturated omega-3 fatty acids.

13.8 Incorporation of long-chain omega-3 polyunsaturated fatty acids in foods

Fortification of commonly consumed food products with n-3 long-chain omega-3 PUFAs in foods is considered an innovative way of providing health benefits to people without major alteration to their dietary habits (Garg *et al.*, 2006). An alternative to increasing consumption would be to supplement with ω-3 daily foodstuffs such as margarine, eggs and their products, pasta, sauces, juices, meat, and milk and dairy products – the so-called functional foods (Gómez-Candela *et al.*, 2011).

There is a restriction in the level of oil fortified in different products such as bakery, dairy, and frozen foods because oils are highly susceptible to oxidation during storage (Willumsen, 2006). Fatty acids present in oil would undergo oxidative deterioration, leading to degradation of the original long carbon chain to yield highly reactive intermediate lipid radicals and ultimately potentially unhealthy small molecules. It has been found that hydroperoxides, which are the primary products of lipid oxidation, are considered to be toxic for human health (Oarada, 1988). As the number of double bonds in a fatty acid increases, so does the rate of oxidation. This makes polyunsaturated lipids such as omega-3 fats highly susceptible to oxidation (Keogh *et al.*, 2001). Oil encapsulation may be useful to retard lipid autooxidation and increase the range of applications where otherwise oil could not be used (Calvo *et al.*, 2010).

Gökmena and colleagues (2011) developed functional bread enriched with omega-3 fatty acids. These authors used high-amylose corn starch to form nano-sized complexes with flax seed oil that was converted to powder of microparticles by spray-drying. The particles were then incorporated into bread formulations at different amounts to investigate their effects on bread quality characteristics. The effects of encapsulation on the formation of lipid oxidation products and thermal process contaminants including acrylamide and hydroxymethyl furfural (HMF) were determined. Encapsulation significantly decreased lipid oxidation as measured by the formation of hexanal and nonanal in breads during baking. Increasing the amount of particles in dough significantly decreased the formation of acrylamide and HMF in breads. Scanning electron microscopic analysis of bread demonstrated that particles added to dough remained intact in the crumb but were partially destroyed in the crust. Compares to its free form, addition of nanoencapsulated flax seed oil increased final product quality and safety by lowering lipid oxidation and formation of harmful compounds in breads during baking.

Rubilar's group (2012) encapsulated linseed oil as a source of omega-3 fatty acids by spray drying, using gum arabic and maltodextrin as wall materials. These authors evaluated the influence of gum arabic, maltodextrin, and mixtures of both in a ratio of 3:2 as wall material, the concentration of wall material (25% and 30% in 100 g of emulsion), and the concentration of oil (14% and 20% in 100 g of emulsion) in the encapsulation of linseed oil. The spray-drying conditions were an air input temperature of 140 °C, an outlet temperature of 95 °C, and a drying airflow of 73 m^3/h and a feed rate of 5.3 g/min. The maximum encapsulation efficiency was obtained with a mixture of both wall materials of 3:2, at a concentration of 30% with 14% of oil. The encapsulated oil exhibited an induction time and an oxidative stability index at 100 °C of 2.83 h and 3.78 h, respectively. According to these authors, the spray-drying conditions (temperature) did not affect the linseed oil's chemical stability. However, the amounts of oleic and linoleic acid decreased by almost 50%.

Microcapsules of linseed oil were added to a soup formulation in a proportion of 14%; this proportion provides approximately 80% of the recommended daily intake of α-linolenic acid (1 g/day) according to the International Society for the Study of Fatty Acids and Lipids. The oxidative stability and the shelf life of oil extracted from the soup exhibited an induction time of 14.85 h, and the stability time was 15.61 h. The determined shelf life was 8.78 months.

13.9 Conclusion

Encapsulation methods such as spray-drying and coacervation have allowed researchers to obtain microcapsules of diverse sources of polyunsaturated omega-3 fatty acids. A variety of other methods are in development including spray-chilling, extrusion coating, and liposome entrapment. The key parameter in any of these processes is the selection of wall material. For spray-dried emulsions and complex coacervates, protein or polysaccharides are primarily used as shell material, although complex coacervation is currently commercially limited to gelatin. When polyunsaturated omega-3 fatty acids are encapsulated, oxidation is reduced, allowing storage for longer periods. Similarly, the composition of fatty acids is not significantly affected. New strategies involving the use of microencapsulation methods along with the use of a combination of novel polymers as wall material and the inclusion of antioxidants, could increase the stability of such products. Polyunsaturated omega-3 fatty acid–enriched foods should be stable and convenient, have an acceptable flavor, and should be without heavy price premiums in order to achieve an effective population-wide increase in consumption of these bioactive fatty acids. Further studies on the use of novel polymers like mucilages in combination with conventional or commercial ones, the interaction of the oils in foods, oxidative stability, bioavailability, and nutritional impact are needed.

Acknowledgments

This chapter forms part of Project 189741 "Aspectos Tecnológico-funcionales de subproductos de chía (Salvia hispanica L.) aplicables al desarrollo de alimentos", financed by Consejo Nacional de Ciencia y Tecnología (CONACYT-México).

References

Abang, S., Chan, E-S., and Poncelet, D. (2012). Effects of process variables on the encapsulation of oil in Ca-alginate capsules using an inverse gelation technique. *Journal of Microencapsulation* 29(5): 417–428.

Agulló, E., Rodríguez, M. S., Ramos, V., and Albertengo, L. (2003). Present and future role of chitin and chitosan in food. *Macromolecular Biosciences* 3:521–530.

Agnihotri, S. A., Mallikarjuna, N. N., Aminabhavi, T. M. (2004). Recent advances on chitosan-based micro- and nanoparticles in drug delivery. *Journal of Controlled Release* 100(1): 5–28.

Aliabadi, H. M., Elhasi, S., Mahmud, A., Gulamhusein, R., Mahdipoor, P., and Lavasanifar, A. (2007). Encapsulation of hydrophobic drugs in polymeric micelles through co-solvent evaporation: The effect of solvent composition on micellar properties and drug loading. *International Journal of Pharmaceutics* 329: 158–165.

Beristain, C. I., Vazquez, A., Garcia, H. S., and Vernon-Carter, E. J. (1996). Encapsulation of orange peel oil by co-crystallization. *LWT – Food Science and Technology* 29: 645–647.

Bouchemal, K., Briancon, S., Fessi, H., Chevallier, Y., Bonnet, I., and Perrier, E. (2006). Simultaneous emulsification and interfacial polycondensation for the preparation of colloidal suspensions of nanocapsules. *Materials Science and Engineering C* 26: 472-480.

Calder, P. C. (2006). n-3 polyunsaturated fatty acids, inflammation, and inflammatory diseases. *American Journal of Clinical Nutrition* 83: 1505–1519.

Calder, P. C. (2001). Polyunsaturated fatty acids, inflammation and immunity. *Lipids.* 36: 1007–1024.

Calvo, P., Hernández, T., Lozano, M., and González-Gómez, D. (2010). Microencapsulation of extra-virgin olive oil by spray-drying: Influence of wall material and olive quality. *European Journal of Lipid Science and Technology* 112: 852–858.

Cárdenas, A., Higuera Ciapara, I., and Goycoolea, F. M. (1997). Rheology and aggregation of cactus (*Opuntia ficus-indica*) mucilage in solution. *Journal of the Professional Association for Cactus Development* 2: 152–159.

Chan, E. S. (2011). Preparation of Ca-alginate beads containing high oil content: Influence of process variables on encapsulation efficiency and bead properties. *Carbohydrate Polymers* 84: 1267–1275.

Cohen, Z., Norman, H. A., and Heimer, Y. M. (1995). Microalgae as a source of omega-3 fatty acids. *World Review of Nutrition and Diet* 77: 1–31.

Cunnane, S. C., Hamadeh, A. C., Liede, L. U., Thompson, T. M. S, and Jenkins, D. J. A. (1995). Nutritional attributes of traditional flaxseed in healthy young adults. *American Journal of Clinical Nutrition* 61(1): 62–68.

De Barros-Fernandes, R. V., Borges, S. V., and Botrel, D. A. (2013). Influence of spray drying operating conditions on microencapsulated rosemary essential oil properties. *Ciência e Tecnologia de Alimentos, Campinas* 33(1): 171–178.

Del Valle, V., Hernández Muñoz, G. A., Galotto, M. J. (2005). Development of a cactus–mucilage edible coating (*Opuntia ficus indica*) and its application to extend strawberry (*Fragaria ananassa*) shelf-life. *Food Chemistry* 91: 751–756.

Desobry, S. A, Netto, F. M., and Labuza, T. P. (1999). Influence of maltodextrin systems at an equivalent 25DE on encapsulated beta-carotene loss during storage. *Journal of Food Processing and Preservation* 23: 39–55.

Devi, N., Hazarika, D., Deka, C., and Kakati, D. (2012). Study of complex coacervation of gelatin A and sodium alginate for microencapsulation of olive oil. *Journal of Macromolecular Science: Pure and Applied Chemistry* 49: 936–945.

Devi, N. and Maji, T. K. (2010). Genipin crosslinked microcapsules of gelatin A and κ-carrageenan polyelectrolyte complex for encapsulation of Neem (*Azadirachta indica A. Juss.*) seed oil. *Polymer Bulletin* 65(4): 347–362.

Domian E. (2005). Physical properties of model food powders in the aspect of the agglomeration method. *Żywność Technologia Jakość* 45: 87–97.

Domian, E., and Wąsak, I. (2008). Microencapsulation of rapeseed oil based on the spray drying method. *Polish Journal of Food and Nutrition Sciences* 58(4): 477–483.

Dzondo-Gaget, M., Nzikou, J. M., Etoumongo, A., Linder, M., and Desobry, S. (2005). Encapsulation and storage of safou oil in 6DE maltodextrins. *Process Biochemistry* 40: 265–271.

Fioriti, J. A., Stahl, H. D., Cseri, J., and Sims, R. J. (1975). Chemical and organoleptic properties of dried emulsions. *Journal of the American Oil Chemists' Society* 52: 395–399.

Garg, M. L., Wood, L. G., Singh, H., and Moughan, P. J. (2006). Means of delivering recommended levels of long chain n-3 polyunsaturated fatty acids in human diets. *Journal of Food Science* 71(5): 66–71.

Gökmena, V., Mogol, B. A., Lumaga, R. B., Fogliano, V., Kaplun, Z., and Shimoni, E. (2011). Development of functional bread containing nanoencapsulated omega-3 fatty acids. *Journal of Food Engineering* 105(4): 585–591.

Gómez-Candela, C., Bermejo-López L. M., and Loria-Kohen, V. (2011). Importance of a balanced omega 6/omega 3 ratio for the maintenance of health. Nutritional recommendations. *Nutricion Hospitalaria* 26(2): 323–329.

Hannah, S. (2009). Microencapsulation of an omega-3 polyunsaturated fatty acid source with polysaccharides for food applications. Doctorate thesis. Virginia Polytechnic Institute and State University, p. 106.

Hirashima, K., Alves da Silva, S., Fernandes-Caruso, M. S., and Aued-Pimentel, S. (2013). Encapsulated specialty oils commercialized in São Paulo state, Brazil: Evaluation of identity (fatty acid profile) and compliance of fatty acids and vitamin E contents with nutrition labeling. *Food and Science Technology, Campinas* 33(1): 107–115.

Hulse, J. (1996). Flavours, spices and edible gums: Opportunities for integrated agroforestry systems. In: *Domestication and Commercialization of Non-timber Forest Products in Agroforestry Systems*, pp. 86–96. R. R. B. Leakey, A. B. Temu, M. Melnyk, and P. Vantomme, eds. Non-Wood Forest Products No. 9. Rome: Food and Agriculture Organization of the United Nations.

Jafari, S. M., Assadpoor, E., Bhandari, B., and He, Y. (2008). Nano-particle encapsulation of fish oil by spray drying. *Food Research International* 41: 172–183.

Kaushik, P., Dowling, K., Barrow, C. J., and Adhikari, B. (2014). Microencapsulation of omega-3 fatty acids: A review of microencapsulation and characterization methods. *J Funct Foods*. doi:10.1016/j.jff.2014.06.029.

Katona, J. M., Sovilj, V. J., and Petrovic, L. B. (2010). Microencapsulation of oil by polymer mixture–ionic surfactant interaction induced coacervation. *Carbohydrate Polymers* 79: 563–570.

Keogh, M. K., O'Kennedy, B. T., Kelly, J., Auty, M. A., Kelly, P. M., *et al.* (2001). Stability to oxidation of spray dried fish oil powder microencapsulated using milk ingredients. *Journal of Food Science* 66(2): 217–224.

Klaypradit, W., and Huang, Y-W. (2008). Fish oil encapsulation with chitosan using ultrasonic atomizer. *LWT – Food Science and Technology* 41: 1133–1139.

Knapp, B. K., Parsons, C. M., Swanson, K. S., and Fahey, G. C. (2008). Physiological responses to novel carbohydrates as assessed using canine and avian models. *Journal of Agricultural and Food Chemistry* 56(17): 7999–8006.

Kshirsagar, A. C., Yenge, V. B., Sarkar, A., and Singhal, R. S. (2009). Efficacy of pullulan in emulsification of turmeric oleoresin and its subsequent microencapsulation. *Food Chemistry* 113(4): 1139–1145.

Kulas, E., Olsen, E., and Ackman, R. G. (2006). Oxidation of fish lipids and its inhibition with tocopherols. In: *Lipid Oxidation Pathways*. A. Kamal-Eldin, ed. Champaign, Illinois: AOCS Press.

Leathers, T. D. (2005). Pullulan. In: *Polysaccharides and Polyamides in the Food Industry*, pp. 387–481. A. Steinbuchel and S. K. Rhee, eds. Weinheim, Germany: Wiley.

Lin, K.-Y., Daniel, J. R., and Whistler, R. L. (1994). Structure of chia seed polysaccharide exudate. *Carbohydrate Polymers* 23(1): 13–18.

Mantzioris, E., Cleland, L. G., Gibson, R. A., Neumann, M. A., Demasi, M., and James, M. J. (2000). Biochemical effects of a diet containing foods enriched with n-3 fatty acids. *American Journal of Clinical Nutrition* 72(1): 42–48.

Mathiowitz, E., Kreitz, M. R., and Brannon-Peppas, L. (1999). Microencapsulation. In: *Encyclopedia of Controlled Drug Delivery*, pp. 493–546. E. Mathiowitz, ed. New York: John Wiley and Sons.

Medina Torres, L., Brito De La Fuente, E., Torrestiana Sánchez, B., and Katthain, R. (2000). Rheological properties of the mucilage gum (*Opuntia ficus indica*). *Food Hydrocolloids* 14: 417–424.

Medina Torres, L., Brito De-La Fuente, E., Gómez Aldapa, C., Aragón Piña, A., Toro Vázquez, J. (2006). Structural characteristics of gels formed by mixtures of carrageenan and mucilage gum from *Opuntia ficus indica*. *Carbohydrate Polymers* 63(10): 299–309.

Medina-Torres, L., García-Cruz, E. E., Calderas, F., González Laredo, R. F., Sánchez-Olivares, G., *et al.* (2013). Microencapsulation by spray drying of gallic acid with nopal mucilage (*Opuntia ficus indica*). *LWT – Food Science and Technology* 50: 642–650.

Minemoto, Y., Adachi, S., and Matsuno, R. (2001). Effect of relative humidity during storage on the autoxidation of linoleic acid encapsulated with a polysaccharide by hot-air-drying and freeze-drying. *Food Science and Technology Research* 7: 91–93.

Miyazawa, K., Yajima, I., Kaneda, I., and Yanaki, T. (2000). Preparation of a new soft capsule for cosmetics. *International Journal of Cosmetic Science* 51: 239–252.

Muzzarelli, R. A. A., and Muzzarelli, C. (2005). Chitosan chemistry: Relevance to the biomedical sciences. In: *Polysaccharides 1: Structure, Characterization and Use*, pp. 151–210. A. Potthast, T., Rosenau, and P., Kosma, eds. New York: Springer-Verlag.

Oarada, M., Ito, E., Terao, K., Miyazawa, T., Fujimoto, K., and Kaneda, T. (1988). The effect of dietary-lipid hydroperoxide on lymphoid-tissues in mice. *Biochimica et Biophysica Acta* 960(2): 229–235.

Phillips, G. O., and Williams, P. A. (2000). Introduction to food hydrocolloids. In: *Handbook of Hydrocolloids*. G. O. Phillips and P. A. Williams, eds. Cambridge England: Woodhead Publishing Limited.

Pokorny, J., Yanishlieva, N., Gordon, M. (2001). *Antioxidants in Food: Practical Applications*. Cambridge, England: Woodhead Publishing Ltd.

Ren, P. W., Ju, X. J., and Chu, L. Y. (2010). Monodisperse alginate microcapsules with oil core generated from a microfluidic device. *Journal of Colloid and Interface Science* 343: 392–395.

Ribeiro, A. J., Neufeld, R. J., Arnaud, P., and Chaumeil, J. C. (1999). Microencapsulation of lipophilic drugs in chitosan-coated alginate microspheres. *International Journal of Pharmaceutics* 187: 115–123.

Rubilar, M., Morales, E., Contreras, K., Ceballos, C., Acevedo, F., *et al.* (2012). Development of a soup powder enriched with microencapsulated linseed oil as a source of omega-3 fatty acids. *European Journal of Lipid Science and Technology* 114: 423–433.

Schubert H., Ax K., and Behrend O., (2003). Product engineering of dispersed system. *Trends in Food Science and Technology* 14: 9–16.

Shahidi, F., Vidana-Arachchi, J. K., and Jeon, Y.-J. (1999). Food applications of chitin and chitosans. *Trends in Food Science and Technology* 10: 37–51.

Simopoulos, A. P., Leaf, A., and Salem, N. (1999). Essentiality of and recommended dietary intakes for omega-6 and omega-3 fatty acids. *Annals of Nutrition and Metabolism* 43: 127–130.

Stamey, J. A., Shepherd, D. M., de Veth, M. J., and Corl, B. A. (2012). Use of omega-3-fatty-acid–rich algae and their oil as a feed supplement for dairy cattle. *Journal of Dairy Science* 95(9): 5269–5275.

Stapelfeldt, H., Nielsen, B. R., Jensen, S. K., and Skibsted, L. H. (1999) Free radical formation in freeze-dried raw milk in relation to alpha-tocopherol level. *Journal of Dairy Research* 66: 461–466.

Stuchlík, M., and Žák, S. (2002). Vegetable lipids as components of functional foods. *Biomedical Papers* 146(2): 3–10.

Taguchi, K., Iwami, K., Ibuk, F., and Kawabata, M. (1992). Oxidative stability of sardine oil embedded in spray-dried egg white powder and its use for n-3 unsaturated fatty acid fortification of cookies. *Bioscience, Biotechnology, and Biochemistry* 56: 560–563.

Torres, L. G., Carpinteyro-Urban, S. L., and Vaca, M. (2012). Use of *Prosopis laevigata* seed gum and *Opuntia ficus-indica* mucilage for the treatment of municipal wastewaters by coagulation–flocculation. *Natural Resources* 3: 35–41.

Torres-Giner, S., Martinez-Abad, A., Ocio, M. J., and Lagaron, J. M. (2012). Stabilization of a nutraceutical omega-3 fatty acid by encapsulation in ultrathin electrosprayed zein prolamine. *Journal of Food Science* 75(6): 69–79.

Uragami, T., and Tokura, S., eds. (2006). *Material Science of Chitin and Chitosan*. New York: Springer-Verlag.

Us-Medina, U. (2015). Microencapsulation of *Salvia hispanica* oil with nutraceutical potential. Master's Thesis. Facultad de Ingeniería Química. Universidad Autónoma de Yucatán, México.

Velasco, J., Dobarganes, C., and Márquez-Ruiz, G. (2003). Variables affecting lipid oxidation in dried microencapsulated oils. *Grasas y Aceites* 54(3): 304–314.

Wakil, A., Mackenzie, G., Diego-Taboada, A., Bell, J. G., and Atkin, S. L. (2010). Enhanced bioavailability of eicosapentaenoic acid from fish oil after encapsulation within plant spore exines as microcapsules. *Lipids* 45(7): 645–649.

Willumsen, R. (2006). Omega-3 in food and beverages. *Agro Food Industries* 17(3): 6–8.

Wyss, A., von Stockar, U., and Marison, I. (2004). Production and characterization of liquid-core capsules made from cross-linked acrylamide copolymers for biotechnological applications. *Biotechnology and Bioengineering* 86: 563–572.

Ye, A., Cui, J., Taneja, A., Zhu, X., and Singh, H. (2009). Evaluation of processed cheese fortified with fish oil emulsion. *Food Research International* 42(8): 1093–1098.

Yilmaz, G., Jongboom, R. O. J., Feil, H., and Hennink, W. E. (2001). Encapsulation of sunflower oil in starch matrices via extrusion: Effect of the interfacial properties and processing conditions on the formation of dispersed phased morphologies. *Carbohydrate Polymers* 45: 403–410.

Yu, D., Qiao, W., Li, Q., and Pei, G. (2012). Preparation and properties of olive oil microcapsules. *Journal of Fiber Bioengineering and Informatics* 5(1): 67–76.

Index

Page numbers in *italics* refer to illustrations; those in **bold** refer to tables

New Polymers for Encapsulation of Nutraceutical Compounds, First Edition.
Edited by Jorge Carlos Ruiz Ruiz and Maira Rubi Segura Campos.

Printed and bound by CPI Group (UK) Ltd, Croydon, CR0 4YY
17/09/2026
14964304-0001